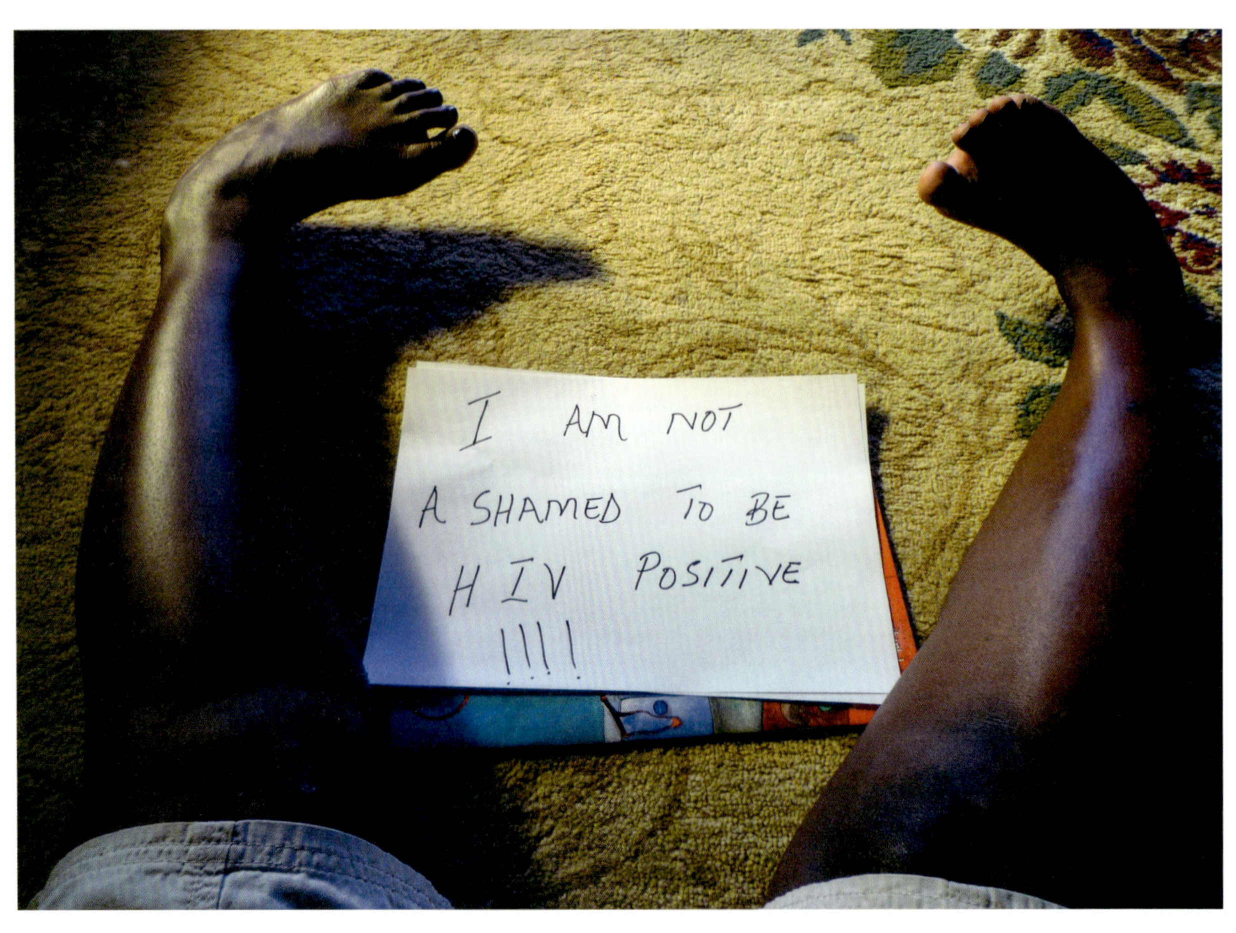

**Edited by
Gideon Mendel & David Gere**

Through Positive Eyes

aperture

In the decade since this project began, ten of the 130 *Through Positive Eyes* participants have died. This book is dedicated to them: Ilián, Magos, Martín, and Roberto in Mexico City; Alcione and Mara in Rio de Janeiro; Betty in Johannesburg; Gemini and Mary in Washington, D.C.; and Priya in Mumbai.

And so they said
Mary Bowman
9

Foreword
Richard Gere
11

Introduction
Gideon Mendel & David Gere
13

Mexico City
17

Rio de Janeiro
35

Johannesburg
53

Los Angeles
71

Washington, D.C.
89

Mumbai
107

Bangkok
125

Port-au-Prince
143

London
161

Durban
179

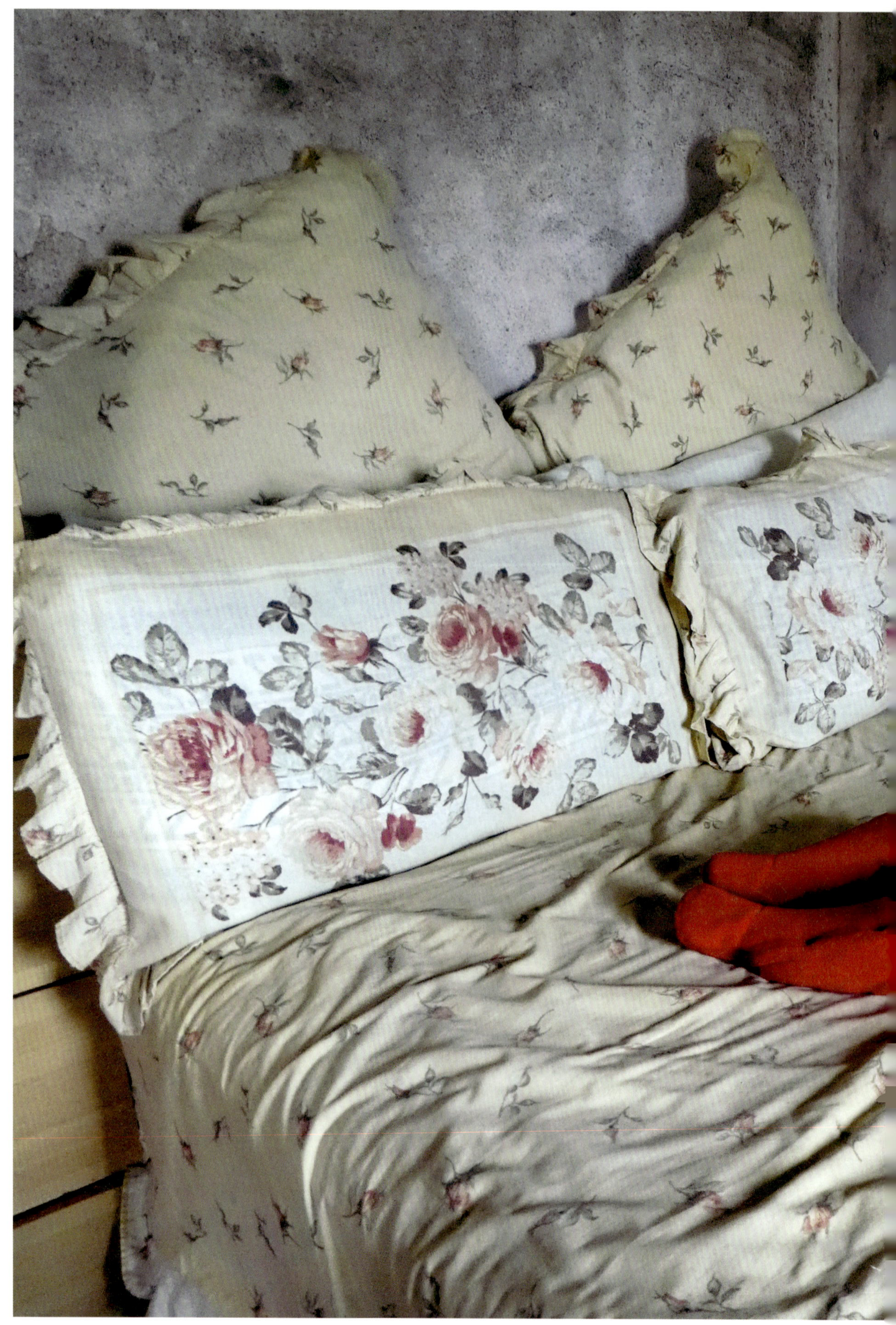

 Xoli/Durban

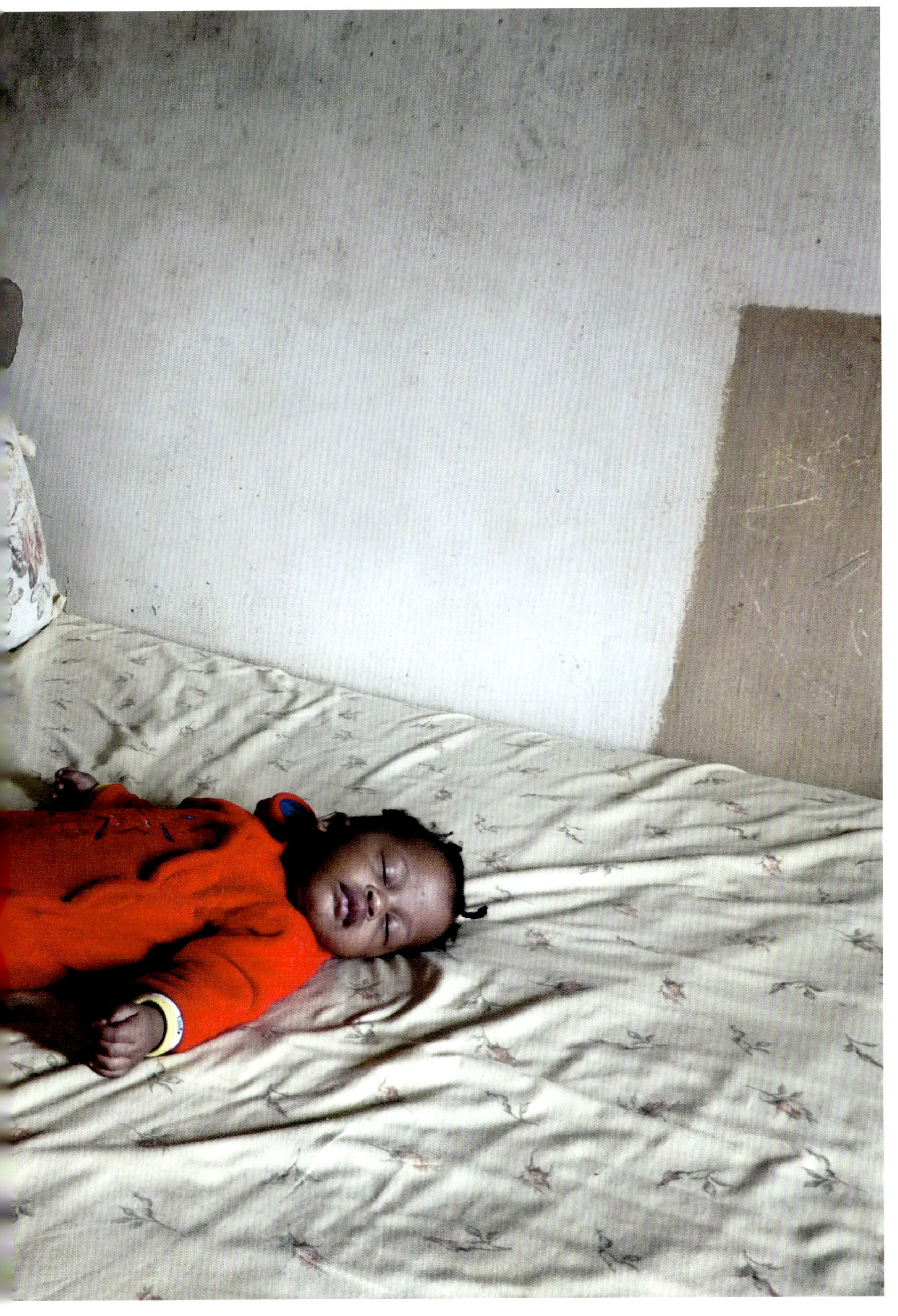

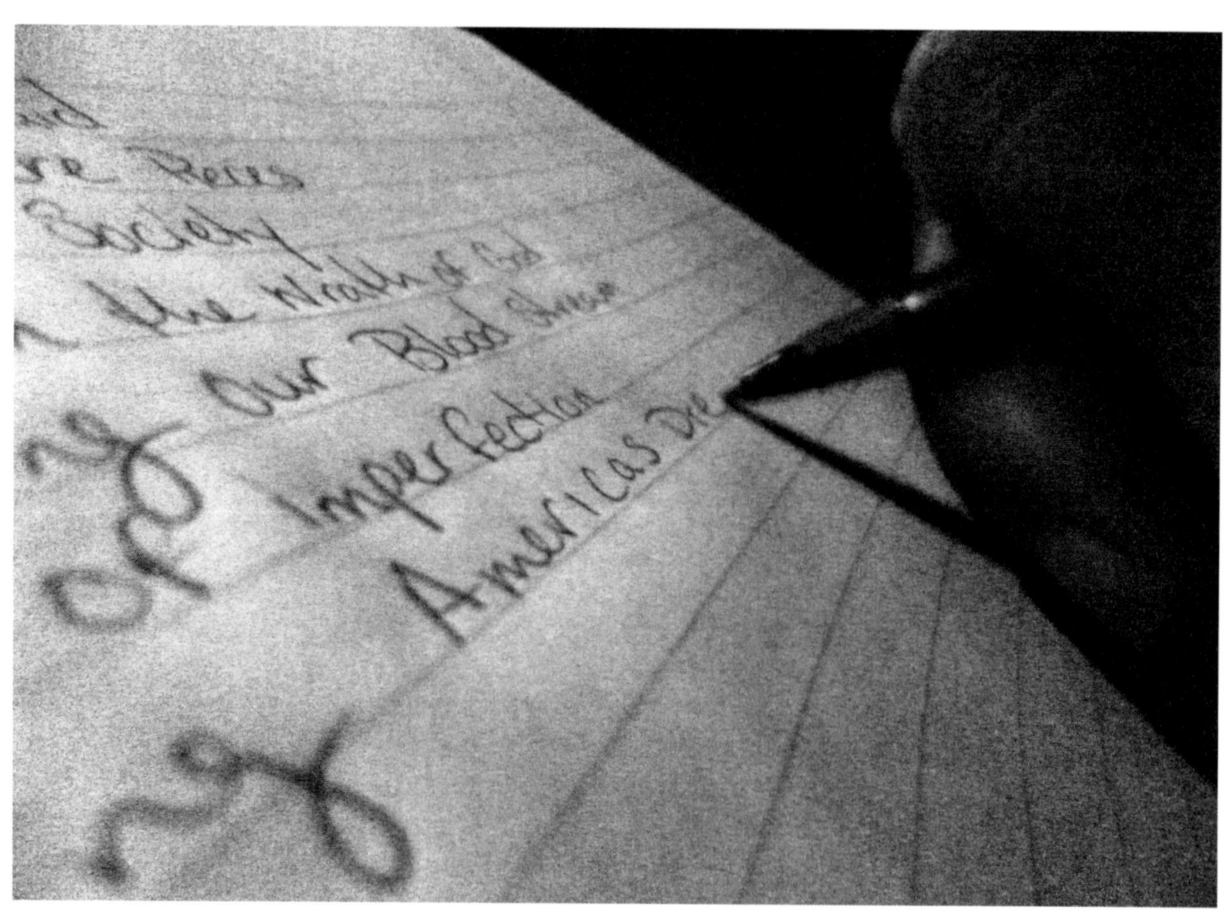

Mary/Washington, D.C.

And so they said
Mary Bowman

And so they said
That we were mere fragments of a broken society
Blotches of imperfection tainting America's dream
God's punishment compromising our immunity

So we snapshot fear, frame our insecurities
Zoom in close so that the world can see that we are alive

Through Positive Eyes the view is beautiful and rare
Taking you where statistics can't go
Deep inside our homes
Where stigma haunts mirrors
And ARVs strut with ego

Who knew that a photo could tell you stories
Of mothers who live for their children's smile
Women full of strength and pride
Men who refuse to die
And youth who choose to be seen as well as heard

We say it loud
Spread the word

We are not fragments of a broken society
We are not blotches of imperfection tainting America's dream
And it is not God's punishment compromising our immunity
It's HIV

We overcome fear through snapshots
Quiet our insecurities within each frame
Zoom in close so that the world can see that
We are very much alive and
Living normal lives
Telling our story Through Positive Eyes

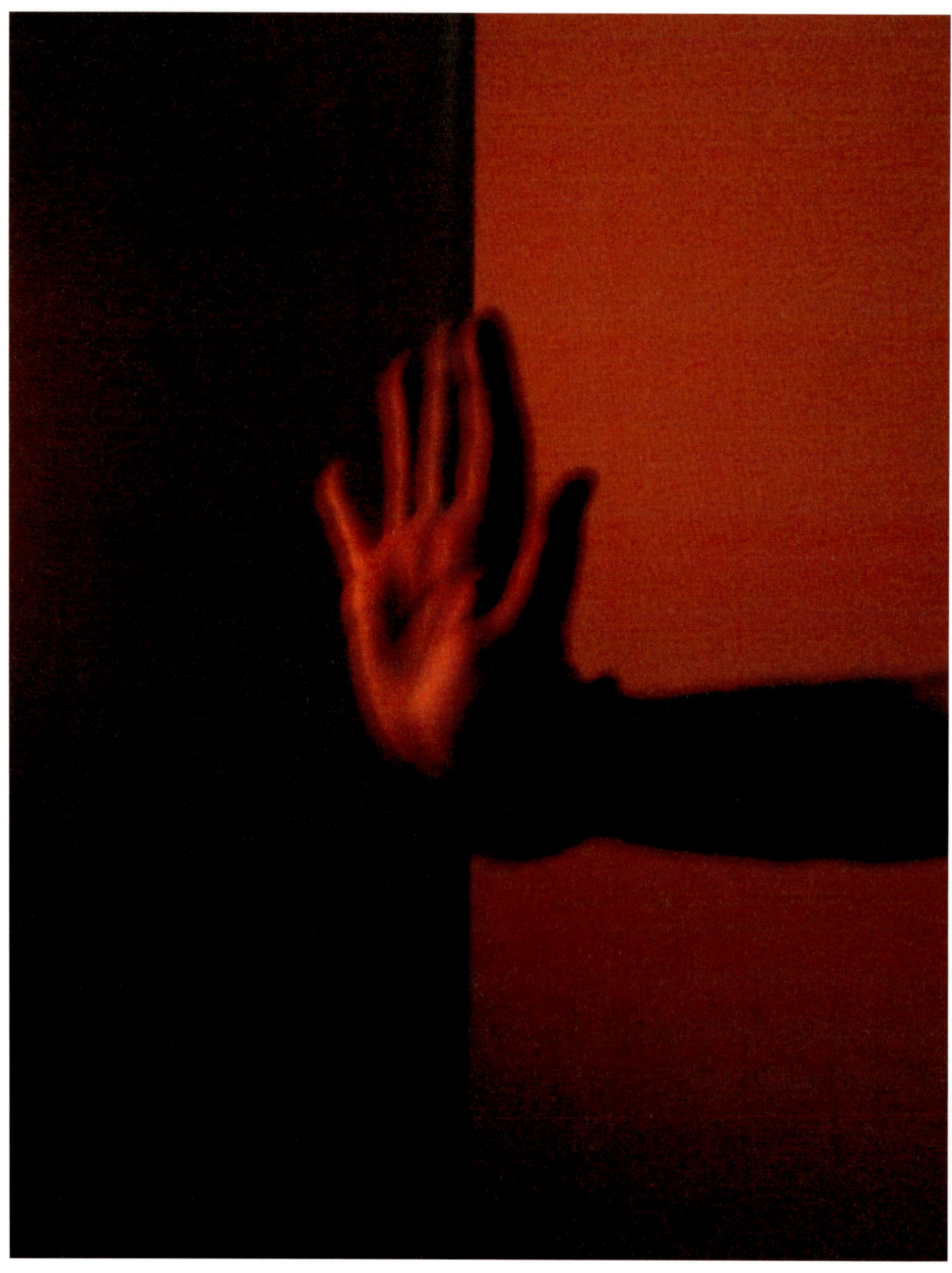

Foreword
Richard Gere

The publication of this book was made possible by The Herb Ritts Foundation. Herb Ritts was a phenomenally successful and influential photographer, probably best known for his fashion and celebrity portraits. He was also my dear friend. We met in 1977, through my then girlfriend. Later that year he took some casual photographs of me that found their way into the pages of major magazines. This marked the beginning of his career as a photographer.

Over the years, we became very close. We would crash at each other's homes, his in Los Angeles and Malibu, mine outside New York. One day he called me, full of emotion, and said, "I took the HIV test. I am HIV-positive." I was stunned. We cried together. At that time there was no effective treatment, and AIDS was considered a long, slow death sentence. Because of the irrational stigma and fear surrounding HIV and AIDS, we both kept his diagnosis secret. Herb was specifically afraid that, if word got out, he would never work again.

To be clear, fear didn't stop Herb from being an AIDS activist, from doing what was right. He would donate photos to AMFAR and other AIDS organizations. He helped raise large amounts of money for research and care. We both contributed to fast-track HIV research, in hopes of a definitive breakthrough, for him and for our other friends, for the world. He was very generous and open with those closest to him. But HIV was his secret.

The Herb Ritts Foundation, created after his death from AIDS-related causes in 2002, supports people living with HIV and AIDS around the world while also advancing the art of photography. Herb's surviving partner, Erik Hyman, heads the Foundation's board. Mark McKenna, Herb's longtime photographic assistant, is the mastermind behind its visionary activities. Together with the board, of which I am a member, the Foundation strives to end the secrecy surrounding HIV, to contribute to AIDS care, and to undo stigma through photography. At this point in the epidemic, no one, anywhere, need die of HIV. Medical advances have been extraordinary. But HIV can't be, shouldn't be, a secret anymore. Photography combined with courageous and intimate storytelling can make a real difference. The photographs in this book represent all of us—brothers and sisters on this small planet.

I want to acknowledge my brother, David Gere, who edited this book with Gideon Mendel. I love him dearly. His tireless and skillful leadership and his international engagement to stop the AIDS pandemic have been a constant inspiration. Through his MAKE ART/STOP AIDS project, minds have been changed. Hearts have been opened. Creativity, compassion, and determination go hand in hand.

Herb would have appreciated and admired this book: the honesty of it, the depth of it, the skill of it. These are powerful photos. The images feel spontaneous but also considered. They are intimate and passionate, as in the best art. Herb would have been deeply proud of this book as a reflection of himself, as an artist and as a responsible and caring human being.

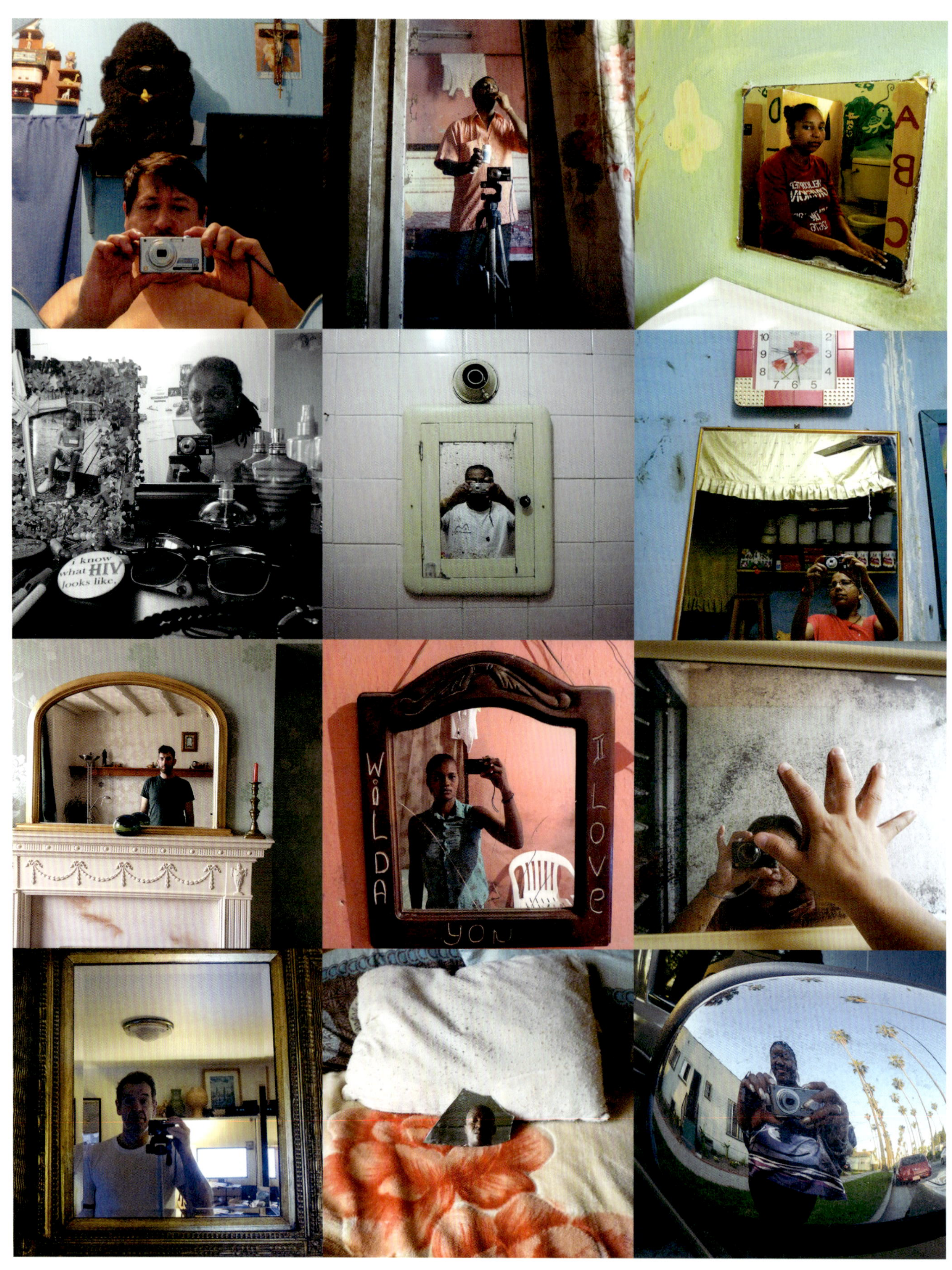

Top to bottom, left to right: Ramón/Mexico City, Sudesh/Mumbai, Elizabeth/Durban; Mary/Washington, D.C., José Luis/Rio de Janeiro, Manisha/Mumbai; Joshua/London, Wilda/Port-au-Prince, Aoy/Bangkok; Chris/London, Pleasure/Johannesburg, Lynnea/Los Angeles

Introduction
Gideon Mendel & David Gere

Through Positive Eyes is a collaborative photo-storytelling project by people living with HIV and AIDS around the world. More than 130 HIV-positive people have participated in workshops led by South African photographer Gideon Mendel and David Gere, director of the Art & Global Health Center at the University of California – Los Angeles (UCLA). Over the past decade, the project has grown, one city per year, to become ambitiously international in scope, now encompassing ten cities in eight countries on five continents. *Through Positive Eyes* paints a vivid picture of the global AIDS epidemic—after its initial outbreak, but before treatment becomes universally accessible—that features insider photography by people living with HIV and AIDS. Many of them are picking up cameras for the first time in their lives.

The project chronicles a very particular moment in the epidemic, when effective treatment is available to some, not all, and when the enduring stigma associated with HIV and AIDS has become entrenched, a major roadblock to both prevention and treatment. The participants in the project have volunteered to tell their stories, in words and in photos, in order to break down stigma and empower themselves. They are identified in this book by their first names, in part to emphasize their humanity and accessibility, but also to protect those who live in cities where stigma can be dangerous, if not life-threatening.

Gideon Mendel As an HIV-negative ally, I have chronicled the epidemic for nearly three decades, in an effort to humanize people living with HIV and specifically to foster empathy and action on the part of individuals and governments. I began in the 1990s when, shooting in black and white, I attempted to show the harsh nature and broad scale of the epidemic. Working in my native South Africa and across seven other African countries, I photographed people wasting from HIV-related illnesses, before there was medication to control it. I photographed clinics and their dedicated staffs. I photographed mothers cradling their sick sons and daughters in their arms. I photographed people dying. And I photographed funerals, too many funerals.

David Gere I arrived in San Francisco, that gayest of American cities, in 1985, and almost immediately became swept up in the AIDS activist movement. I was a young HIV-negative gay man experiencing the darkest days of the epidemic in the United States firsthand. As a writer of dance and music criticism for Bay Area newspapers, I was also witnessing an amazing outpouring of activist creativity, born of anger and mourning. The epidemic catalyzed my belief in arts activism as a method for addressing the epidemic and for seeking to end it. MAKE ART/STOP AIDS, a project I cocreated with Robert Sember, became a slogan to live by.

GM After some major exhibitions and the publication of my first book, *A Broken Landscape: HIV & AIDS in Africa* (2003), I felt it important to respond to critiques I had received from some HIV-positive people: that I was one of many photographers who were essentially "vultures," portraying them as helpless victims. Moreover, with the advent of antiretroviral treatment, the politics around the representation of people living with HIV was changing, because more and more people were rising up like Lazarus, to become healthy and active again. At that same time, I was searching for a way to respond to what I saw as the harsh divide between those in the global North, who were able to access life-saving treatment relatively easily, and the millions in Africa who were condemned to horrific illness and painful deaths. I began working in color, to render my images more accessible, and I became much more of an activist. I identified strongly with South Africa's Treatment Action Campaign and collaborated with TAC on a number of initiatives, making new tools of visual advocacy in the crucial struggle of the early 2000s for global treatment justice.

DG It was in the early 2000s when I first read Gideon's *A Broken Landscape*, which was placed in my hands by a South African friend and colleague. Not only did I find the photographs to be extremely vivid and alive—and beautifully composed—but I loved that they were presented side by side with concise first-person narratives, always told in the present tense. "I wake up in the morning and drink my tea," writes Joseph Gabriel of Tanzania. "I like listening to the radio." In important ways, Gideon's approach refigured the expectations that held sway at that time: Joseph has AIDS, and he is also enjoying his life, the simple things that bring texture to everyday existence. Joseph is rendered as someone familiar, a next door neighbor, a potential friend. In the classroom, my students at UCLA responded viscerally to Gideon's layering of image and words, recognizing in his approach a particularly potent strategy for banishing stigma.

GM One day in 2007, David called me in London, where I live with my family. He asked if I would consider collaborating with his Art & Global Health Center to develop a photo-storytelling project about HIV in Los Angeles. I was keen to expand my work beyond the African context. A few months later, I found myself teaching a workshop class to UCLA students, during which we developed the basic concepts that have informed *Through Positive Eyes* to this day. Within a year, we had developed our own new approach—a variation on my prior practice—which we continue to adapt and improve as we take the workshop to new cities.

DG At each new location, my staff and I always begin by establishing a relationship with a local HIV organization, which agrees to assume responsibility for convening a diverse group of people living with HIV and AIDS. As partial payment, we provide small digital point-and-shoot cameras as well as a modest honorarium. Throughout, the participants must be willing to show their faces publicly, because, in our view, this is fundamental to overcoming the stigma associated with HIV. Selfless and courageous action is required to counteract stigma.

GM First and foremost, the members of our group must be willing to explore photography as a serious artistic medium. With *Through Positive Eyes*, we strive for images capable of cutting through the visual noise that surrounds us. While the process is important—for many, the workshop is a transformative experience—we also feel that the final product is crucial. In order to be effective as advocacy, the work needs to stand as art. So I always push our participants to achieve the highest possible photographic standard on every level.

My friend and colleague Crispin Hughes, whom I have long known and worked alongside in London, plays a key role as primary photo educator. Together, Crispin, David, and I have developed a ten-day workshop sequence, starting from the basics, such as how to turn off the flash in favor of available light, but advancing quickly to equip our group with the sophisticated knowledge required to use their cameras to make their own personal visual statements. The conclusion of the workshop consists of an intensive group editing session, during which each photographer—with support from the group and input from Crispin, David, and me—chooses a set of twelve images as well as a single "signature" image. This raucous session is a highlight for me.

DG From the beginning, the story-sharing part of the project has been weighted as heavily as the photography. Each person sits for an extended interview in their home language, with a translator if needed. After transcription, the interviews are condensed to focus on a central theme or element of each person's story, which is then posted at throughpositiveeyes.org, alongside their set of twelve photographs. In my experience, something powerful begins to happen when images meet words. The impact is most evident in our work with high school students, who tell us that they begin to identify with the photographers as fellow humans, as a version of themselves. They cross the divide. And, as a result, stigma begins to fall away. As an acknowledgment of this magical chemistry, we refer to the participants as "artivists," a term adopted by Brazilian artist Adriana Bertini, as a portmanteau of "artist" and "activist" together.

GM Early in the project, I thought of my portraits, taken of our HIV-positive subjects, as central. But as the years went by, we realized that the artivists' self-representations were much more interesting. We wanted to encourage this. So we refined our teaching process and began providing a small tripod with each camera kit, and took special care to teach the participants about the self-timer, encouraging them to be the documenters of their own lives. This approach led to many deeply considered self-portraits.

As we continued to develop *Through Positive Eyes*, I began to recognize the limitations of my own photographic practice in relation to HIV and AIDS. Where HIV was concerned, I realized I would always be a compassionate outsider, composing my images from a distance. When I saw these images, of lives lived by HIV-positive people, I recognized a level of intimacy and personal revelation that I could never hope to achieve. It was time to hand over the camera.

Mexico City

The inaugural *Through Positive Eyes* workshop, in June 2008, was held during the build up to that year's XVII International AIDS Conference, which emphasized continuing breakthroughs in antiretroviral treatment in relation to the epidemics in Latin America. On the intimate level of the workshop, however, the Mexico City participants focused on fundamental human issues—loving and being loved; the impact of HIV on the transgender community; the sexual expression of women with HIV; and the desire to be radiantly, defiantly, muscularly healthy, even while taking HIV medication.

Mexico's AIDS epidemic, as of 2008

Number of people living with HIV:	200,000

HIV prevalence

Adults (15–49 years):	0.3%
Female sex workers:	5.5%
Men who have sex with men:	9.9%
People who inject drugs:	2.8%

Treatment

Universal access to antiretroviral drugs through national social security program since 2003.

Numbers on treatment:	31,000
% of those in need of treatment who are receiving it:	54%

Key events

2003	*Discrimination on the basis of sexual orientation outlawed.*
2005	*National anti-homophobia campaign launched.*
2007	*Supreme court rejects dismissal of HIV-positive soldiers from military.*
2008	*Needle exchange programs in six states.*
2008	*XVII International AIDS Conference in Mexico City: "Universal Action Now."*

Update 2019

230,000 Mexicans are living with HIV. HIV prevalence has risen to 20.7% in men who have sex with men. 62% of people living with HIV are on treatment and 46% of these have no detectable virus in their blood. AIDS-related deaths have decreased by 3% since 2010.

Through Positive Eyes in Mexico City—*Una Mirada Positiva*—was organized in partnership with Letra S, with major funding from The Ford Foundation and the University of California Institute for Mexico and the United States (UC MEXUS).

Alejandro

I decided to fight to remain in the best physical, emotional, and psychological condition I could during the time I had left on this planet. I decided to be tough.

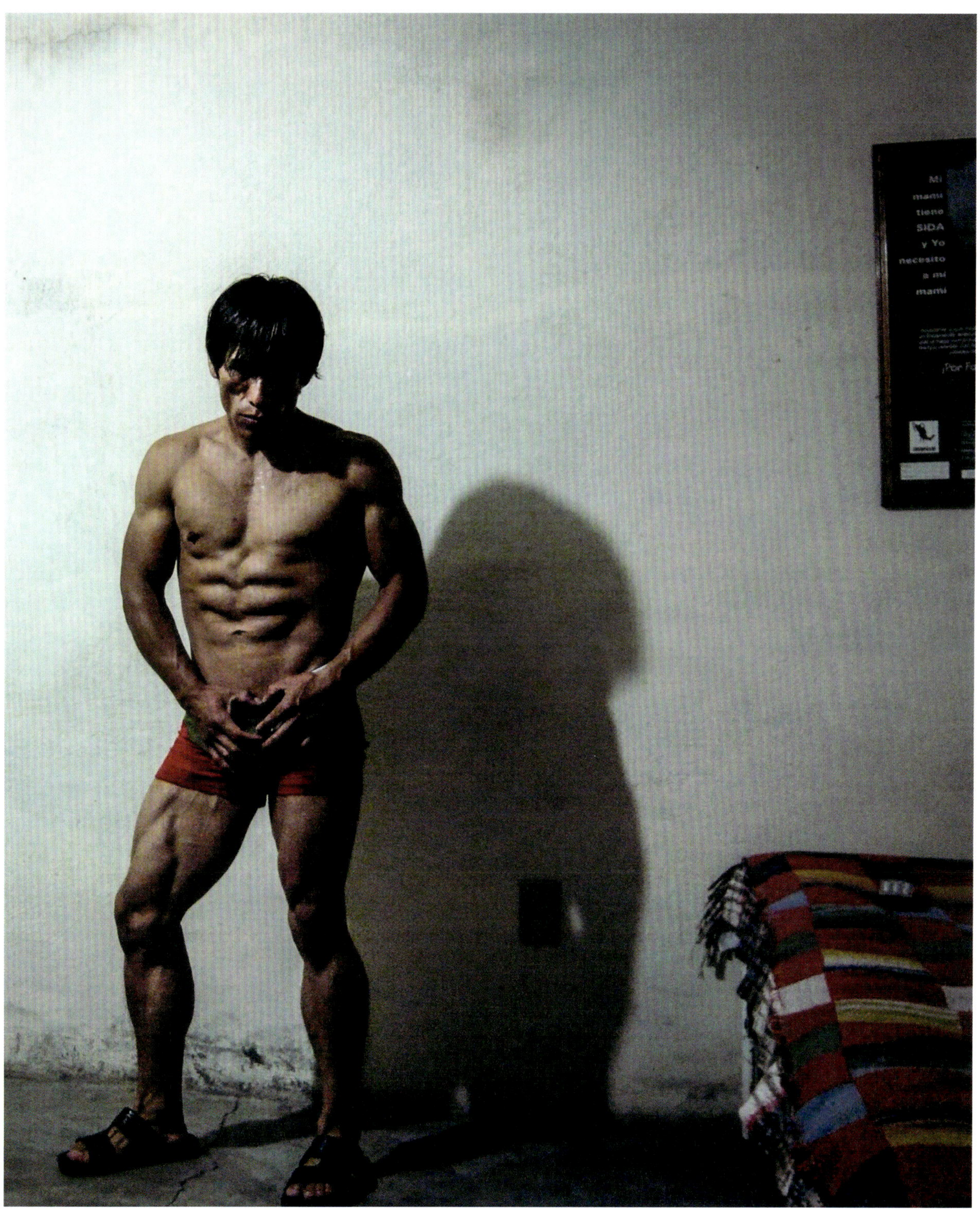

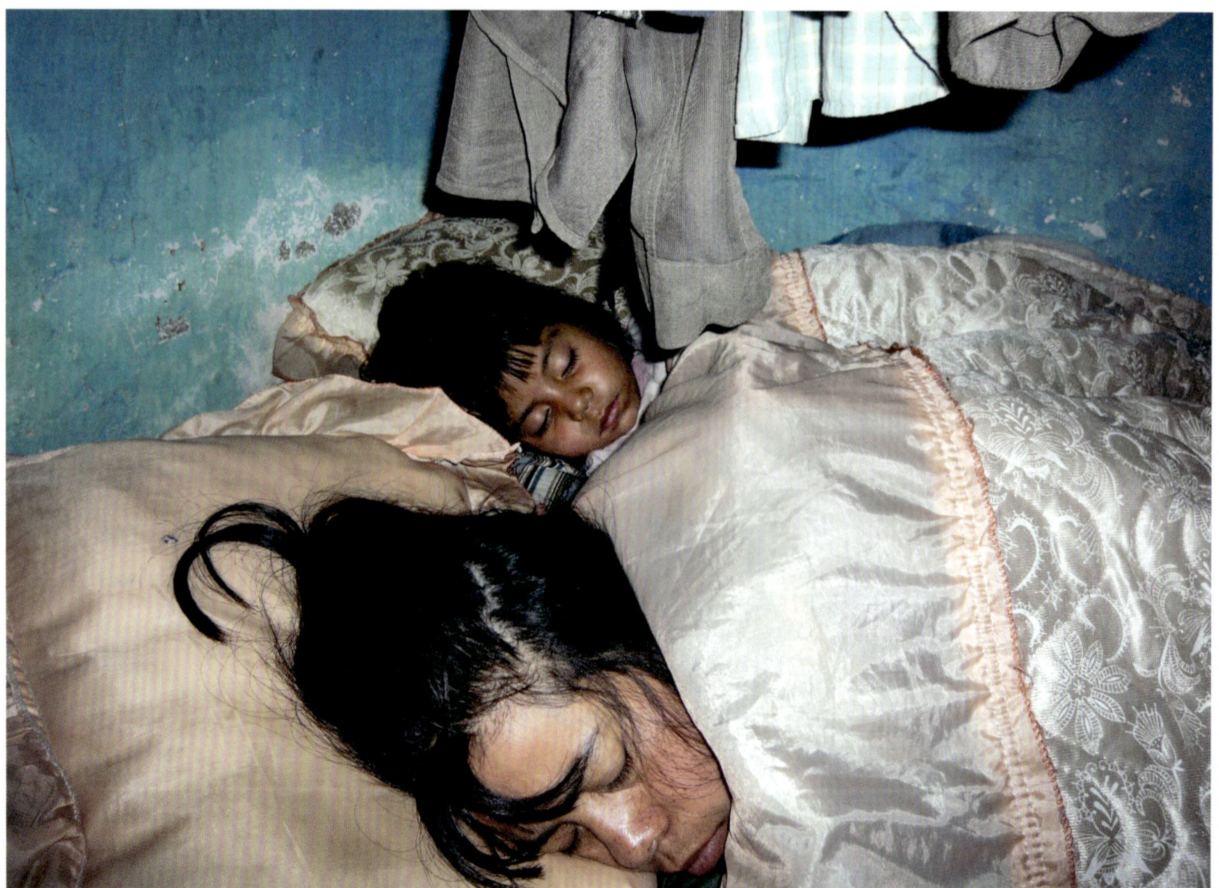

I am an electrician and I have been living with HIV for the past fifteen years. That afternoon when I got the news, I was in shock. I left the doctor's office and wandered aimlessly along the streets, all night long. When I finally came to my senses, it was dawn.

I decided to fight to remain in the best physical, emotional, and psychological condition I could during the time I had left on this planet. I promised myself that the virus would never defeat me. I decided to be tough.

It doesn't matter if the virus came to my life or if I went out looking for it. I just live like anybody else. I love to exercise, not only because it is good for my health, but also because I always wanted to have the body of a wrestler.

The years I have spent living with HIV have taught me to be more humble, respectful, and humane. My greatest satisfaction now is to help other people get medical care. We who live with HIV do not ask for special privileges, only that our rights be respected.

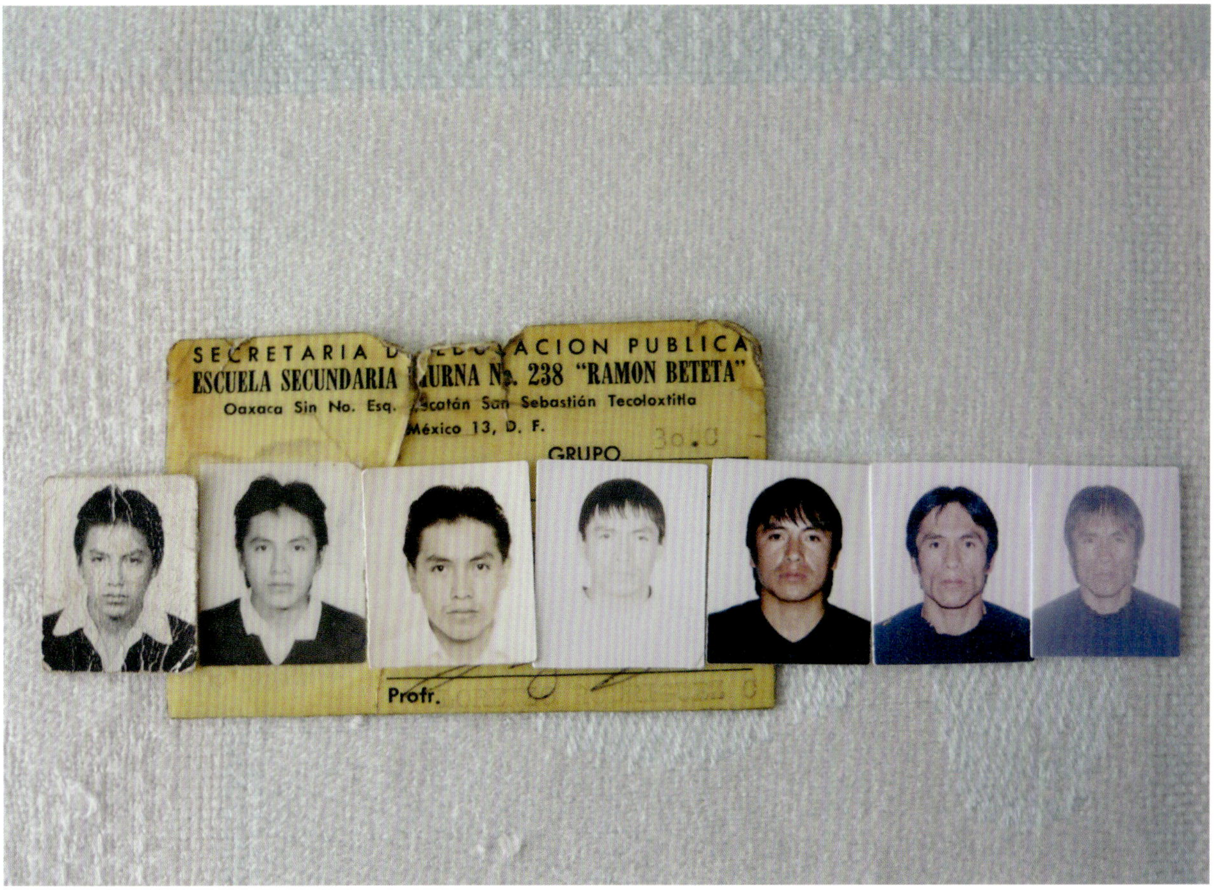

ACION PUBLICA
ESCUELA SECUNDARIA
238 "RAMON BETETA"
Oaxaca Sin No. Esq.
San Sebastián Tecoloxtitla
México 13, D. F.
GRUPO
Profr.

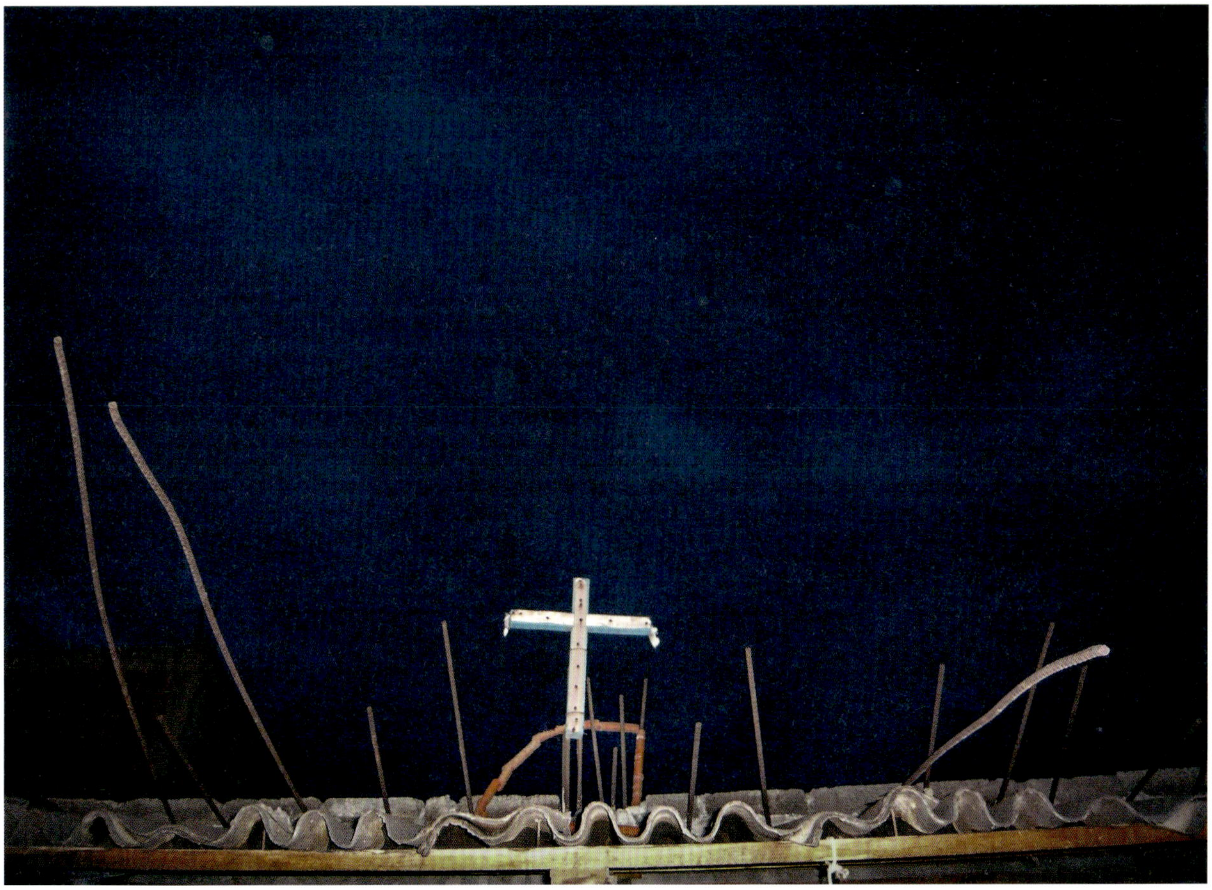

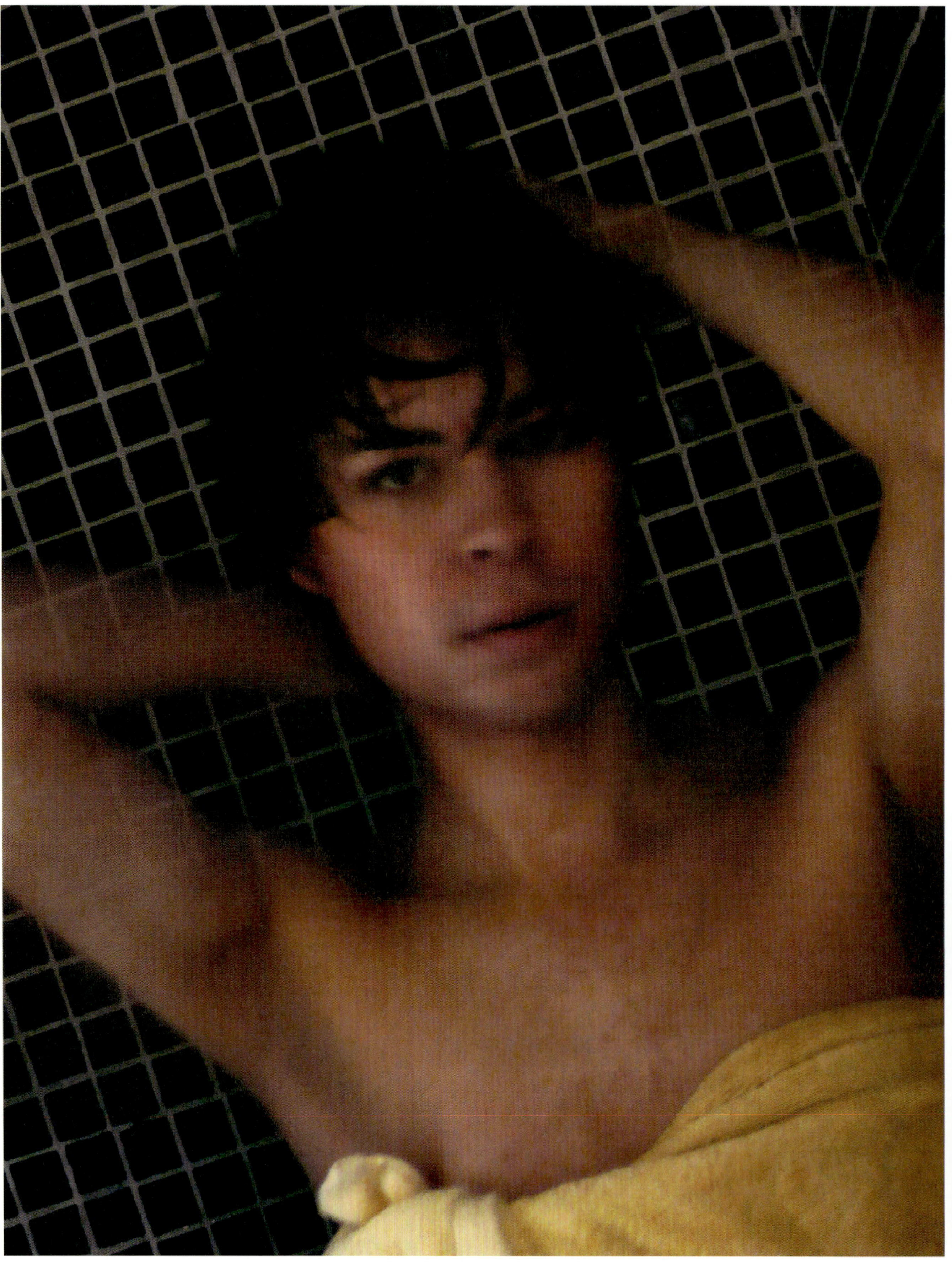

Ilsa

The first time I dressed as a woman I felt I was another person. My gestures no longer provoked laughter. I don't care any longer about the way others react. No matter what I do, I am a person who matters.

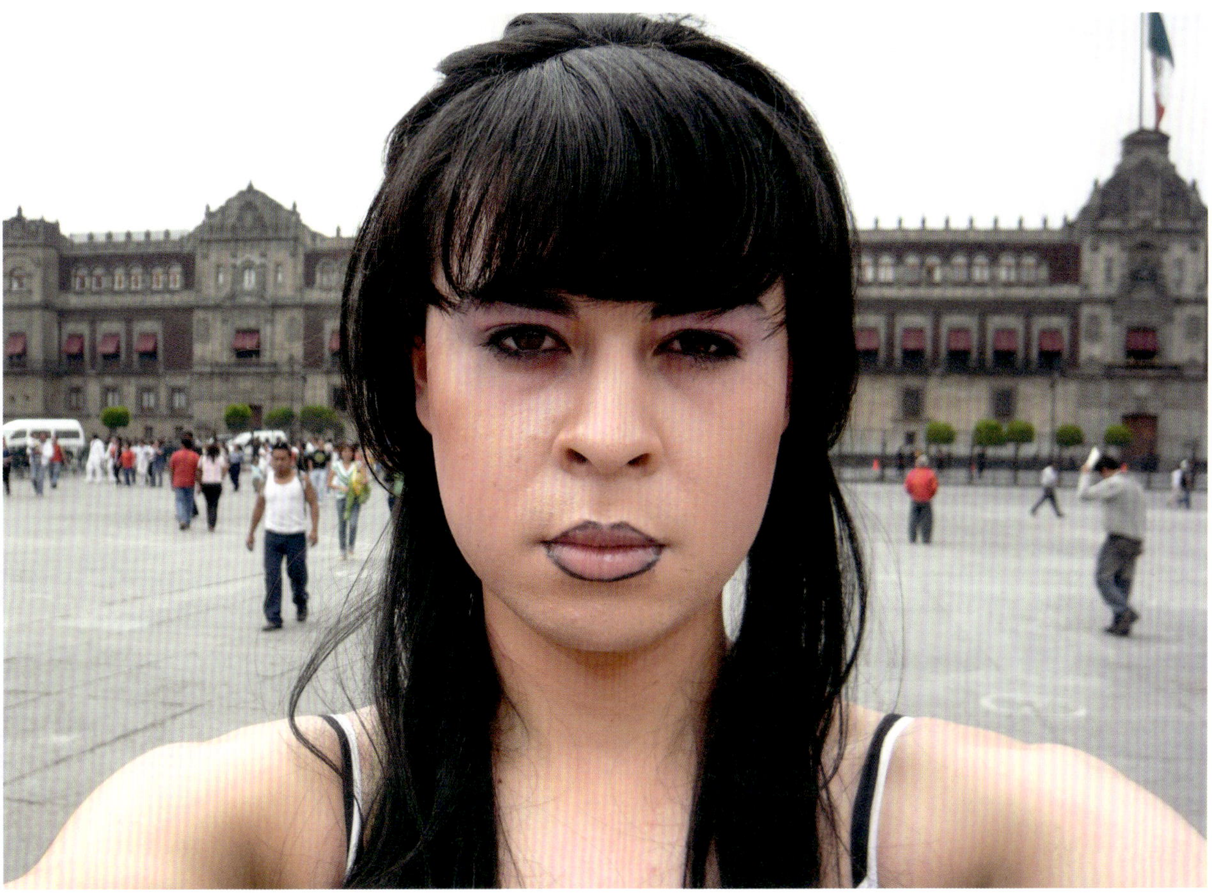

Ilsa is the name I have given myself. Now that I am eighteen years old, I feel empowered and my decisions are legally recognized. What I want is to feel fulfilled and productive, in order to take the next step toward becoming a transgender woman.

I wish my family understood me better, but we became distant from each other when I told them I was gay and that I liked to dress as a woman. At that time, I didn't want to live anymore, I didn't take care of myself. That included not wearing condoms, but also not feeding myself. I felt I was just causing problems.

I lost weight until I got sick and ended up at the hospital, where they administered an HIV test. I was sixteen years old. The doctor informed my parents of the diagnosis. To them it was harder to learn that I had HIV than to learn that I was trans, although they think that one thing led to the other.

The first time I dressed as a woman I felt I was another person. My gestures no longer provoked laughter. I don't care any longer about the way others react. No matter what I do, I am a person who matters.

Magda

If they tell you that you have a disease about which you know nothing, and then they tell you that you are dying from it at age forty, with small children, the blow is devastating.

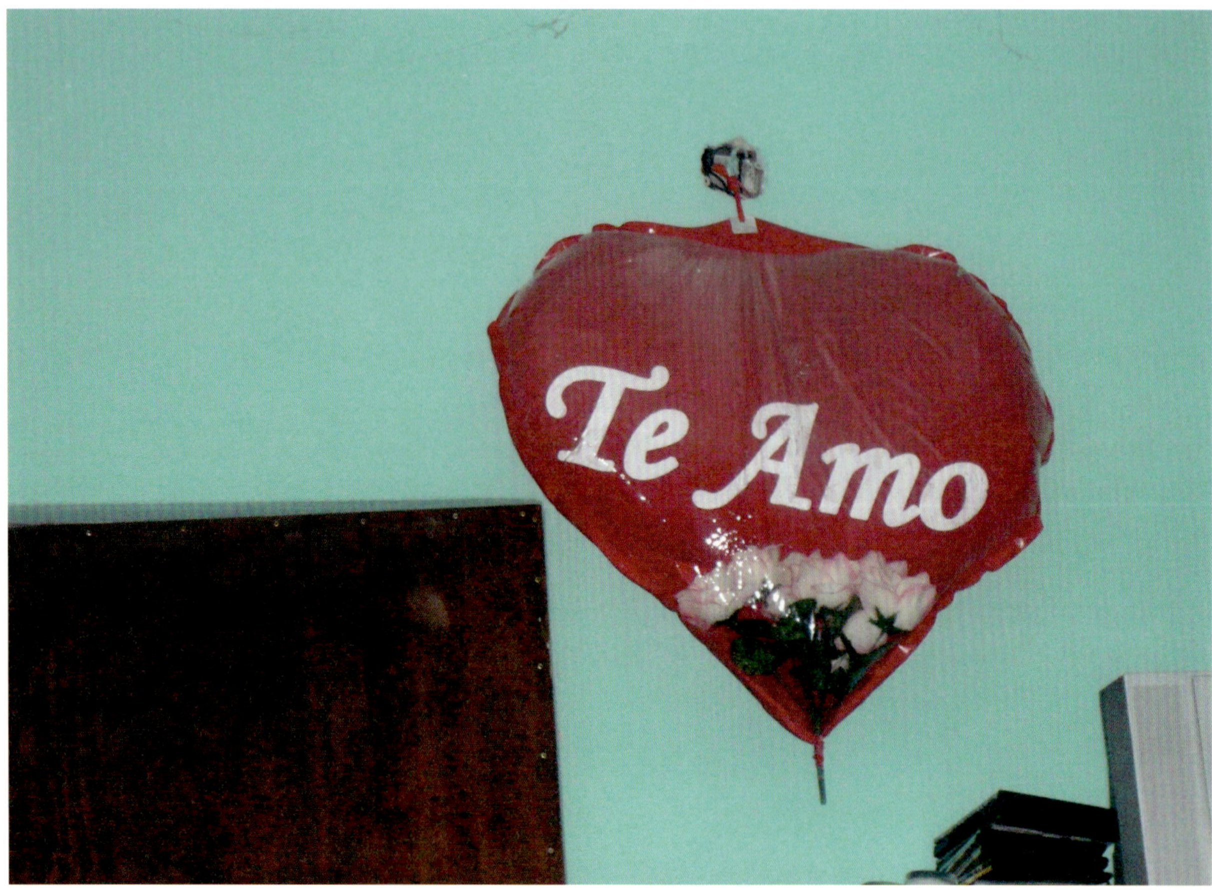

I was diagnosed with HIV over five years ago. Before then my life was no different from that of any other housewife. I consider myself to be a strong woman, but if they tell you that you have a disease about which you know nothing but the name, and then they tell you that you are dying from it at age forty, with small children, the blow is devastating.

My husband is a truck driver. From the very first moment he gave me his full support. He said: "If you are infected, so am I. We're going to get out of this together, the way we have overcome every other problem."

Once the initial fears and symptoms passed, I became aware of deficiencies in the available medical services. This "discovery" turned me into an activist, which means something more than distributing condoms. We have to re-educate ourselves in the knowledge of our fundamental rights.

It was at this moment that I realized all the potential I have as a woman. My life is a continuous learning experience. I did not know that having a camera in my hand would prove lethally orgasmic for me. I feel fulfilled.

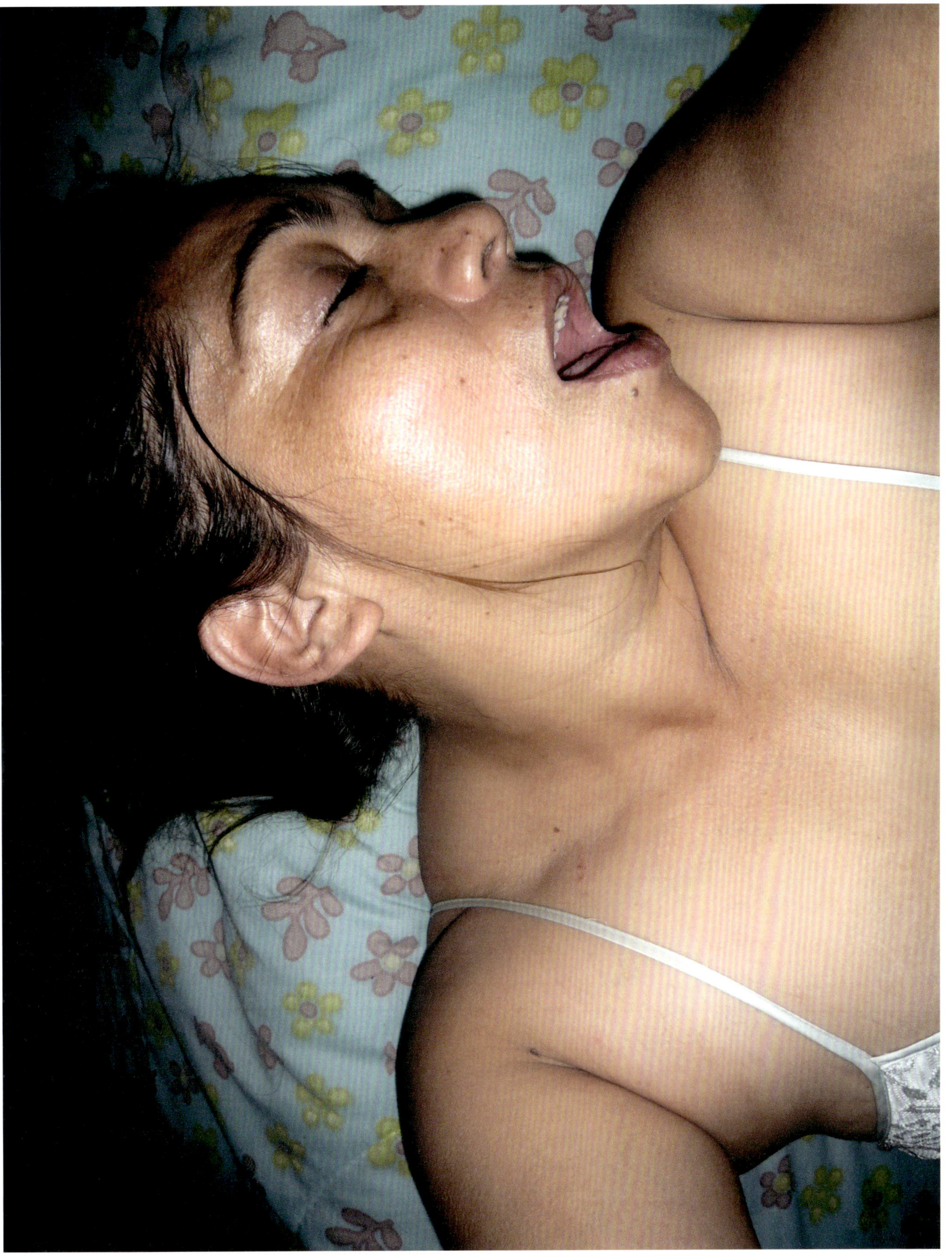

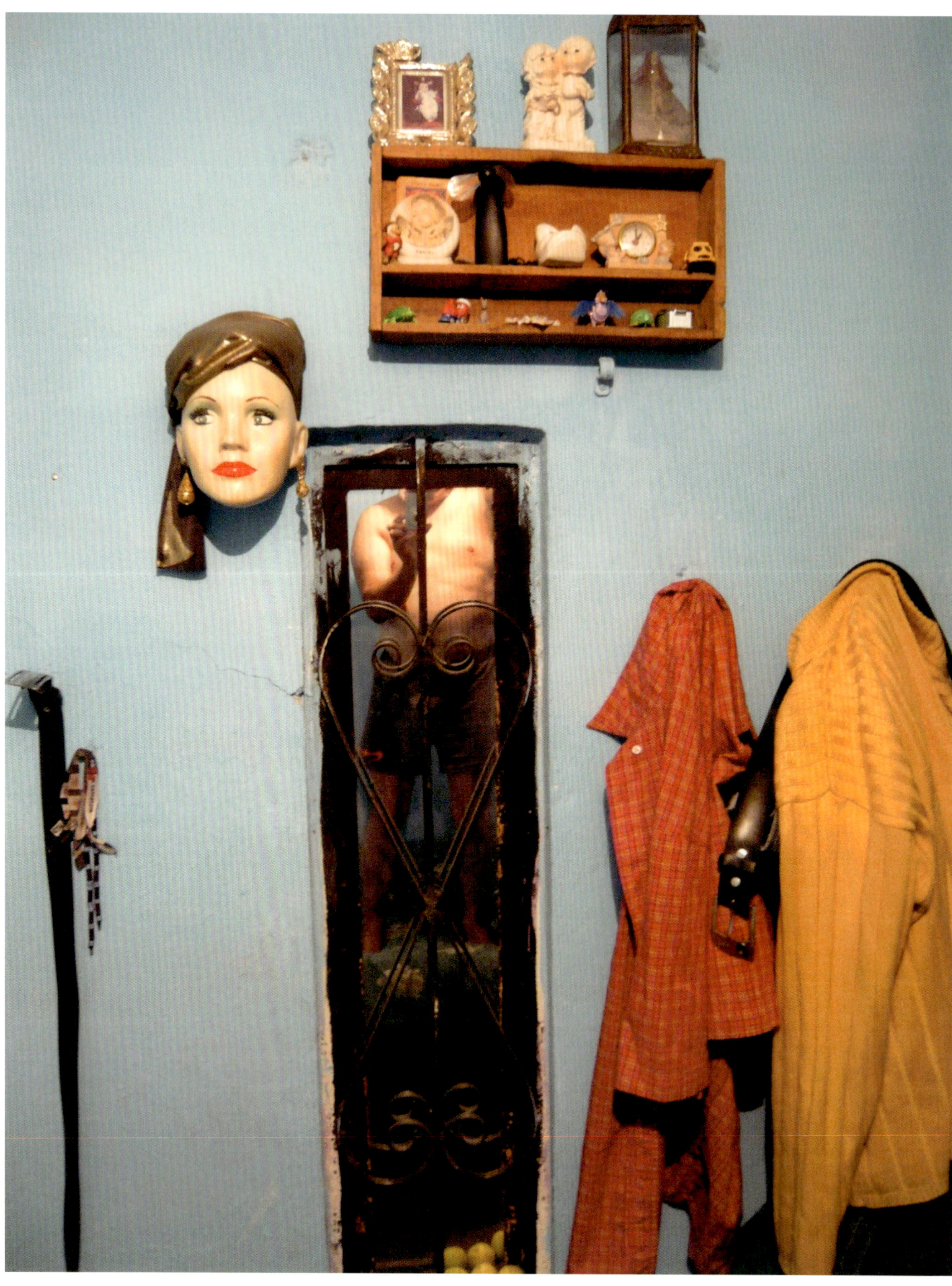

Ramón

All these years of living with the virus have taught me to become more mature and to work on my feelings. Among my future plans, I want to enter the university, study chemistry, and then teach.

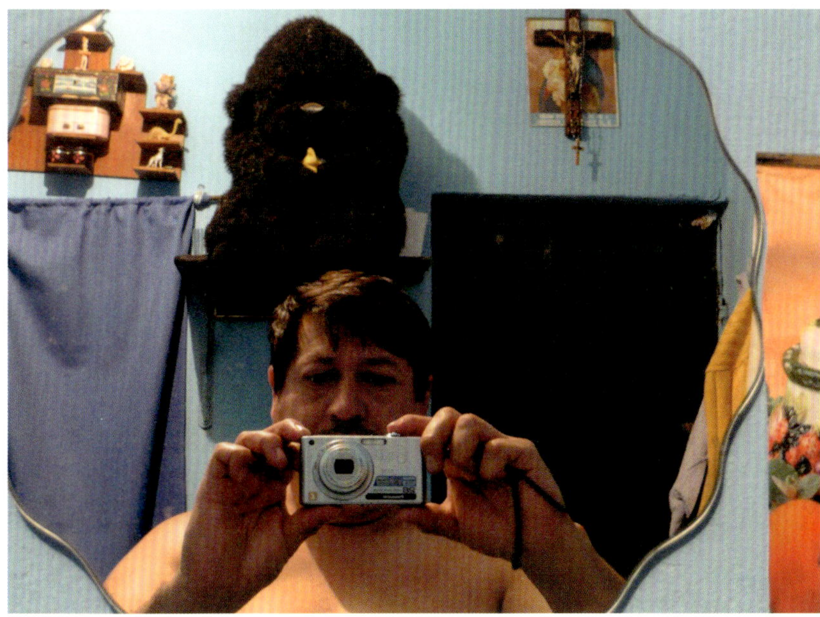

Eighteen years ago I was working in a laboratory, and it was in that very place that I tested myself for HIV. The result was positive. It was hard for me to accept the news.

The hardest thing to accept was my family's behavior. They value money, and since I used to have plenty of it, they treated me well. I even took care of their expenses. Now they refuse to give me their support. I find their attitude painful, particularly since I never ask them for money, neither for my studies nor my medicines. I get by financially by helping high school and university students with their homework.

Some time ago, in Coatzacoalcos, Veracruz, the drug gang Los Zetas kidnapped one of my brothers. My family asked me to go and negotiate with them. I didn't know what to do, I was very much afraid. Finally they released him, and when I came back I learned that they all had agreed to send me, since nobody else wanted to take the risk. At any rate, they gathered that I was doomed to die soon.

All these years of living with the virus have taught me to become more mature and to work on my feelings. Among my future plans, I want to enter the university, study chemistry, and then teach. I am standing right here, happy that I am going to succeed in everything.

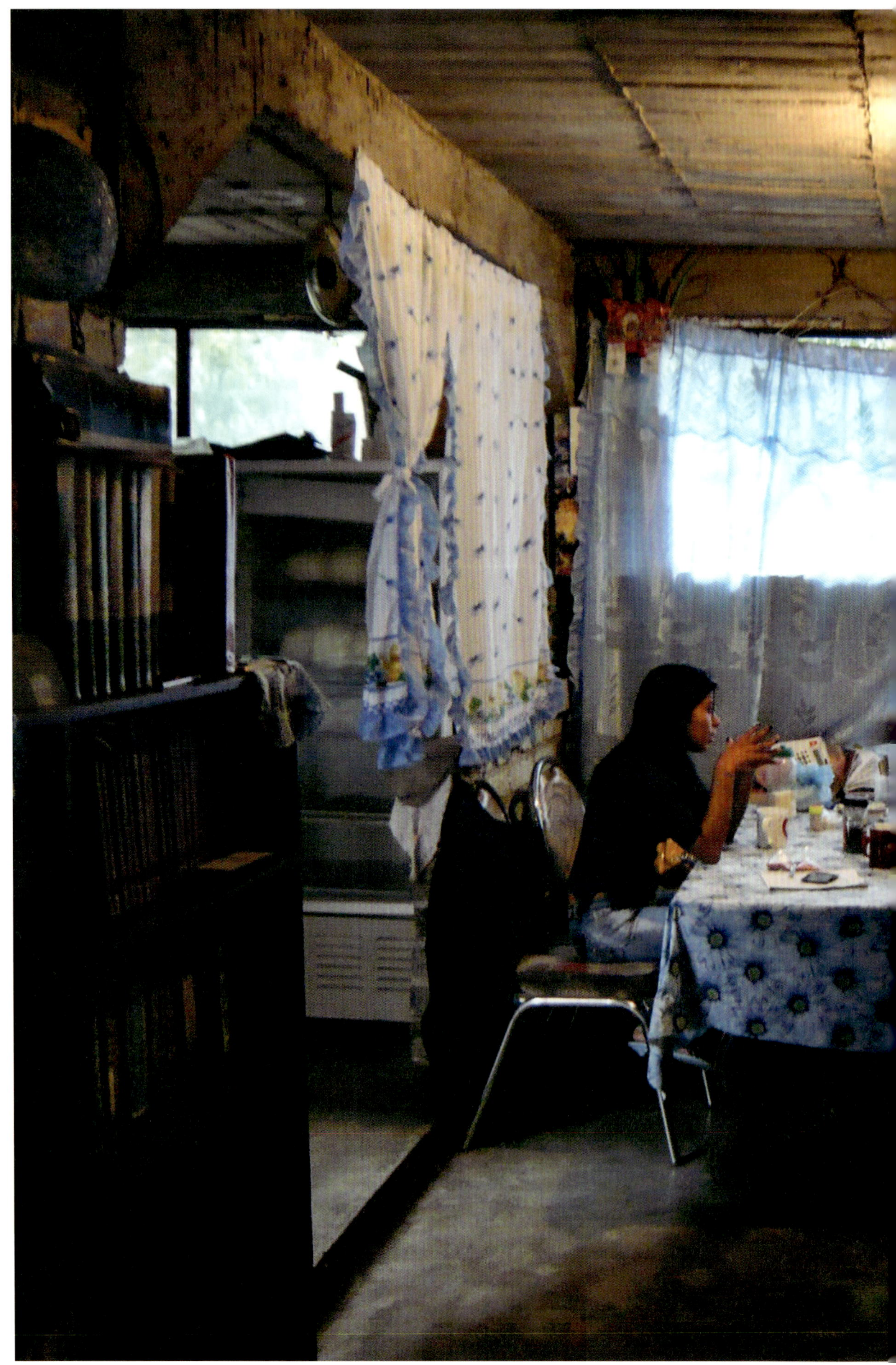

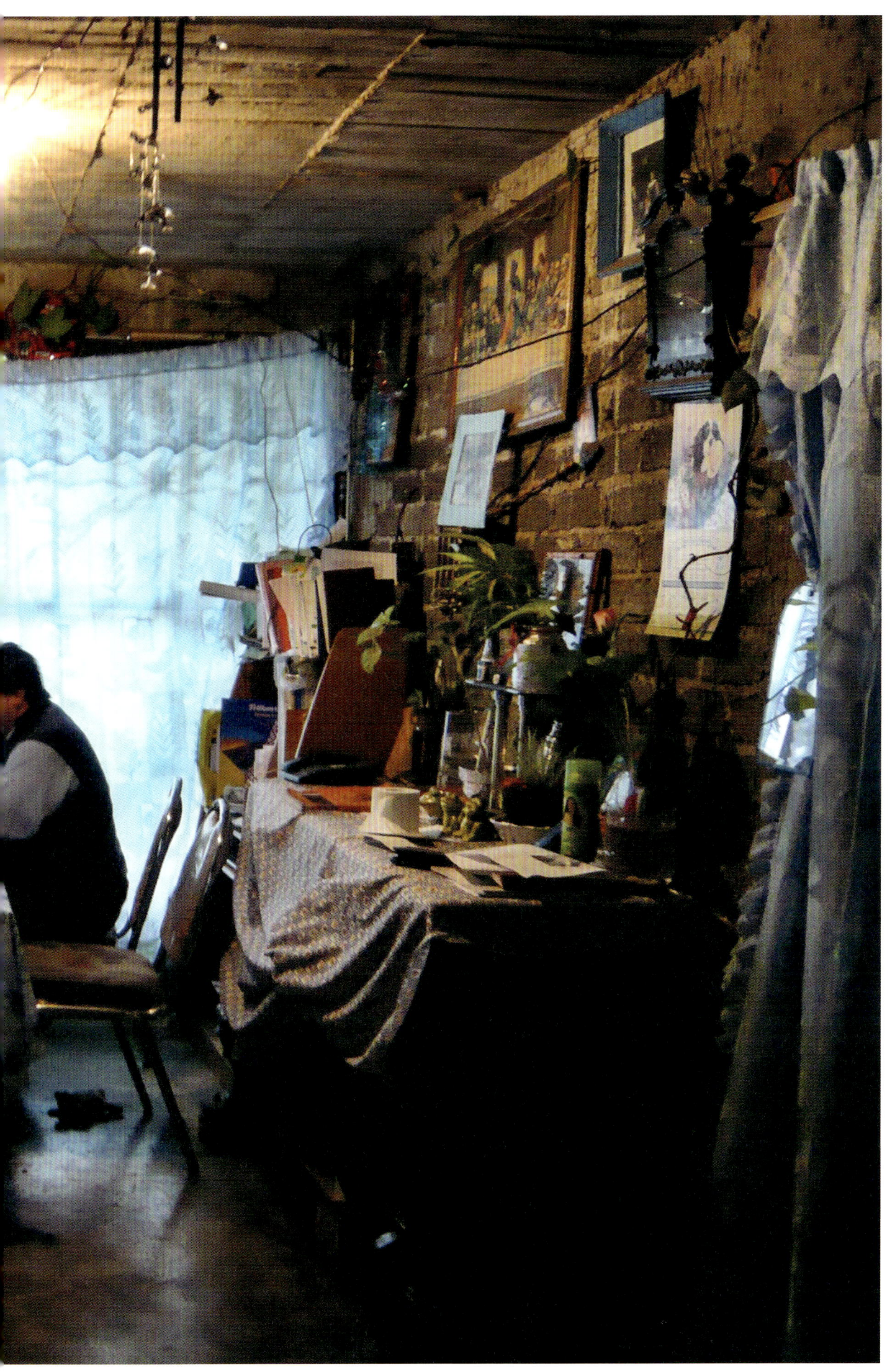

Martín

Each of our actions leaves a mark, sometimes on ourselves, sometimes on others. If I can influence at least one person to change his or her perspective about HIV, then I also will have left my mark.

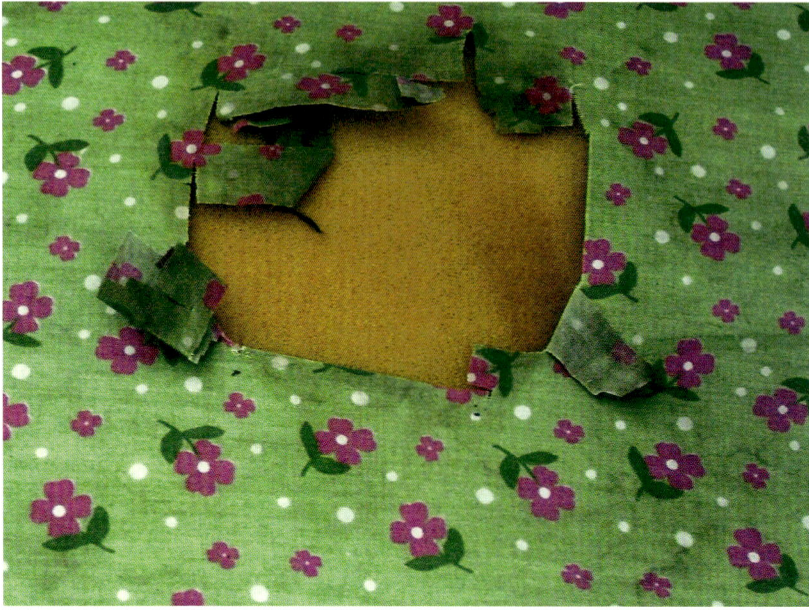

When the doctor told me we needed to discuss the results of my blood test, I already knew I was positive. I guessed it because Alfredo, my lover, had been diagnosed already. It was a hard blow for Alfredo. He felt really bad.

But the disappearance of Alfredo was even worse than learning I was HIV-positive. We had lived together for five years. One afternoon he called to tell me he was coming home. He never arrived. His family, friends, and colleagues at work never knew what happened. Seven years have gone by and we still haven't heard a word from him.

I have never suffered from living with HIV. My daily life has not changed and I'm still working. The only difference is that I have to take my meds. For some time, I was a professional dancer, but the struggle between dancing and working forced me to abandon this intriguing career.

Each of my images depicts a footprint in time, a mark left by the environment or by society. The cars, houses, and trees in my photographs keep their essence despite these marks. Their condition may not look appealing, but we cannot change it. What we can change is how we see.

Just as these images cannot be modified, neither can my HIV status. However, with a good attitude and by facing the facts, I can help people take a different view of this pandemic.

Each of our actions leaves a mark, sometimes on ourselves, sometimes on others. If I can influence at least one person to change his or her perspective about HIV, then I also will have left my mark.

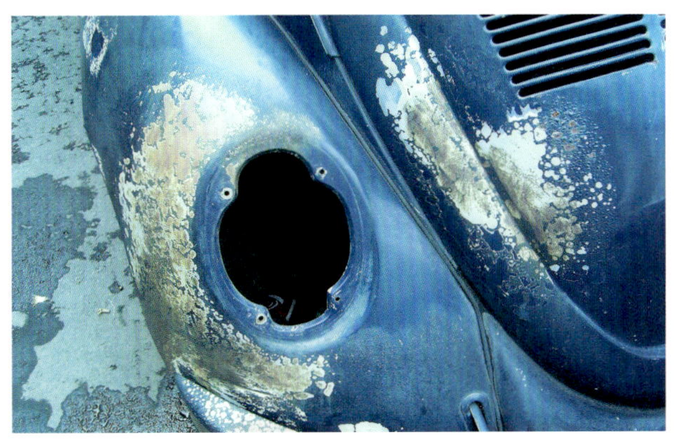
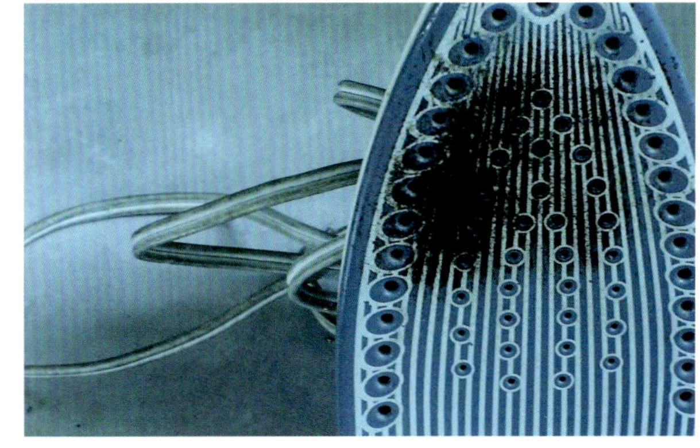
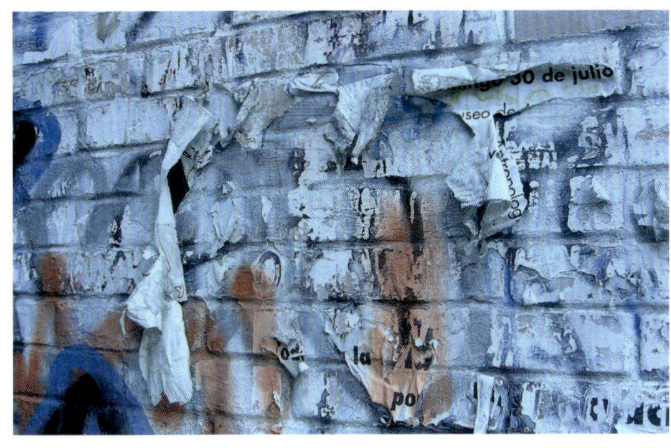
30 de julio
la
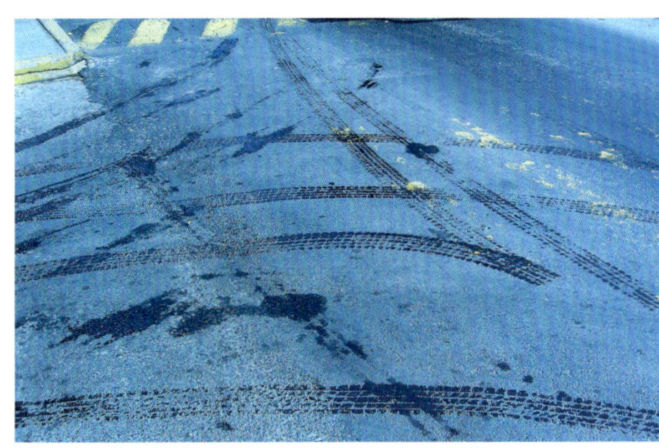
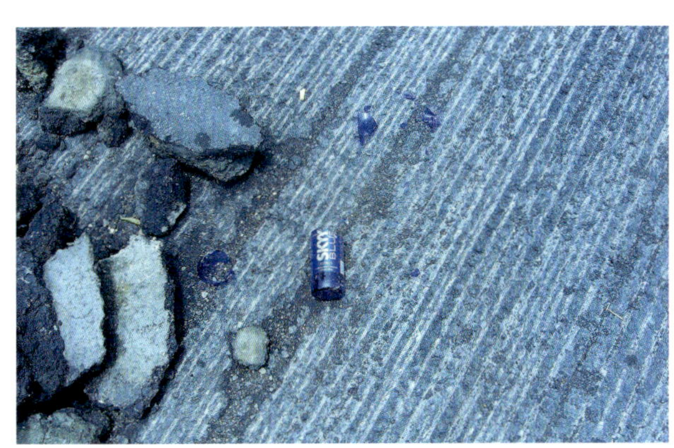
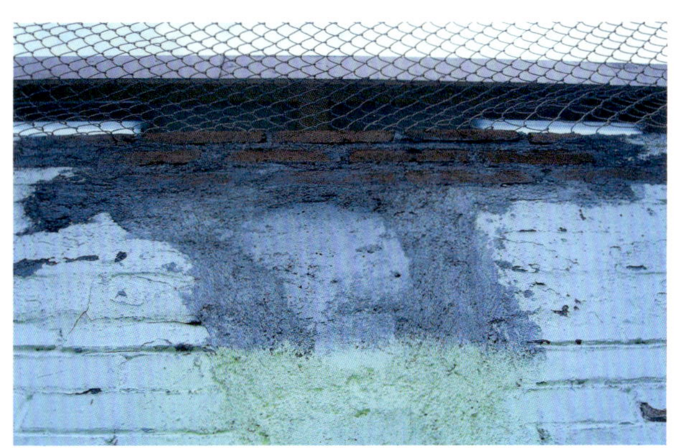
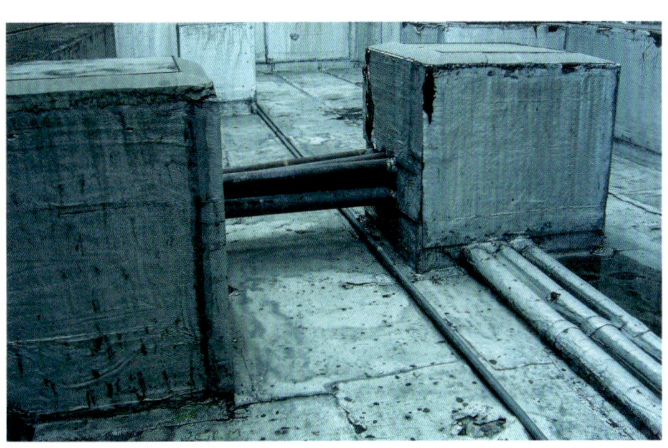
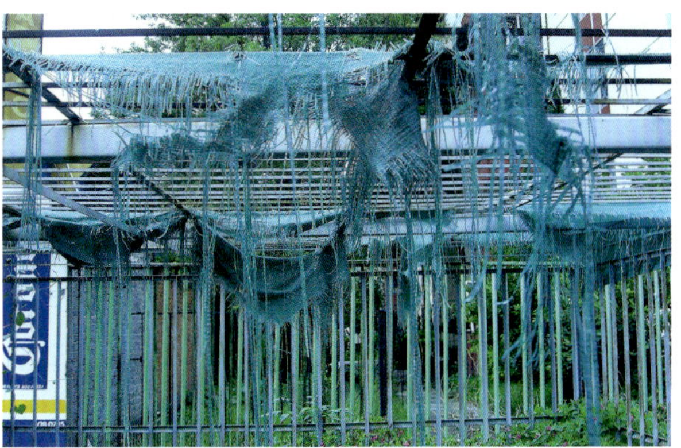

Eduardo
I am twenty-four years old and I love rainy days. As raindrops fall, I am reminded of the place where, ten years ago, I started understanding myself as a homosexual. It was the first time I ever shared something special with another man.

When I was diagnosed HIV-positive, I already had some information on the subject. One of my best friends lives with the virus. What immediately concerned me was how advanced the infection was and, from that point on, how to make the best decisions I could about my health. The moment when I contracted the virus is still very clear in my mind. The condom ripped when I was with a guy. He said nothing would happen, that HIV didn't exist.

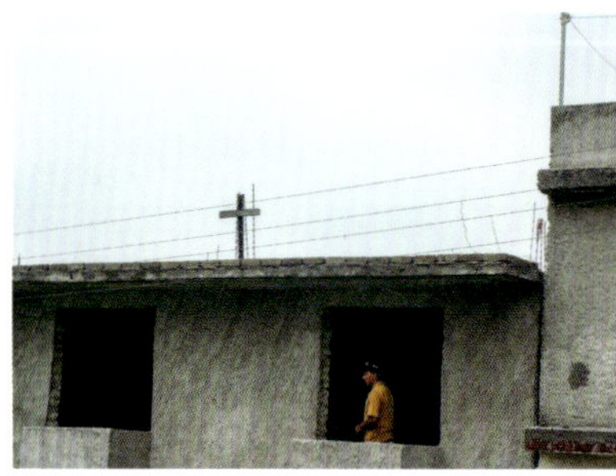

I'm dedicated now to providing psychological support to others in a community organization, but I do not consider myself an activist, only a community fighter. I think people are capable of judging what is best for them, and henceforth of fighting for what they want. By contrast, activists tend to pose themselves as starring actors in their own cause.

I have decided to show my face in this project to convey that I work, that I have a sexual life, that I am a son, and that I contribute to the betterment of our community. I have weaknesses, but also strengths. I am not an alien. I do not want any special privileges. I just want my rights to be respected.

Flor
I am not sure if I contracted HIV through a blood transfusion or by contact with contaminated medical instruments. But when I was diagnosed twelve years ago, I was sure it was God's punishment.

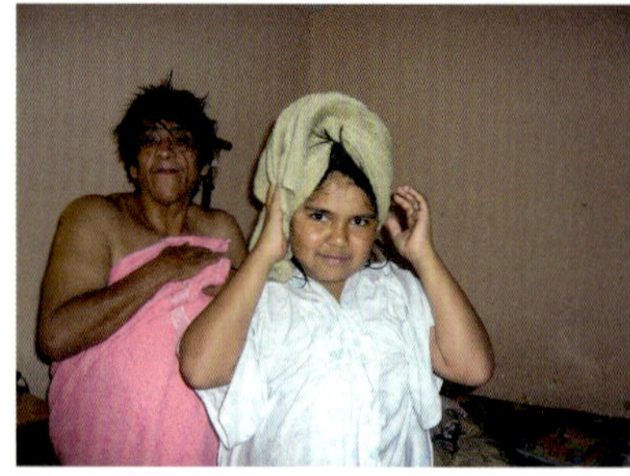

I was frightened by the idea that my husband would think I had been unfaithful. Fortunately, he always gave me his support, and so did my daughters and sisters. As far as other people, I preferred to remain silent. I didn't know how to share my story with them.

I was a union leader for a long time and I transferred this experience to the field of health. Now I represent patients in the hospital where I'm receiving medical care, and I demand respect for our human rights.

In the future, I hope to create a shelter for people affected by the epidemic who have no relatives or are rejected by them. I want to leave a trace, just as the leaders of the Mexican Revolution did, with the hope that my life would serve as an inspiration for others.

At the age of fifty-six, I feel happy that I have finally removed the stigma I had earlier imposed on myself. Now I expect to get a good response from those who would otherwise have ignored that I live with the virus.

Ilián
When I learned I had HIV, I thought that all feelings and emotions and doors would now be closed to me. After a while, I learned that HIV is only one part of me, that I have no reason to fall apart, that I have many other life options.

I am a hairdresser. I love combing and cutting hair, and making people up. The beauty shop where I work stands between a mechanic workshop and a ceramics factory. At the beginning I felt a bit afraid in such a masculine environment, but little by little people grew fond of me.

I have a strong character, but there's a part of me that feels very bothered and hurt, because I thought I could count on all my family's support. Nevertheless, today I see an Ilián who is more sure of herself, who wants to face the world and say that HIV is just one more experience that can be transcended. The world is quite large and there is room in it for all of us.

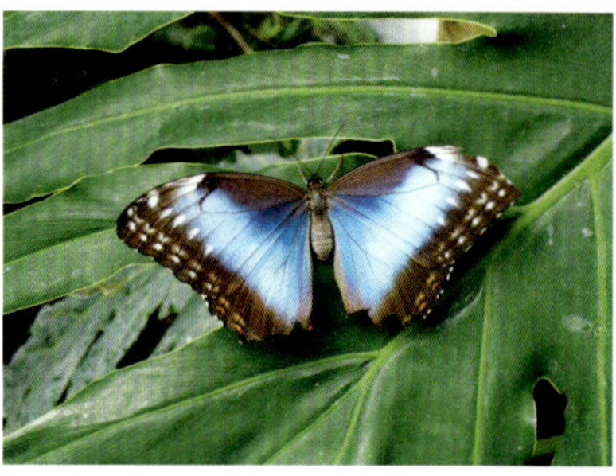

Photography awakened my consciousness and my sensitivity to the things that surround us. I noticed shapes, colors, and diversity. But above all I became aware of my inherent empathy with nature, with butterflies. I am very drawn to them because of the metamorphosis I initiated in myself, to finally be free.

Magos
I am forty-one years old, I've been married for nineteen years, and I have been living with HIV for the past seven. Before being diagnosed I was another woman, the typical housewife who takes care of her husband and children. This has changed, since although I still do the same things, I'm now also a vendor. I sell candy on the street. I also give talks to fellow HIV-positive people.

I was diagnosed in 2001. It was a very bitter moment. My doctor was on vacation and the hospital refused to give me the results. I fought against that. I told them it was my right to know my health condition. If I hadn't done that, I'm sure I would have died of sheer frustration.

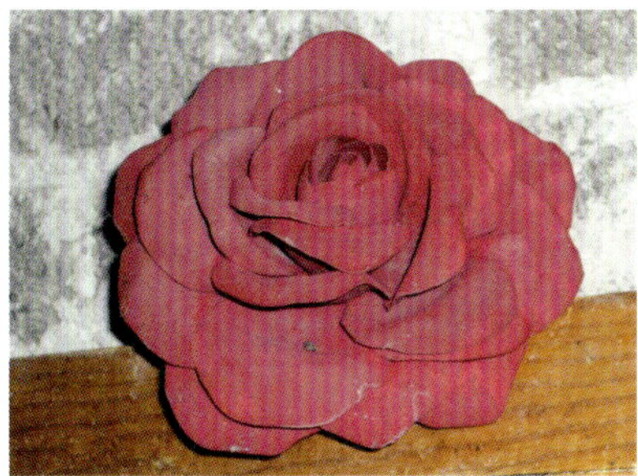

HIV has taught me that life goes on and there's always a tomorrow. I give thanks for all the good and bad things that have happened to me. I pray for my family and to sell lots of candy. I don't pray for my health, because I'm not going to relinquish to anyone else the power that is in my own hands.

I know it is my obligation to fight discrimination, against me and against the upcoming generation. This is why I give a face and a heart to AIDS. I want people to see that we are all equal, that we should not be judged or discriminated against, and that everyone should be informed.

Octavio

My HIV infection was the consequence of a gang rape. When the doctors gave me the diagnosis, I felt my life was over. What else could happen to me? I had been a very abused child. My mother was homophobic. So I left home.

For a long time, I indulged in sex work and kept fooling around. When I got sick, I ran away from the hospital because I didn't want to die there. Suddenly I got a message from a community group that helped me a lot. They encouraged me to make a commitment to myself and to life.

I am now a sexual health advisor. We promote a quick HIV test, alongside which I offer counselling. In addition, I work for a company where I am in charge of preparing and organizing events.

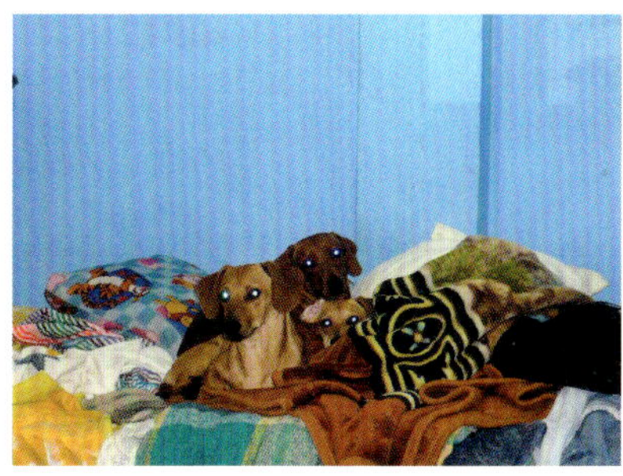

It is very important for me to be public about my HIV status, because I am not just a number, and I'm not falling apart. I am a passionate man, committed to what I do. And passion is a lifestyle. It's what keeps me going. Photography is one of my passions. I am very daring in all aspects of my life, and my pictures reflect that.

René

I was diagnosed with HIV just a year ago. I was not surprised. I always took care, but then on one occasion I didn't protect myself. I became seriously ill and there seemed no hope I would live. My family was fully supportive. They were by my side, night and day.

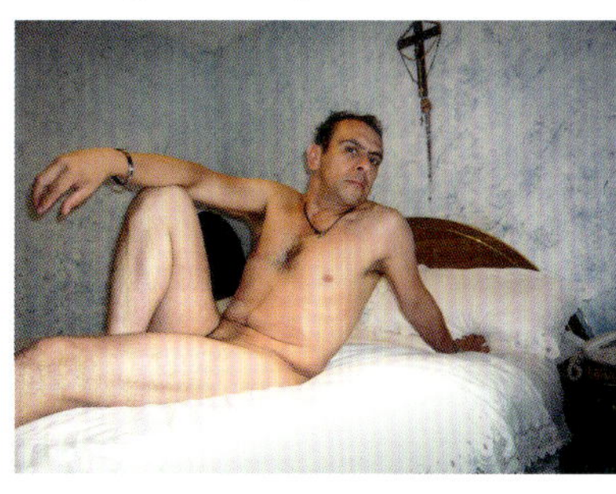

I'm now under treatment, and people are amazed at my recovery. I do a lot of sports, I'm a spinning instructor, I work at three gyms.

I don't pretend to be an example. All I want is to open people's eyes, because anyone can be in this situation.

I'm a very happy person, because if you have a good sense of humor you can achieve lots of things. You transmit joy to other people and help them endure their problems.

I identify a lot with this thought: "Don't fall asleep thinking that something is impossible to achieve, because you might be woken up by the noise made by someone who is achieving it."

I always make jokes about my situation. HIV lives with me, I don't live with it. I'm not going to let it defeat me. I laugh at it, I have fun, I have it, and I'm still here.

Roberto

When I learned the results of my HIV test, I asked myself if I could live with the infection. At that moment, all my prejudices and internalized stigmas came to the surface, because although I knew about AIDS—thanks to my job as a journalist—I still had to go through a period of denial.

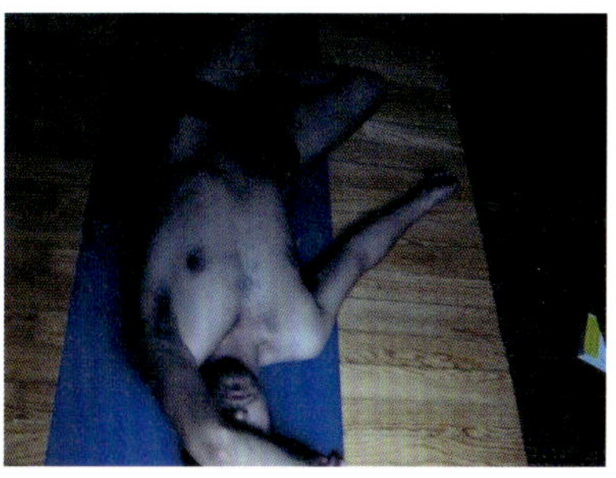

I am very committed to my health now because my recovery was difficult. I have learned the value of life. I have learned that in spite of the infection, it is not so difficult to live if you really put your mind to it.

I'm a very lucky guy because I've always had the support of my relatives, friends, and colleagues at work.

They know HIV is a viral, not a moral, infection.

My favorite singer is Eugenia León. In one of her songs she sings, "God made me unlucky, but I am not in the mood for that." With this, I mean to say that I'm still alive, that I can love and give pleasure, because although happiness is not forever, neither are sadness and depression.

Through photography I have been able to reflect on myself and my relationship to my body, this companion that is going to be with me until the day that I die.

Salvador

My reaction twelve years ago, when I learned I was HIV-positive, was to feel I had been so stupid, because I had the information and didn't use it. I played with fire and look at the result.

My lover also turned out to be HIV-positive. We didn't reproach one another, but we made a pact to let the disease advance unimpeded. Each of us wanted a quick death, with little suffering. It was a fatalistic decision made out of fear. But we were wrong, because by 1996 there were new treatments. We took the drugs and we're still here.

I was originally a medical transcriber, but I now work as a clinical file clerk at the National Institute of Nutrition. At the Institute, I provide support and information to people who do not know what to do when they come in for HIV treatment. I facilitate their admission to the hospital and help them get quick medical care.

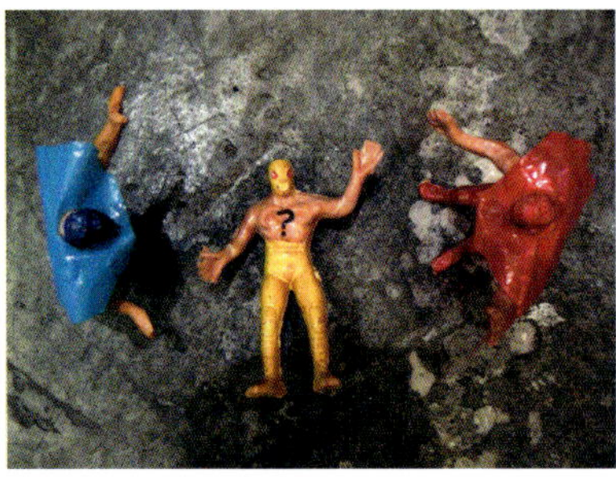

Being sound and healthy helps me to encourage people: "Don't give up so easily. Just think, you can be as healthy as I am." There are people who have died from ignorance, from having a fatalistic attitude, from not taking HIV as just a new step and opportunity in life. These people have to be told that there is still a long road to go, that they have many years ahead of them.

Silvia

I am thirty-nine and have been living with HIV for fifteen years. When I received the diagnosis, I felt like I was already dying. I thought of my three children and imagined I was losing them. I was the typical downtrodden housewife. I had endured my husband's machismo and bisexuality, but I said to myself: "Silvia, you have to move on. You can't just stand still, waiting for death to come."

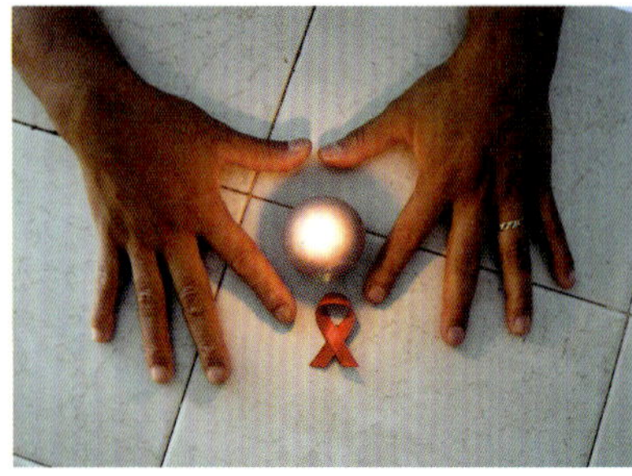

Over time, I have become an activist, helping people at the hospital. I work mostly with women, building on my own experience as a bold, fighting woman. When I negotiate with authorities at the hospital, I often tell them, "Either you stick to your word or I'll sue you." That is what gives me strength, fighting for the rights of people living with HIV.

I photographed myself alone and with my children, because they give me hope. And I took one photo of a candle with the HIV symbol because in the past fifteen years I have seen a lot of people die. I send them light so they can rest.

And to tell you the truth, I am very happy, for I now understand HIV and have myself as the best reason for living.

Rio de Janeiro

Health is ensconced in the Brazilian Constitution as a fundamental right. Consequently, Brazil is known for offering some of the most comprehensive treatment options in the world, including low-cost generic medications. However, by June 2009, when the *Through Positive Eyes* workshop was held in Rio de Janeiro, it was already clear that AIDS care in Brazil, while among the best in the world, remained less than perfect. Workshop participants specifically referenced the lack of HIV testing facilities in the early days, the frequent misdiagnosis of women, and the difficult side effects caused by early generations of antiretroviral therapy. Another theme that emerged loudly was the heightened vulnerability of young people and sexual minorities. Notably, almost all the project participants were infected with HIV not as adults but as teenagers.

Brazil's AIDS epidemic, as of 2009

Number of people living with HIV:	630,000

HIV prevalence

Adults (15–49 years):	0.61%
Female sex workers:	4.9%
Men who have sex with men:	12.6%
People who inject drugs:	5.9%

Treatment

Universal access to treatment since 1996.

Numbers on treatment:	197,000
% of those in need of treatment who are receiving it:	95%

Key events

2003 *First generic antiretroviral medications (ARVs) produced domestically.*

2007 *First compulsory licence to import low-cost generic ARVs.*

2009 *National strategies to combat HIV-related stigma directed to LGBTQI citizens.*

Update 2019

860,000 Brazilians are living with HIV. 64% of these are on treatment and 59% of those in treatment have no detectable virus. HIV prevalence among men who have sex with men has declined to 10.5%.

Despite anti-stigma programs, in 2017 it was estimated that 12.1% of sex workers and 62% of men who have sex with men avoid health care due to stigma and discrimination.

Brazil's progress on HIV is now under threat from the newly elected conservative president, Jair Bolsonaro. In 2019, he removed LGBTQI rights from the purview of the Human Rights Ministry, and he opposes state-funded treatment for people living with HIV.

Through Positive Eyes in Rio de Janeiro—*Olhares Posithivos*—was organized in partnership with the Brazilian Interdisciplinary AIDS Association (ABIA), with major funding from Brazil's STD/AIDS Prevention Department, housed within the Ministry of Health, and The Ford Foundation.

Cleverson

The fear I had on account of the stigma associated with the disease—that I was going to get thinner, wane, and die—suddenly dissipated. Today I live a normal life like any other person.

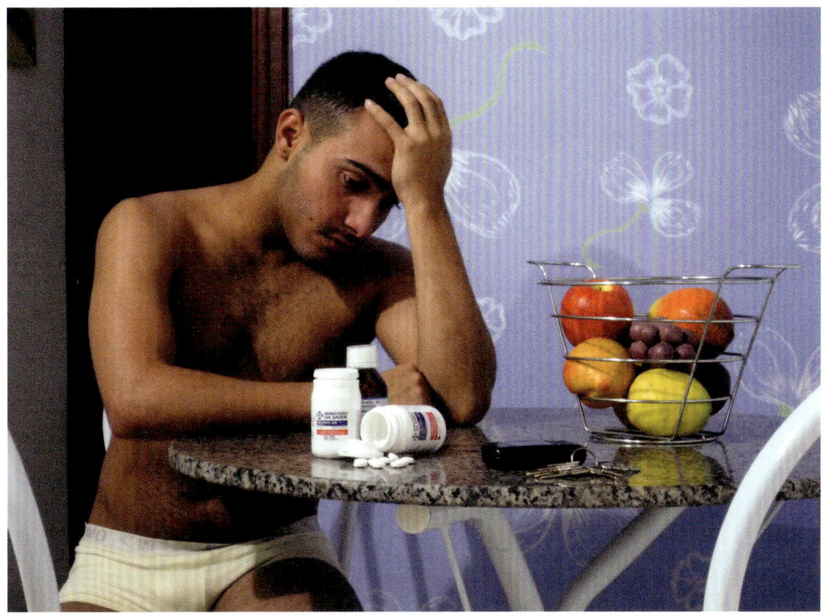

I realized I was gay when I was nine years old. But actually understanding it took some time. At twelve, I had a friend who was openly gay and I wanted to find out more about it through him, to get to know the lifestyle. He took me to parties, introduced me to friends. I used fake IDs to go to nightclubs. I had my first sexual experiences when I was thirteen or fourteen years old. I never used a condom—in my mind STDs and HIV did not exist.

My life followed its natural course until I joined the Army when I was eighteen. I took preliminary exams to see what it would be like. When I passed, I had a perfect moment—a night with a beautiful moon. I knew I was going to earn a good salary, that I would be able to buy a house. I was celebrating and there were fireworks somewhere. It was like a film.

When I completed the mandatory health checks in the Army hospital, the syphilis test came back negative, but the HIV results took a long time to be delivered. I was in the middle of exams when a lieutenant told me that I could not proceed, because I was HIV-positive. My life was over. I started to cry, but no one knew why. I considered shooting myself, but I knew this would not make any difference.

Three days after I found out about my status, I met Guilherme on the Internet, in a chat room of people living with HIV/AIDS. He invited me to visit Pela Vida, an HIV support organization. I got to know more about HIV and things changed. The fear I had on account of the stigma associated with the disease—that I was going to get thinner, wane, and die—suddenly dissipated. Today I live a normal life like any other person.

Guilherme and I started living together about six months ago. We have some disagreements, a few scuffles sometimes. But it's a good life. Guilherme is a sweetheart. He is my love, and he takes care of me.

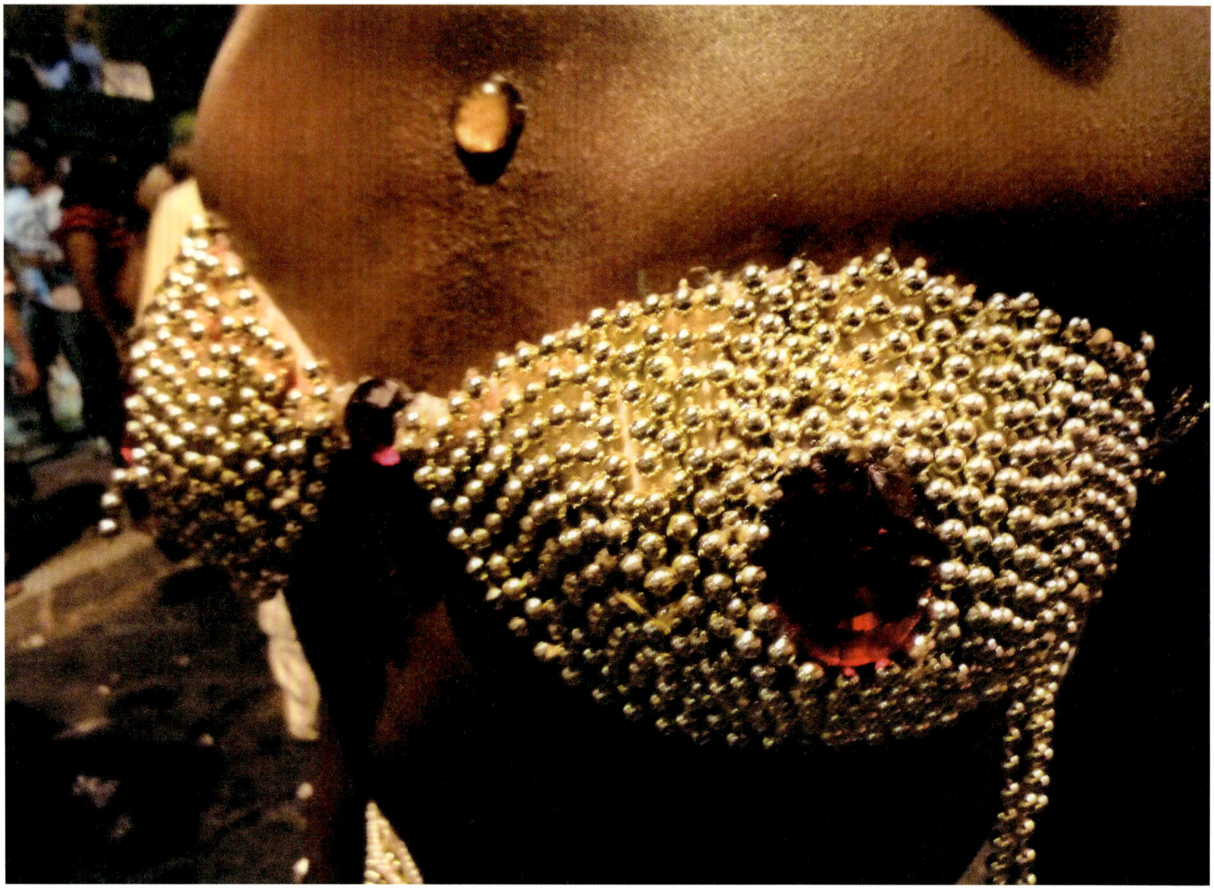

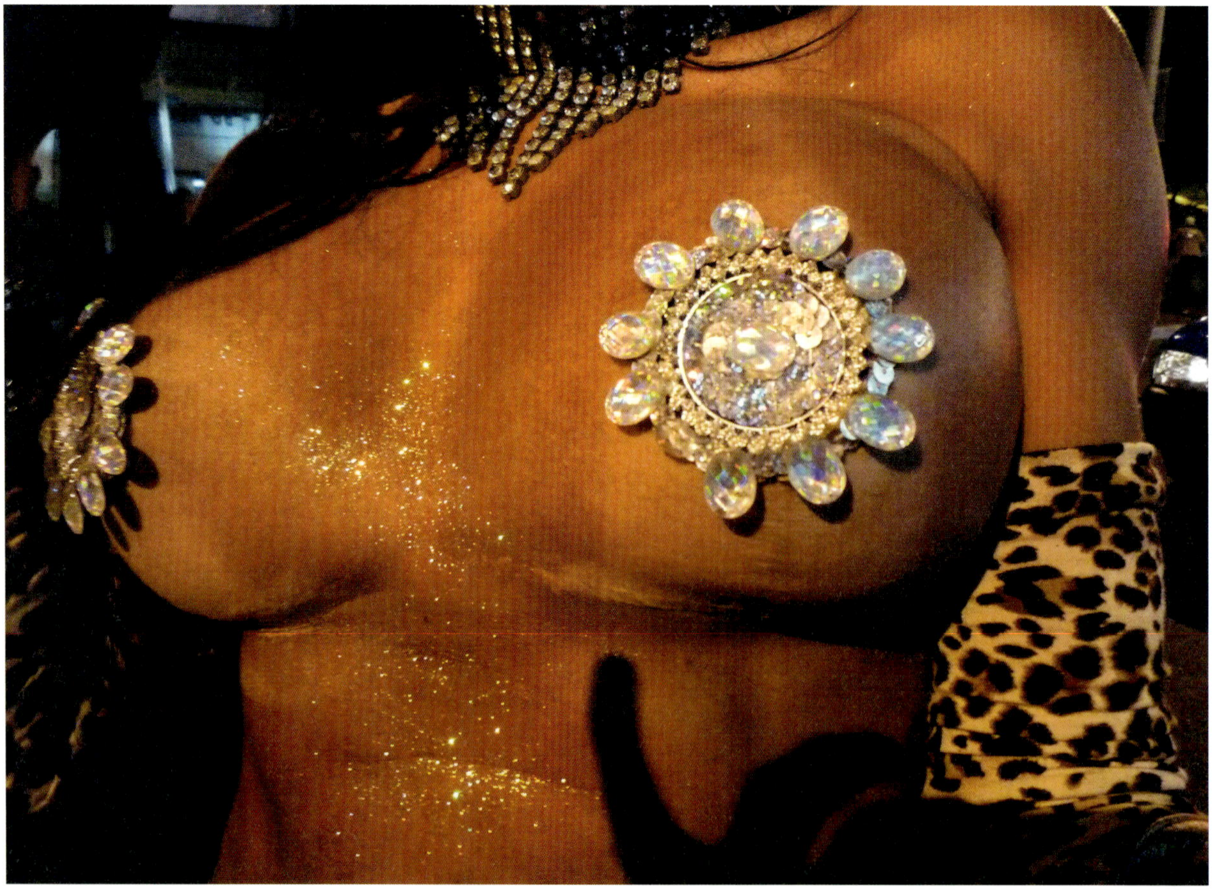

Albany

For a time, I lost my eyesight, I couldn't talk, I lost my sense of touch, I couldn't hold things. I almost died, but God gave me everything again.

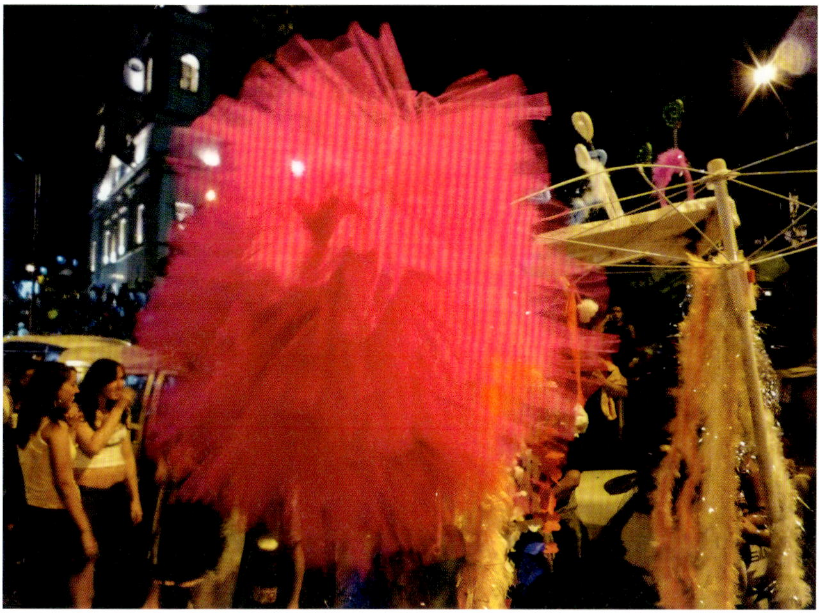

I used to be a very naughty person, very crazy and totally irresponsible. I had no love for my body. I had no love for myself. When I discovered my diagnosis I was very fragile. The doctor told me I had contracted HIV about eight or ten years before. He said, "Albany, today you're a person living with AIDS."

What got me down the most was meningitis, an opportunistic disease that affects many people living with HIV. For a time, I lost my eyesight, I couldn't talk, I lost my sense of touch, I couldn't hold things. I almost died, but God gave me everything again. The doctors gave me all their support, moral and ethical. I knew then that I had to be different, that I couldn't live with the mistakes of the past. I couldn't waste any of this life.

So I have had to change my story, my life. I have suffered a lot with HIV, but today I am sure that I have changed. I have balance, and I have goals to live by, because I contracted something very serious.

Today I'm an AIDS militant. I left the nightlife, the nightclubs. I'm not dating anymore, but I'm always with my activist friends. This is how I survive. This is how I live, how I love those close to me, how I'm coherent, and how I'm patient. I am open, I show my cards, and I'm much better now, thank God.

Jorge

In the beginning I thought I had an expiration date, that I was being told, "You're going to die." But when I started going to self-help groups, people showed me that you can live a long time with HIV.

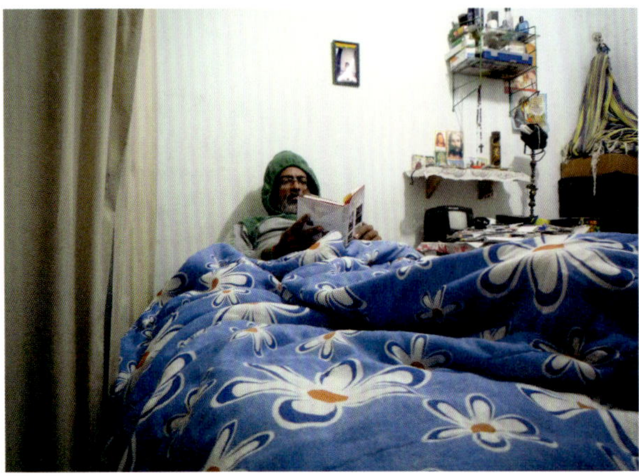

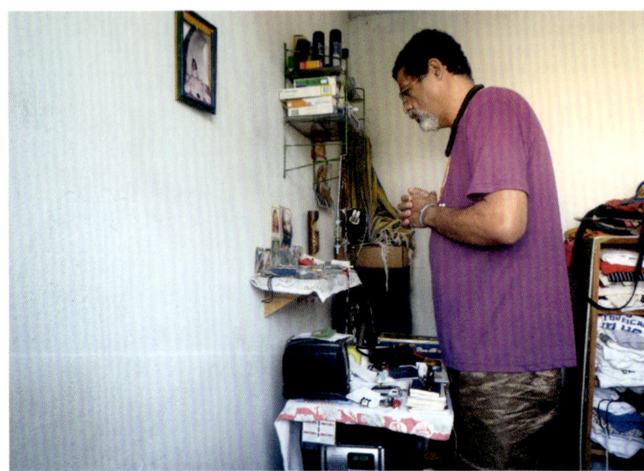

HIV changed my life a lot, but it had a good side too, which is that I started doing prevention work, raising awareness so that other people don't become infected with HIV.

In the beginning I thought I had an expiration date, that I was being told, "You're going to die." I thought like that. But when I started going to self-help groups, people showed me that you can live a long time with HIV, many many years.

Nowadays the government assists patients with adequate medication. The government is helping a lot by financing the treatment—a compromise on their part, for this is much easier for them than allowing hospitals to become packed with HIV patients, turning it into an epidemic. They would have to spend much more money if that happened.

I do not know for sure how I got infected. I was involved in many risky situations. I needed a blood transfusion for a surgery I had on my leg. Blood was not yet tested for HIV at the time. And I had extramarital sex without protection, even though I was aware of the need for condoms.

When I found out about my infection, my wife was pregnant with my son. My greatest happiness was finding out that she wasn't a carrier of the virus, and neither was my son. Today I don't live with her, but we're friends, and my son is always here with me. He is thirteen years old. He is a strong boy. He plays football in Cabo Frio. Who knows, he might be the next Caca.

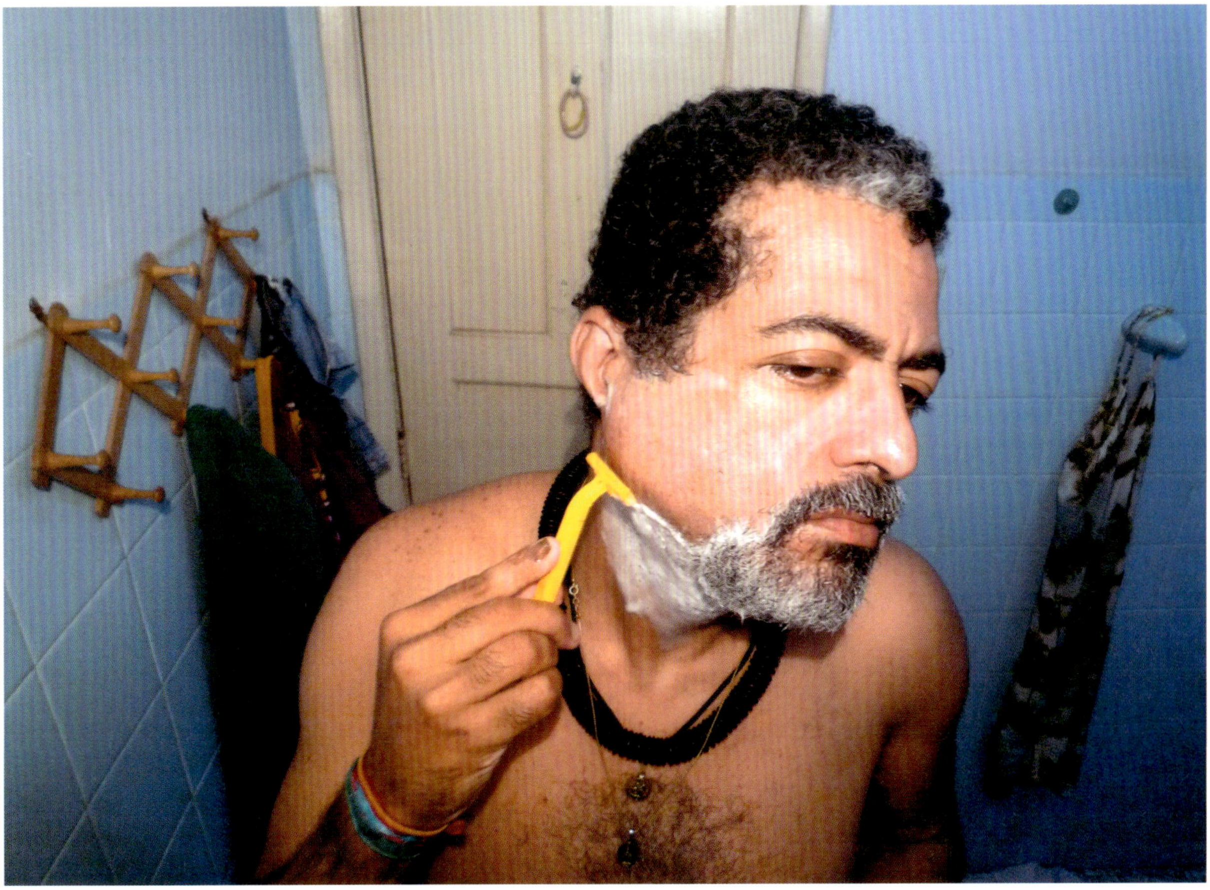

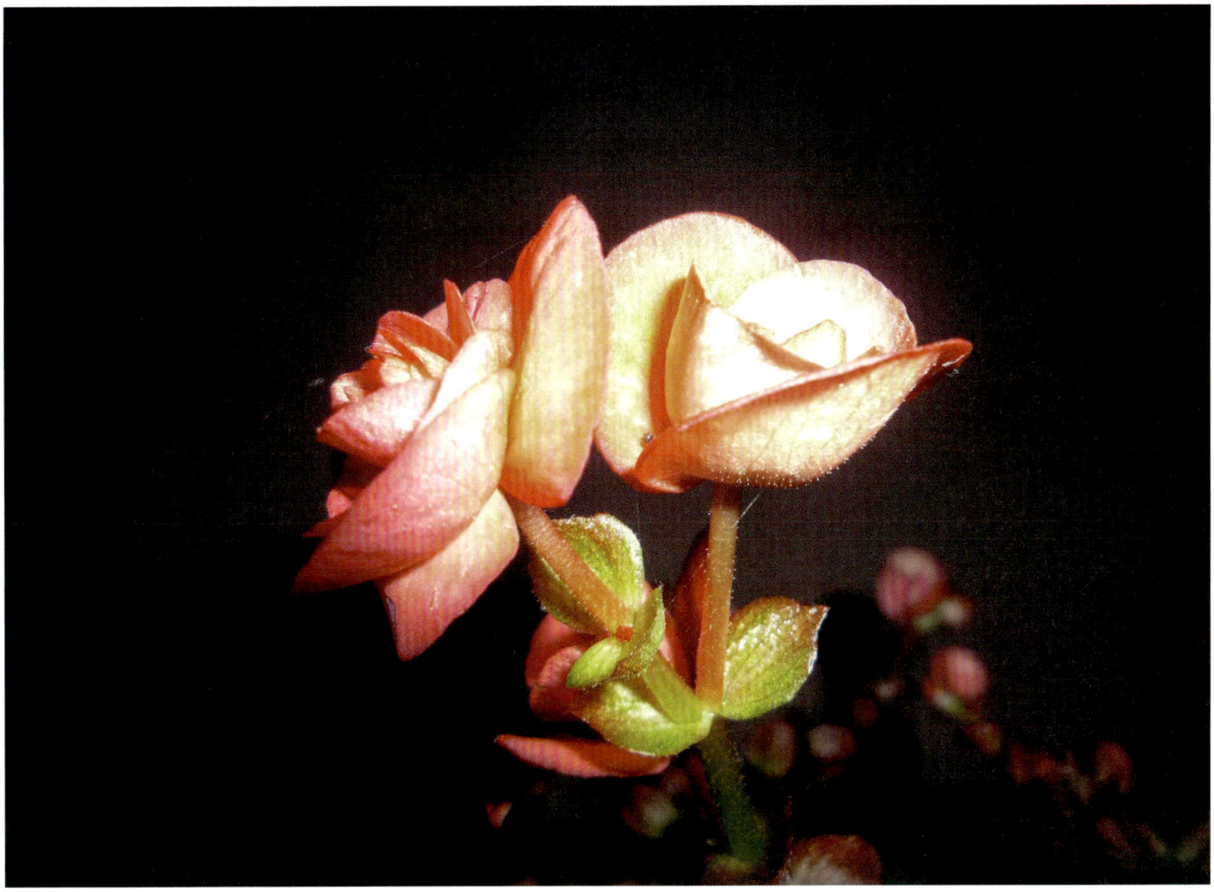

Cazu

HIV didn't fundamentally change my way of life. Sure, I now have to practice the discipline of taking medication. But I started living more after HIV.

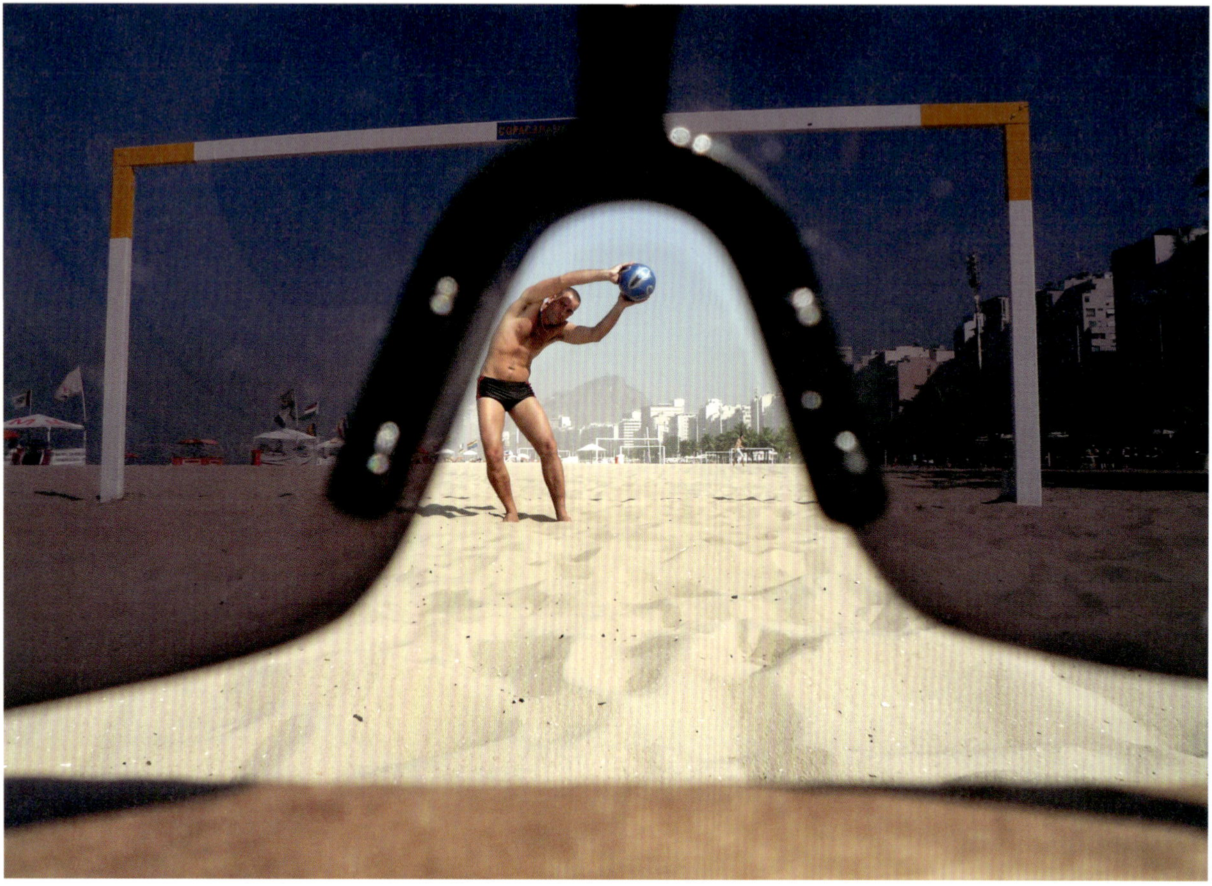

Living with HIV, I have achieved many things that I never thought possible—public recognition, great roles both in the cinema and in the theater— all since I became HIV-positive. This has given me the strength to encourage more people with HIV to take the same stand: "I am HIV-positive and I won't give up on my goals. If something is not working out, I can change it and find a way forward." That is what I did.

What made me go public about AIDS was the need to break the stigma that people living with AIDS are ugly, that they are unproductive, and that they must be isolated or treated like wretches. People living with AIDS will remain who they were before HIV, independent of it. Those who were good people will remain good people, and the same goes for those who weren't. Independently of having HIV or not, people are still human beings. They still have feelings. They love, suffer, cry, and laugh.

HIV didn't fundamentally change my way of life. Sure, I now have to practice the discipline of taking medication. Death left my subconscious and entered my conscious mind. But in no way can HIV get in the way of my life. In fact, I started living more after HIV. May people live life independently of being positive or negative, may they be happy, build their life projects, continue their studies, continue working, continue loving. Because HIV shouldn't be stronger than life.

Francisco

I am speaking here, from the place where I was attacked yesterday. I even have a broken arm, but that's not going to stop me from fighting.

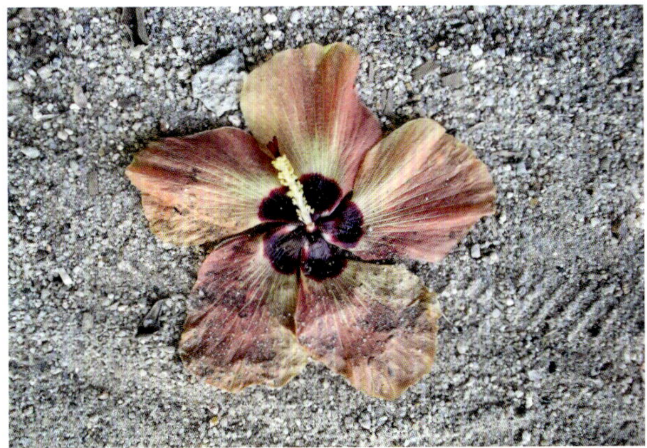

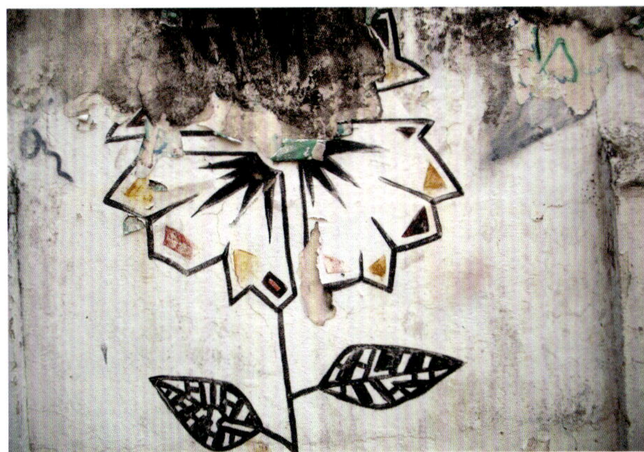

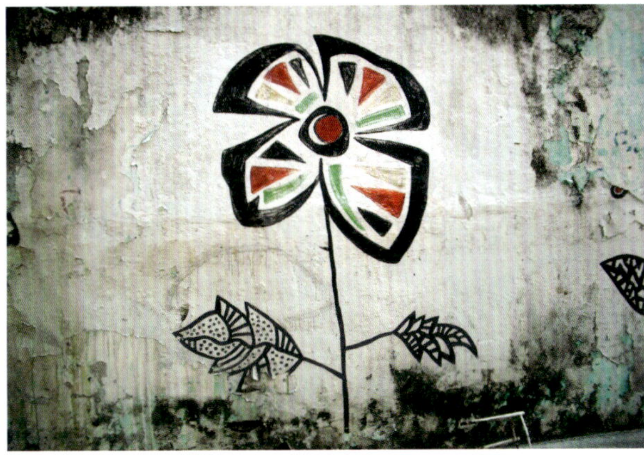

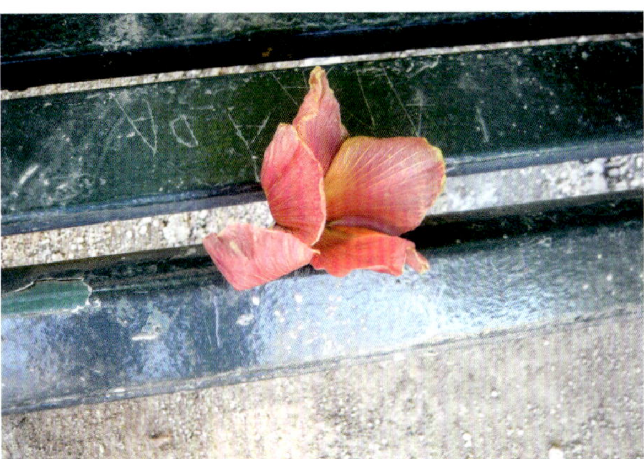

My name is Francisco. I live in Rio de Janeiro. I have AIDS.

I traveled from Recife, through Natal, through Paraíba. I was kicked out of my house. I am like a nomad. I started traveling, traveling, traveling.

I have family here in Rio de Janeiro, but they have rejected me, because I am HIV-positive.

I have shown that I am a fighter against the disease. I take my medication. I am speaking here, from the place where I was attacked yesterday. I even have a broken arm, but that's not going to stop me from fighting.

Prejudice against homosexuals is a terrible thing. I am fallen, psychologically, mentally. I have nothing else to say.

I am a fighter, maybe even a warrior. That's it.

Aninha

My greatest joy was when I opened the result of my son's exam and there it was, "negative." I cried. I laughed. I ran and told my friends. And then everyone cried and laughed with me.

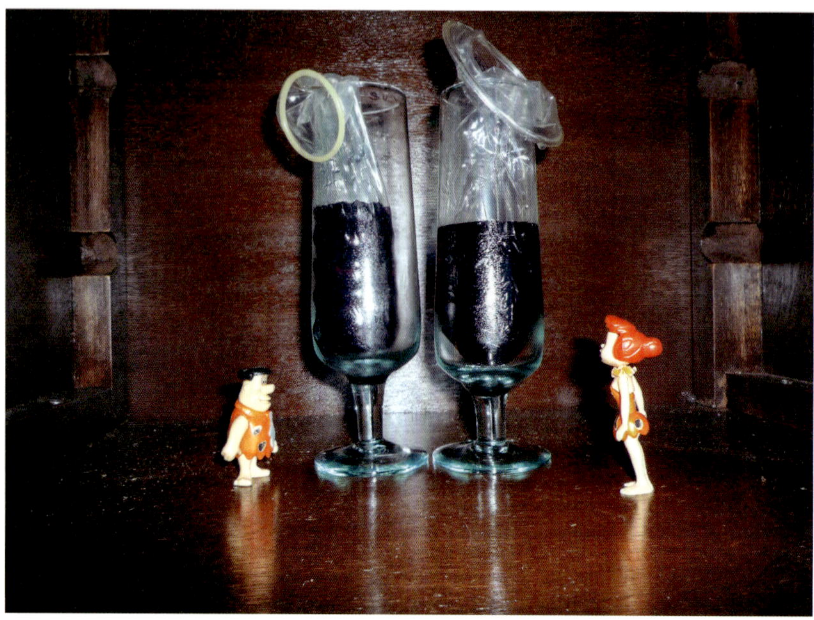

I am a happy person, but it hasn't always been like this. I was rebellious. I didn't want to take the medication. I was sick with AIDS, bedridden, in a wheelchair. I almost died but didn't, thanks to my will to live, the Brazilian Unified Health Care System, and the medications. I have trouble with speech and memory loss. What bothers me the most is to have forgotten things from my past. It's not easy to live like this.

The most difficult moment of my life was discovering that I was pregnant and I had HIV. I suffered for months. I even tried to have an abortion, but the doctor said there was no need for one, that I was very sick and the baby wouldn't survive. To my surprise and to the surprise of all, the baby was born. He was sick, but in time I found out he was HIV-negative. My greatest joy was when I opened the result of my son's exam and there it was, "negative." I cried. I laughed. I ran and told my friends. And then everyone cried and laughed with me. It was the greatest emotion I have felt in all my life.

My son is a teenager now and recently has suffered prejudice at school. In recent years, I have suffered serious prejudice as well, as a result of which I have been hiding myself. I could not protest without showing my face, so I went quiet. It is so annoying to have to hide.

My message to my son is that I don't want AIDS to cause such discomfort in people. I want my son to live in a better world. The people I know did not go looking for AIDS. AIDS showed up in their lives. I have heard of people who were killed for having AIDS, for being gay. We cannot go on in a world like this.

José Luis

I used to have friends with well-established jobs, and I used to go on holidays with them everywhere around Rio. But when they found out I was positive, they walked away.

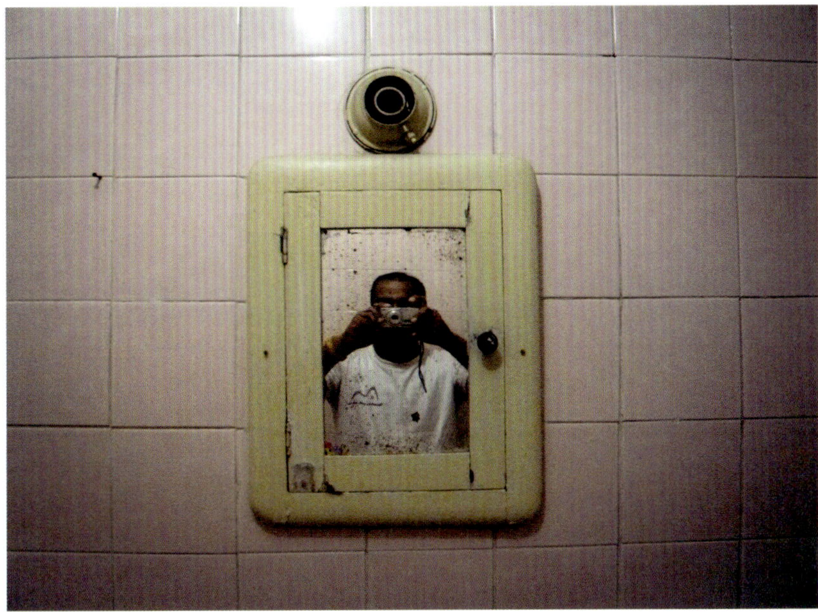

When I found out that I was positive, my only fear was my partner's reaction. I went out, got drunk, and went home. I couldn't sleep. When my partner woke up, I told her. She stared at me for ten minutes. She didn't say anything, didn't cry.

I asked her, "So?" She said, "Paqueta Street, number 72." That was our address. I asked her what she meant by that and she said, "We are together to the end." But I didn't really feel that she meant it.

The next day I went out to think everything over. I just knew she would not be able to adjust to the news. Sure enough, when I got home that night all my clothes were in the guest room.

That was on a Thursday. The following Tuesday she told me she could not cope, socially and emotionally. When people would start to see that I was losing weight, that I had AIDS, she would be discriminated against in her hometown. She asked me to leave. All my savings had been spent on her. I had no resources left. She did not even help me pack. I ended up staying in the Novo Rio bus terminal in Rio for thirty-six days.

I used to have friends with well-established jobs, and I used to go on holidays with them everywhere around Rio. But when they found out I was positive, they walked away.

Nowadays I am on the other side of Rio. It's different of course. It's hard to live in the Republica area. I live in a support house located between the communities of Mangueria and Tuiutí, and drug traffic is in charge over there, not the state. There, instead of buying food, people buy alcohol. Me, instead of buying alcohol, I buy a newspaper. I enjoy going to the library, to the theater, to the movies. Before, when I could afford them, I used to buy a book a month in the various subjects I am interested in: law, social sciences, and anthropology. Nowadays I cannot afford them, but I see this as my motivation to overcome all these obstacles.

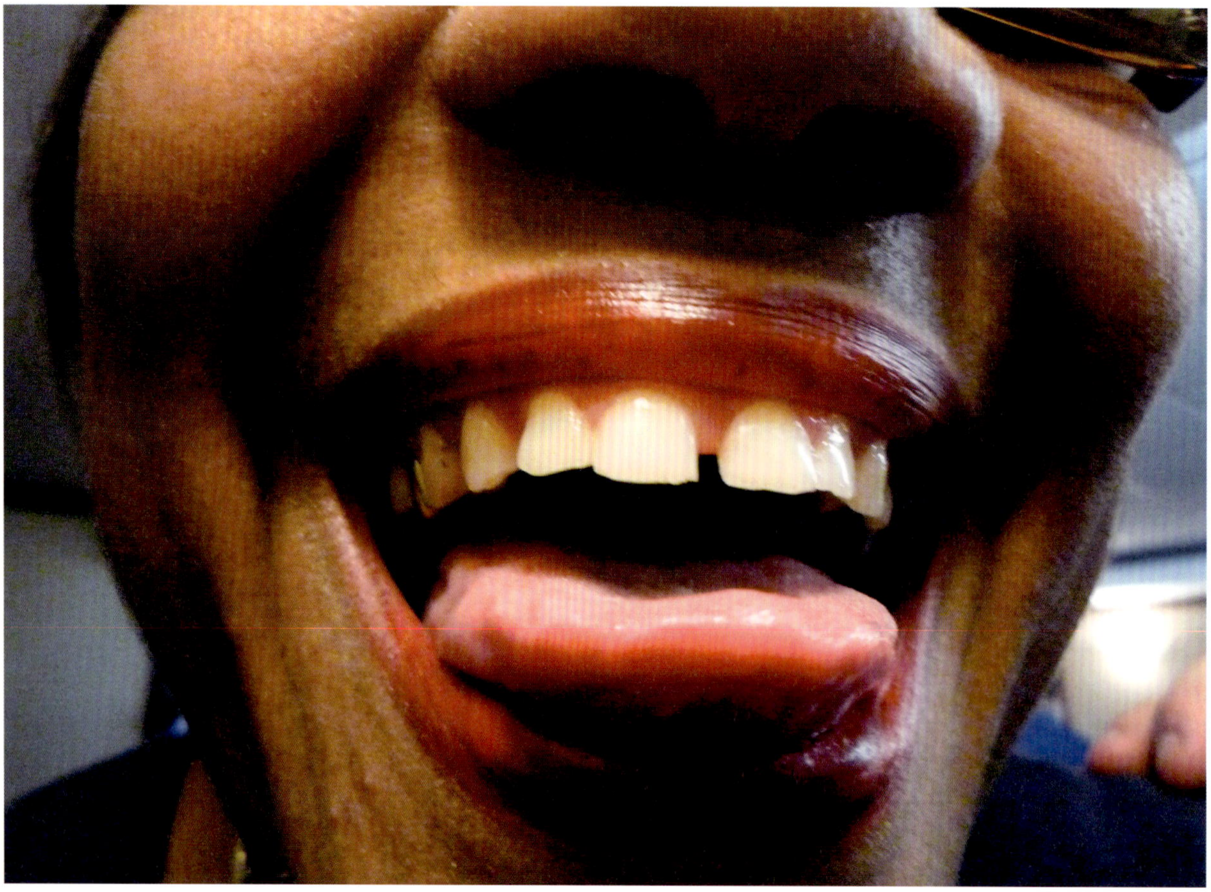

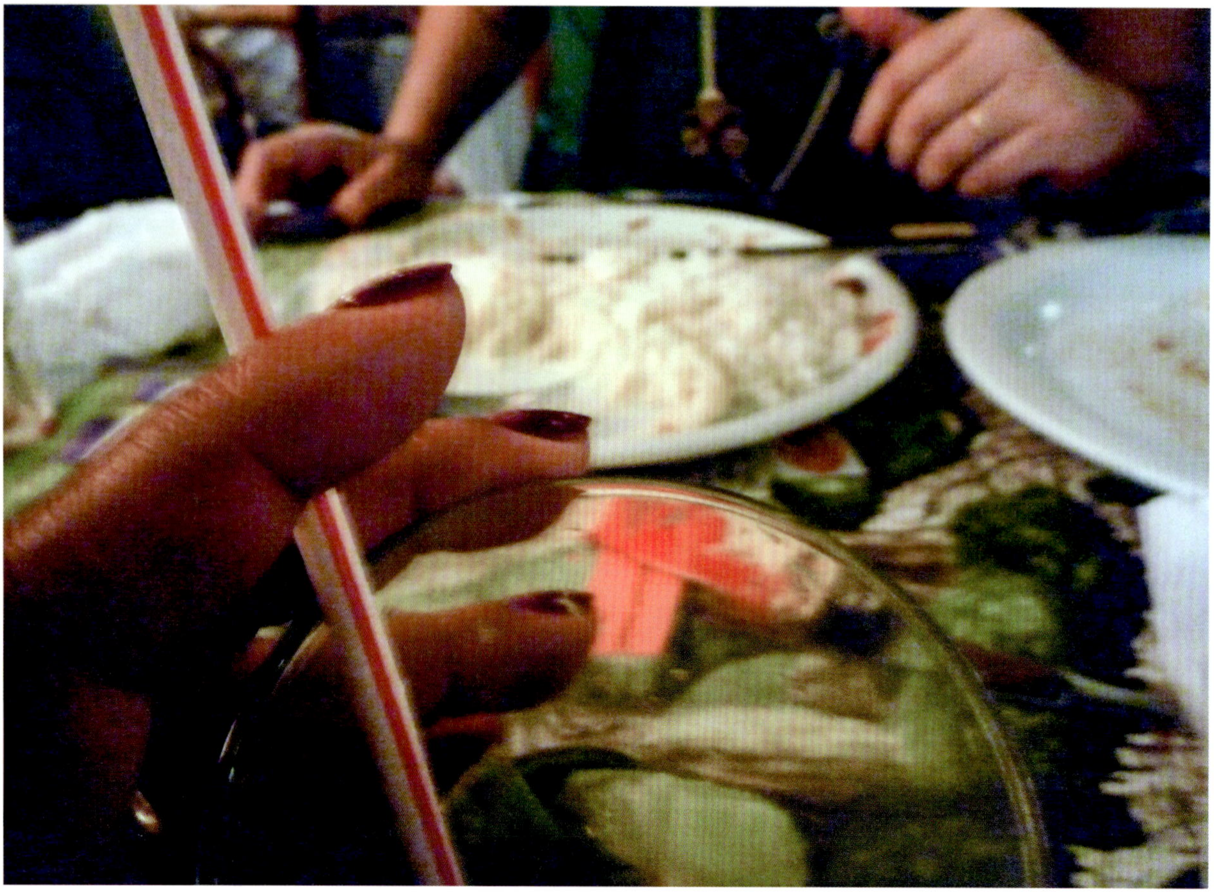

Cida

Yesterday I was taking pictures with a friend, and people stopped to look, saying, "A blind person taking pictures?!" I had help at times, but I did it myself.

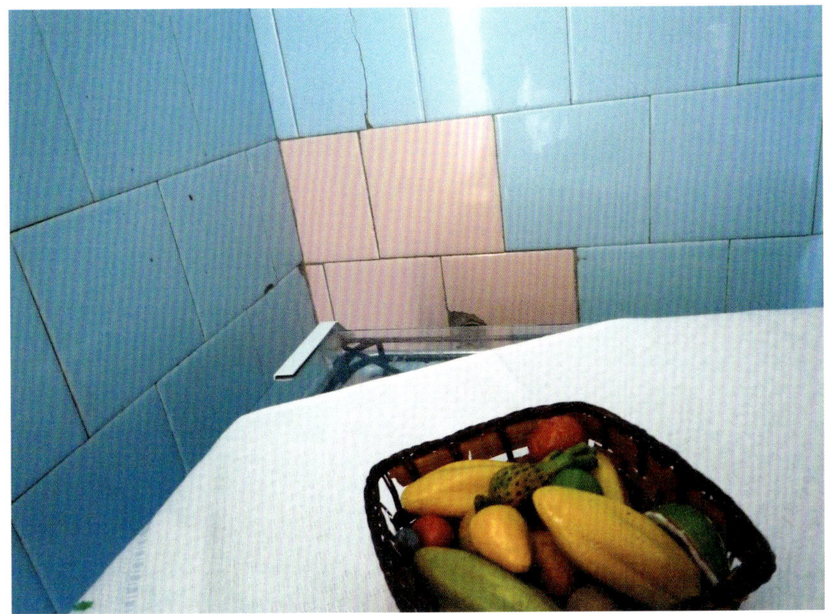

I never thought that AIDS could one day be part of my life. I am a retired teacher, and I always guided my students to take care of themselves, to get tested and treated. I thought I was immune. When we have little information or knowledge, we end up not believing that some things can happen to us. I was forty-five years old when I was diagnosed and, up to that point, I had never met anyone who had AIDS. I thought only artists got it, or other people—but it happened in my house, in my bed.

A year after diagnosis, in 2001, I went blind due to an opportunistic disease, a cytomegalovirus that attacked my retina. I lost my eyesight after having five surgeries in each eye. From the moment I went blind, everything changed.

In those first moments, when I reached out to others, I thought I would only be seeking help. But I discovered I could also offer help. And it was really good for me, because the more I said to people, "You're going to get better. Take care of yourself," the more I heard it too. I heard it and I got better.

Yesterday I was taking pictures with a friend, and people stopped to look, saying, "A blind person taking pictures?!" I had help at times, but I did it myself.

I am often told how strong I am. People invite me to give talks about my life experience. But I don't have any other option. I can sulk, or I can raise my head and fight. For a year I stayed at home crying, but that didn't take me anywhere, so I decided to get up and do it differently, to seek new challenges. I can say I make myself proud at times.

Paulo

I was born by the sea. I go there to relax, to talk to people, or just to stay by myself and go for a swim. Because if I'm stuck at home alone, I get kind of down.

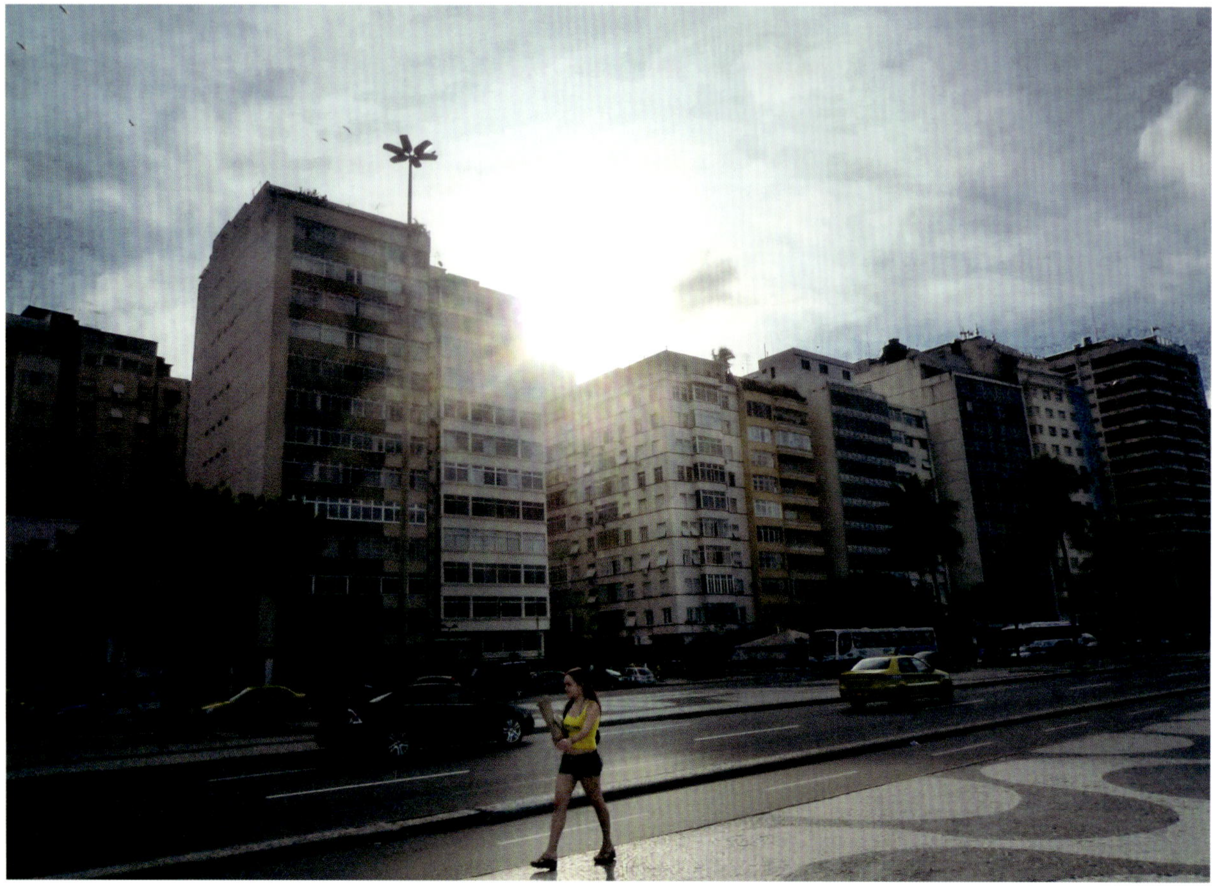

When I received my diagnosis in 1988, I wasn't nervous. I never had any opportunistic diseases, never had anything. I simply went and got tested because I thought I should. I had no symptoms. The doctor expected me to have some kind of crisis and wanted me to look for a psychologist. I said, "There is no need, everything is OK." I got my results and left. She expected me to throw myself under a car or something. But I got the results and went to the beach. After two years, I told my sister about it.

Sometimes I think, "I caught it so fast," because I was never a promiscuous guy. I thought it was unfair because I never used any drugs, never took part in any sort of orgy, and I thought this happened only to promiscuous people. I have done nothing wrong. I was a bit upset about that, but I do not moan about having AIDS. I don't know how it happened, but I don't spend the whole day thinking I'm going to die. I let life take me, and that's it.

I started taking the drug cocktail in 1996. These medications have really bad side effects, nausea, you get shaky. So to get away from all this, I go to the beach. I was born by the sea. I go there to relax, to talk to people, or just to stay by myself and go for a swim. Because if I'm stuck at home alone, I get kind of down. I have to go out and see people so I can feel better and so I won't have time to think about negative things. I go on with my life.

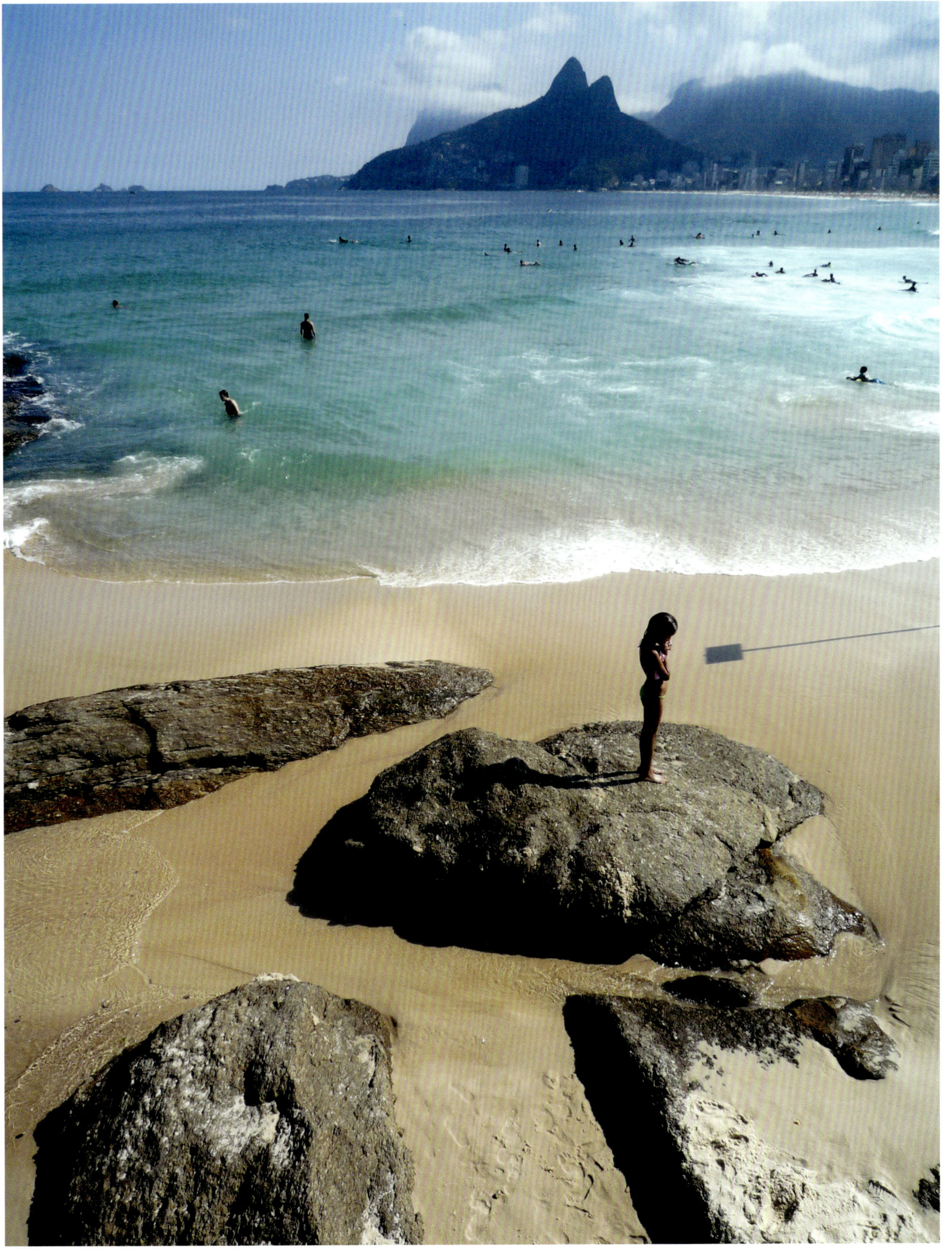

Alcione

I used to live in a guesthouse, where I paid rent daily to the madam. Not paying meant having to sleep in the streets. I didn't want that. So I slept during the day and hustled at night to be able to have a place to live. I wanted to fuck. I didn't even think about protecting myself. At that time the Unified Health System didn't give out condoms. You had to buy them. I had no money for that. I was young and pretty, and it was my heyday, with all these men after me.

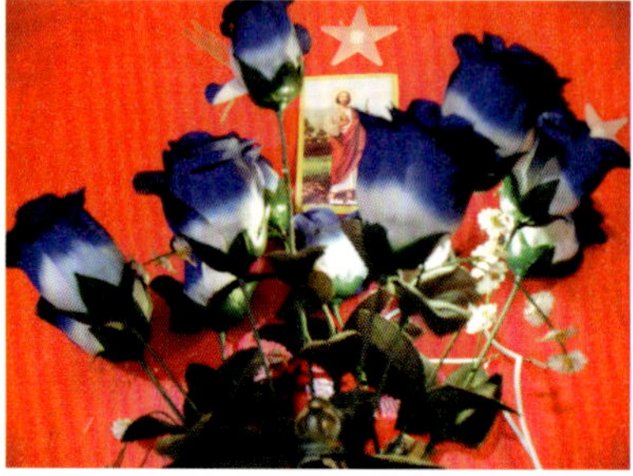

I got infected, but I don't know by whom, because they were many. I was a whore. The thugs saw me, so young and pretty, and took me to have sex with them. I lived with their boss. The police did not bat an eyelid when they saw me, but thugs, they were drawn to me.

I don't have anything against those who have, or don't have, the disease. We are in this not because we want to be, but because of destiny. I wouldn't want to have HIV, but since I have it, I am here.

I don't live from working the streets anymore. I don't disagree with those who do. They don't do it because they want to. It's because of necessity. I take all my medication at the right time. I go to the doctor every time the doctor recommends it. I want all to follow my example, no matter if you are a man, a prostitute, bisexual, or transsexual. Protect yourselves, use a rubber.

Artur

I was diagnosed when I was nineteen. I went to a local health center to have an anonymous test done. I was sick, throwing up. When I passed by the place where everyone else had their HIV tests done, I felt something, some sort of warning, a fear and an apprehension. Eventually I gathered the courage to go. I made up a story and got my results straightaway.

My reaction was utter despair. The first thing that went through my head was that my life was over, it was the end of it all. I thought I was condemned, outcast, bound to die.

In the beginning I was being treated for psychological reasons. I tried to commit suicide. It was a side of me I had not known before. I was hearing voices, thinking about death, having hallucinations.

But the storm passed, I pulled through. Over the years I regained my self-esteem and am stronger now. And no one can tell that I have HIV.

Why live in secrecy? Because there is prejudice. I share my experiences with other people who are HIV-positive, but not with my family. I live with my grandparents and my mother. They know my sexual inclination, but that's it. They accept it, although my grandfather is a bit homophobic. I get my treatment, I keep the tests in a safe place, and my medication is hidden in my wardrobe. I am man enough to go through this on my own. I do not make a fuss about it.

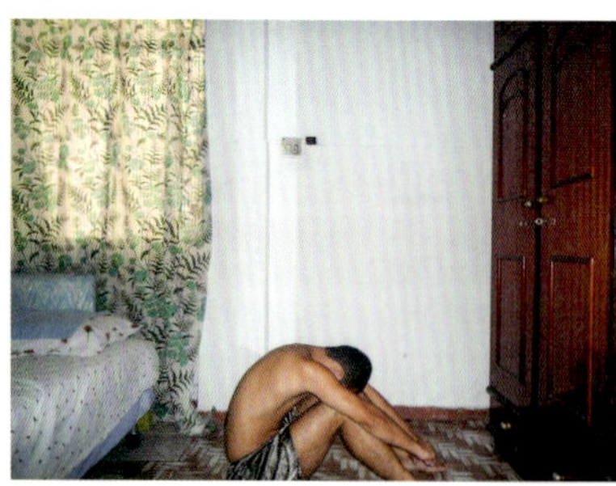

Sometimes I have little setbacks and get sick. But I do it all on my own. I go by myself to the hospital, and no one has to know about it. People think we are aliens, animals, beasts, as if we could infect them just by walking down the street. It is prejudice, of course. This makes me stop and think, "Shall I do this all on my own?" And my answer is always the same: yes.

Gladys

I learned I was HIV-positive in 1991. How I caught it, I don't know. When the doctor told me about my status, I went home and locked myself in for a week. I didn't want to go outside, didn't want to see anybody, didn't want to talk to anybody. All I did was cry and say that I wanted to die. It was a whole week. When I realized I wasn't dying, I said, "OK, the only thing to do now is live."

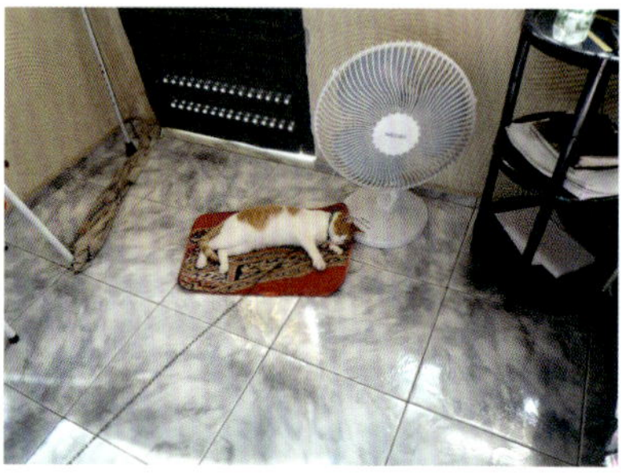

The truth is that I didn't have any friends, anyone to guide me. I discovered my HIV status around the same time I separated from my ex-husband, so I received two very difficult blows at once. It was a hard life.

And then, in 1993 I had a stroke, which left me unable to walk very well, plus I have trouble using my arm. My doctor said that HIV was not the cause of this stroke. He said it was from nervousness. I was completely lost.

Around that time, I met a man named Francisco who decided to take control of everything. I told him I had HIV and he turned to me and said, "I want to take care of you." I said to him, "Wherever you go, I'll go. But there is a problem. I can't walk." "No problem," he said, "I'll carry you." And he walked from Rio de Janeiro to São Gonçalo carrying me in his arms.

He had rented a small room where I stayed with him. This was where I started proper treatment. He would say to me, "You can't surrender.

You're beautiful, you're intelligent, you have everything ahead of you. You can have everything you want."

Today I do physical therapy. I swim to increase my mobility. But all this has been a slow process. Because of the stroke I was in bed for a year, but today I walk. I live in my own house and I have chores. I pay my bills. I can say I am a happy person, because I have a home and people who love me. I thank God for being here.

Jonatha

My partner and I met at a nightclub when I was fifteen years old and he was sixteen. I fell in love with him at first sight. He looked healthy. I could not tell he was ill. It was when I was clearing his things away nine years later, after he died, that I found the test results. I got the test myself and the results showed that I too am positive.

His last words were, "Death is not the end, but the beginning of a new journey." I am not scared of dying anymore. I believe that life goes on. I miss him very much.

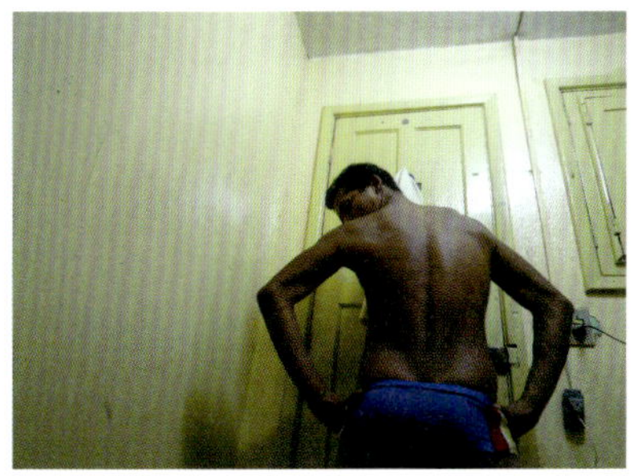

My mother never accepted the fact that I am homosexual, my father even less. After my partner died I tried to move in with her, but she did not let me. She was the first person I wanted to tell that I was positive. I thought she would look after me, but she didn't. My father wanted to beat me up when he found out about it.

Today my life is part happy and part sad. During the hardest time of my life, I found the love I did not get from my family in ABIA, the AIDS support organization. They are my family. I have a roof over my head thanks to the goodwill of friends. I know I won't have my family's support, so I must move on. Still, I hope one day my mother can hug me like a mother should.

Leonardo

In the late 1980s, a lot of my friends were dying. I thought to myself, "I will not have the test done, because if I have it, I will be dead in six months, one year's time. I will let the bomb drop."

I eventually moved to Germany, graduated from circus school as an acrobat, and went on to work as a performer. I worked over there for four years and completely forgot about the whole HIV thing.

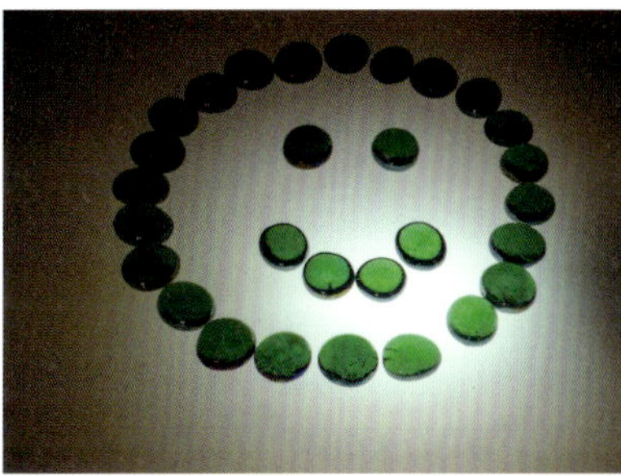

Around 1998, I became very ill. As I lay on a stretcher, the doctor asked me whether I would like to have an HIV test done. When the results finally came, I was worried about my partner. That was my sole concern. I myself was somewhat aware that I might have the virus anyway.

I see now how important it is to get tested because I could have died. In my case, I had a break in my life, a cut, of five years until I regained my health. Because of advancements in medicine, if you get tested as soon as possible, you can have better results.

What got me out of this really bad state of affairs was the support I received from my family, from my friends. Having a very rule-bound life, eating well, practicing meditation, also helped. I think it is very important for HIV-positive people to not just take their medication, but to be surrounded by a whole support network: friends, family, and a life that has meaning, some kind of goal. Today I have this goal through working with HIV-positive people to lift their spirits, and to make them see that there is hope, a light at the end of the tunnel.

I have been taking the same medication for ten years. My viral load, which was four million back then, today is at zero, undetectable, which means that the treatment is working. Not that today I'm free from suffering, from problems. That is part of being human. Life as a whole has its difficulties, with or without HIV.

Leotino

I came to Rio from the central western region of Brazil, bordering Bolivia, to grow as a gay man, to come out, because with my family I couldn't do this. I also came to Rio to get a better job and to get ahead in life.

I found out about my HIV status in September of last year. It is difficult to live with HIV, facing discrimination and prejudice. We are already stigmatized for being homosexual. Being HIV-positive is something completely different. To be gay is to discover oneself, it is to be what we want to be, whereas being HIV-positive is a cold, hard fact.

I really believe in scientific evolution. I believe that one day there will be a cure. I live with HIV, but I hope for a cure, a complete cure, a scientific cure. I think one day there will be a definitive cure for AIDS.

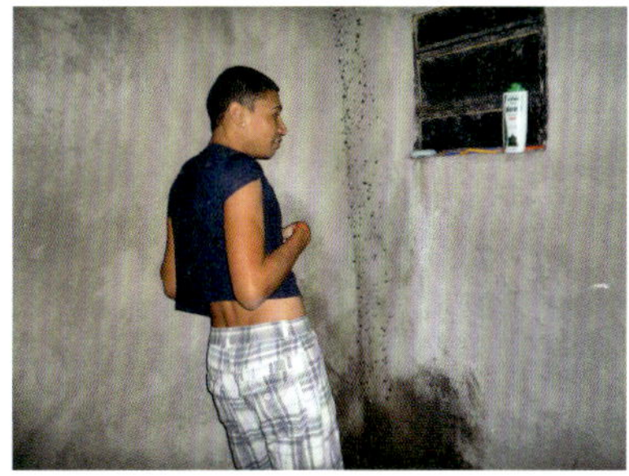

I am a member of ABIA, an HIV organization based in Rio, which sponsors events for interaction and integration. They show gay films every Friday, and there are outings to cultural centers. There is a fulfillment in this coming-together of reading and leisure—this interaction completes me. HIV-positive people need information, need to interact, need to develop, and ABIA gave me the structure that I really needed.

Our true treasure lies within ourselves, and the introspection that I practice in my life brings me a certain balance between being HIV-positive and being gay. I want to pass on to every HIV-positive person in the world that they should explore all the internal resources that exist within them, because the true solution of physical healing and emotional healing lies within oneself. I don't know whether at some point I will come down with an opportunistic disease. I have not had one yet. But if I do I will handle it by looking for my personal power.

Mara

I was infected with HIV during my first relationship, at the age of eighteen. I thought I was outside the risk groups, that AIDS was only found among homosexuals and drug users. I thought that I—who married as a virgin, and who practices evangelical Christianity—was immune from this epidemic.

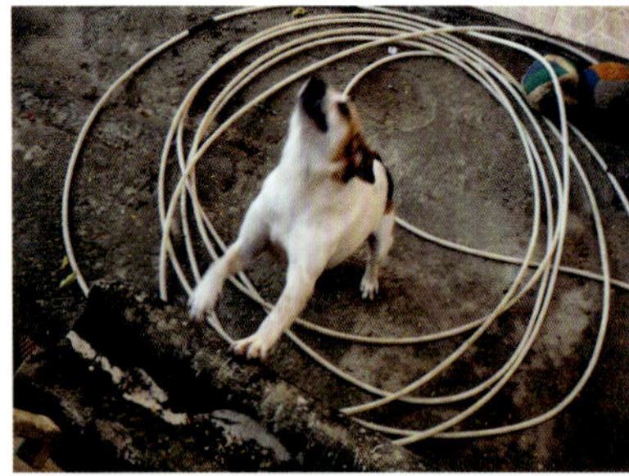

Three months after my wedding, my husband became very sick with pneumonia and we discovered that he was HIV-positive. He died a year later. Suddenly, there I was, at nineteen, a widow.

My husband had been sexually active. We had STD tests done before our wedding, but we were not asked to do an HIV test. I never thought for a second that my husband could be HIV-positive. For contraceptives, I used only the pill, not condoms. I should have used both.

It took three months for me to receive my own test results. I wasn't afraid because, as an evangelical Christian, I have no fear of dying. My reaction wasn't the usual one. But I understood that this would be my reality from then on: I had AIDS.

In Brazil there are many churches that offer no support to people with HIV. Some preachers demand that their followers stop taking the medication, telling them that God alone will heal them. These people then stop taking the medication and die, because of the ignorance of their preachers.

I do believe God can heal us, but through medicine. If I take the medication at the right time and do my bit, God will do His bit through the medication. That was the kind of psychological and emotional support I received from my church.

We who live with HIV cherish every minute. We see life in a different, precious way.

Marcos

I started in the gay scene as a rent boy. My father was a preacher, and my whole family is Christian. I never had to tell my family about my homosexuality, but I never had to hide it either. They accepted it in a completely normal way. But I did not accept my own homosexuality. I started going out with this friend who was a rent boy and I started doing it too. I did it for less than a year, because I knew that was not me. It was only a way to hide my homosexuality. Since I was paid for it, in my mind I was going out with other men for the money. It is very likely that I got infected during this period.

After a year, I stopped doing it because my mind got clearer. I understood I did not do it for the money. I did it because I enjoyed it.

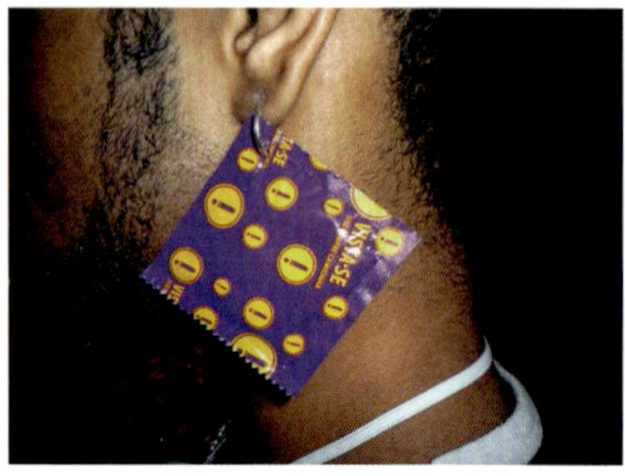

There is still a lot of prejudice against so-called "promiscuous" people, but I have abolished this word from my vocabulary. I talk about vulnerability instead. There are vulnerable people who have sex more often than others, but they are not doing anything wrong. I don't have hang-ups about anything—to me everything is fine as long as it is done properly, with protection.

There are many educated people who pick up condoms but do not know how to use them. I have given workshops in big corporations where, at the end, we ask someone to volunteer to put a condom on a rubber penis. You find that there are well-educated people who make the silliest mistakes, tearing it the wrong way, putting it on without getting rid of the air. And there are particular groups of people who need to be focused on, like housewives who cannot negotiate the use of condoms with their partners, or young people who still do not use protection for various reasons.

Most probably, I caught the virus when I turned tricks on the street. Today I work there, trying to help gay boys who prostitute themselves not to become positive, to use prevention, to have a better quality of life and health.

Johannesburg

The March 2010 *Through Positive Eyes* workshop in Johannesburg, South Africa's populous economic center, brought the AIDS epidemic's most pressing issues into sharp relief. The politics of heterosexual relationships emerged as a leading topic, with a focus on masculine power and the problematic dynamics associated with it. The tension between Western medicine and traditional medical practices was a recurring theme. Recent information about how to prevent mother-to-child transmission was also addressed in many of the participants' stories.

South Africa's AIDS epidemic, as of 2010

Number of people living with HIV:	5.3 million

HIV prevalence

Adults (15–49 years):	17.8%

In 2010 there was no national data for HIV prevalence among female sex workers, men who have sex with men, or injecting drug users.

Treatment

Antiretroviral treatment available in the public health sector since 2003.

Numbers on treatment:	971,566
% of those in need of treatment who are receiving it:	36%

Key events

1994	*South Africa's Constitution is the first globally to outlaw discrimination based on sexual orientation.*
1998	*Treatment Action Campaign formed to fight for universal access to treatment.*
2000	*President Mbeki questions whether HIV leads to AIDS and a decade of denialism begins.*
2006	*Civil Union Act provides for same-sex marriage.*
2009	*The new Minister of Health pledges to accelerate treatment access.*

Update 2019

By 2017 there were 7.2 million South Africans living with HIV and 61% of HIV-positive adults were on treatment.

National HIV prevalence among sex workers, MSM, and injecting drug users is estimated at 57.7%, 26.8%, and 17% respectively. National plans to combat HIV among sex workers and LGBTQI communities were launched in 2016 and 2017, but stigma and discrimination are still barriers to treatment and prevention programs.

Through Positive Eyes in Johannesburg was organized in partnership with Positive Convention, with major funding from the U.S. President's Emergency Plan for AIDS Relief (PEPFAR) and The Ford Foundation.

Betty

Here are some of the reasons people become sex workers: Because they need money for their kids. Because they have no family. Because they never went to school. Because the money is easy.

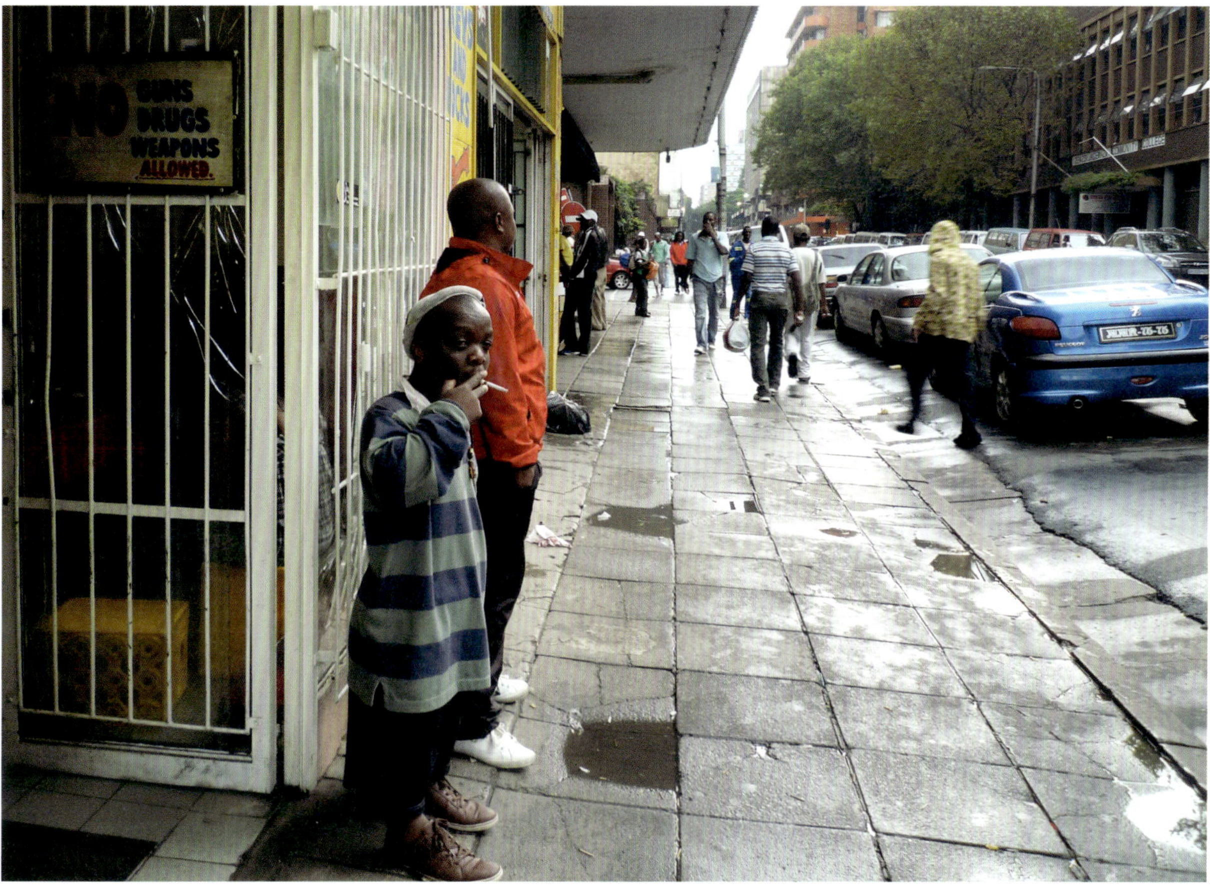

I used to visit an HIV organization to get my medicines and counseling. One day the assistant asked me, "Are you working?" I was not. "Would you mind having a job here?" They were about to start a five-day training, so I joined it. That's how I became a peer educator teaching sex workers how to use condoms, how to put them on, how to have safe sex, and how to get treatment for HIV and STIs—sexually transmitted infections. I'm proud to be an HIV counselor focusing on sex workers because I have HIV too.

I encourage sex workers to get tested every three months and to know their status. Sometimes condoms break. Sometimes they have a client who won't use a condom. The sex workers charge extra money for that. I say, "Come to us. We'll give you treatment. And we can test for your HIV status. I'm here to help you."

Here are some of the reasons people become sex workers: Because they need money for their kids. Because they have no family. Because they never went to school. Because the money is easy.

Once I was assigned to follow up on a sex worker. I looked for him at a hotel but I didn't find him. Turns out he passed away. I'm sure he was killed by a client.

My message to sex workers is that you're vulnerable to so many things: HIV, AIDS, being killed. It's not safe for you. It's better to volunteer for an organization. I'm sure that in three months' time you can get a job.

Mgladzo

I was determined to have HIV-negative kids. So I went to the clinic and they informed me about PMTCT—prevention of mother-to-child transmission. Now my two kids are healthy.

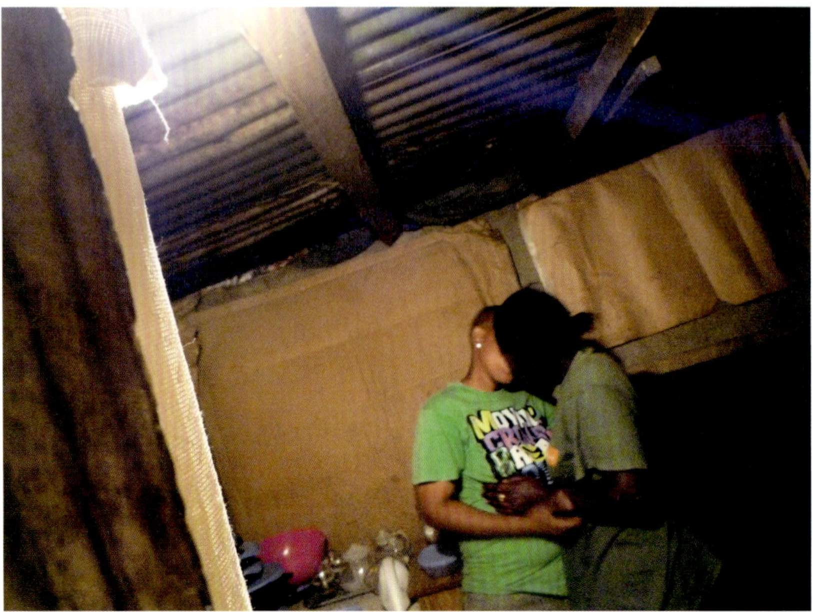

Some people said I was possessed by demons because I'm a lesbian. So I decided to grow my hair and get a boyfriend. That's when all these things started. I got the boyfriend and we slept together, and that's when I got HIV. And I became pregnant at the same time. I was fifteen years old.

When the child was born, she got sick and then they decided to test my blood. When the doctor told me I had AIDS, I said, "Fuck you." I didn't take it seriously. The child died at four months. I myself was still a kid.

When I grew up I decided to try having kids again. In 2004, I went back to the very same man, we slept together, and I got pregnant. My son's name is Mpendulo, which means "answer," because God gave me a child—my prayers were answered. In 2007, we had another baby. I named him Asibonga, "thanks." As the father of my kids and I became closer, I disclosed my sexuality to him and he was supportive. Unfortunately, my kids' daddy was HIV-positive. He died two weeks ago. He loved his kids very much.

I was determined to have HIV-negative kids. So I went to the clinic and they informed me about PMTCT—prevention of mother-to-child transmission. I went through that process. I attended every appointment and they gave me Nevirapine. I followed every precaution. Now my two kids are healthy, they know my HIV status, and they know my sexuality.

In 2007, my colleague, an open lesbian, was murdered. They stabbed her, they shot her, and they took her underwear and put it in on her head. I was so confused and scared. I'm proud of myself, but going out and saying it loudly—"You know what, I'm a lesbian and I'm proud!"—is very difficult.

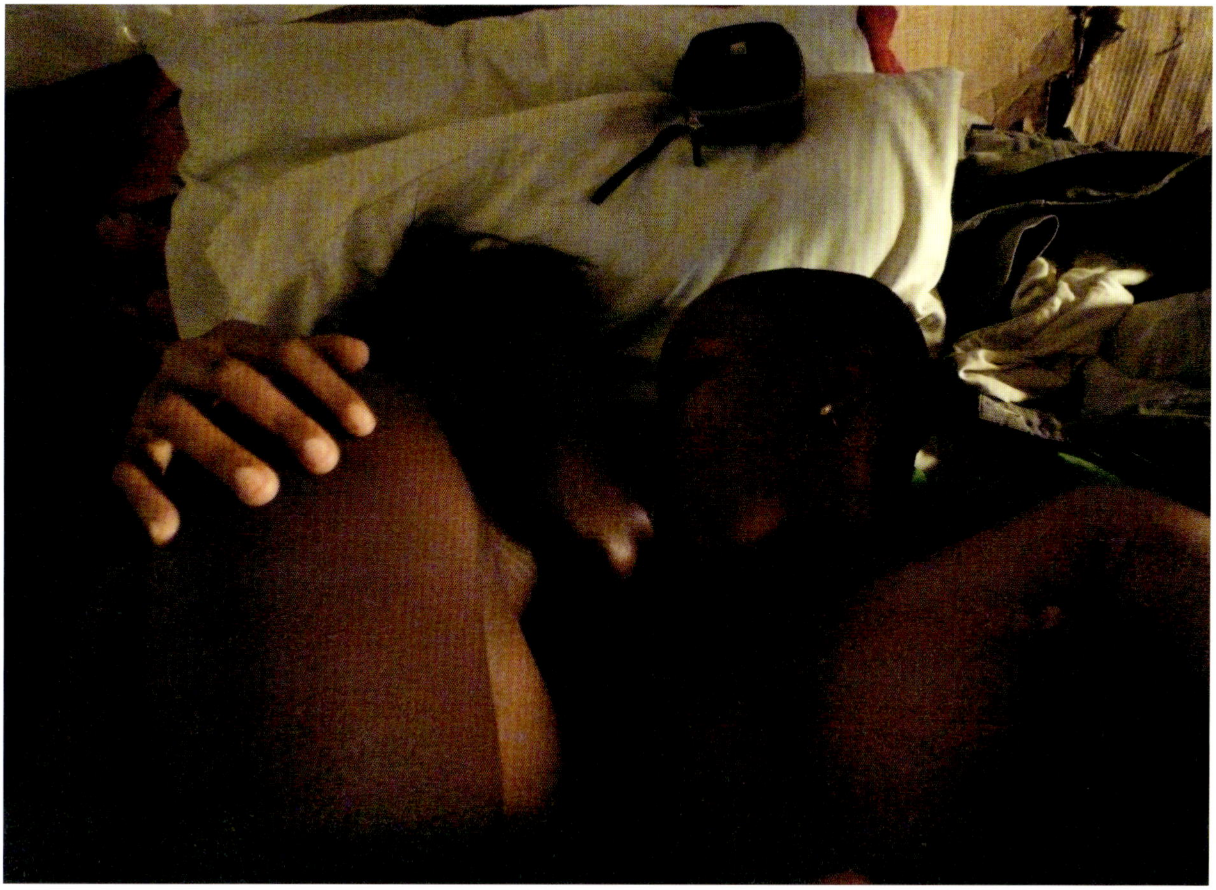

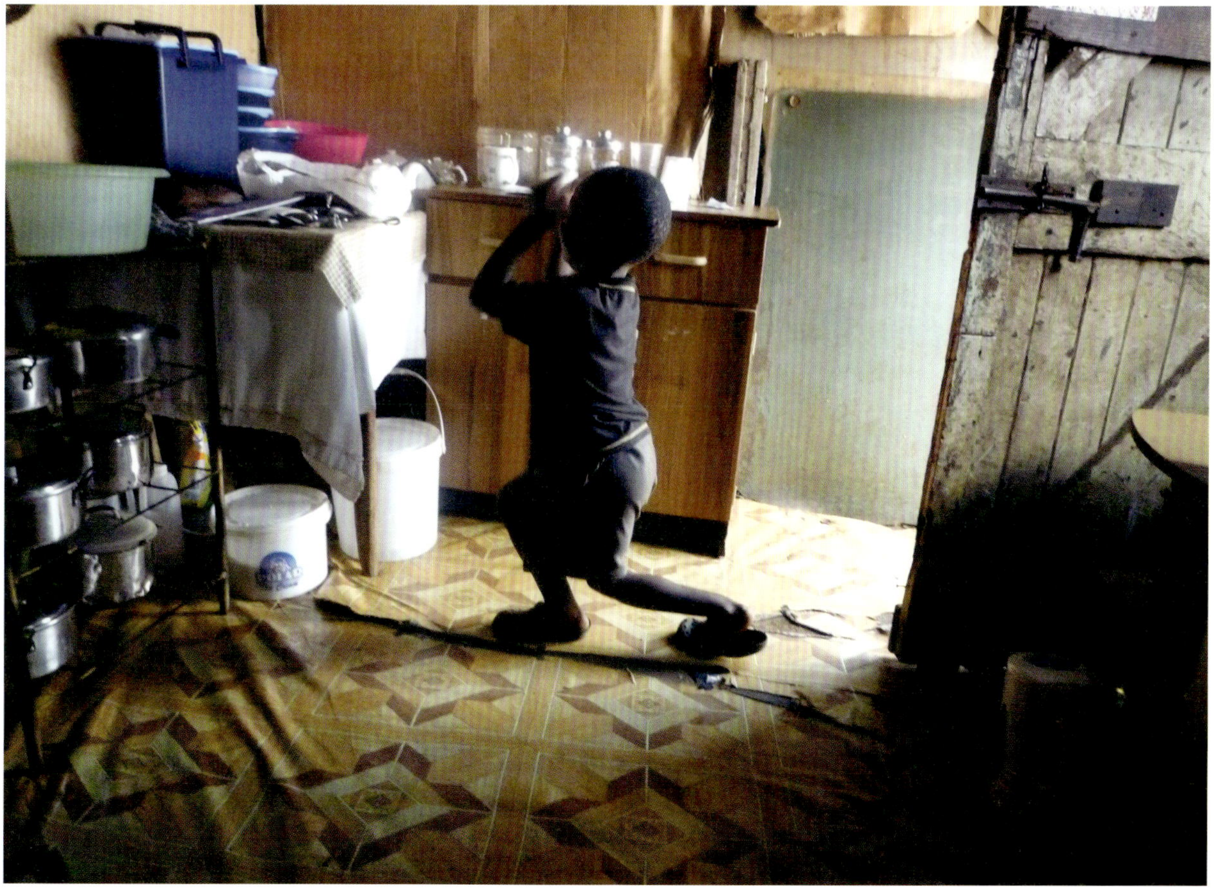

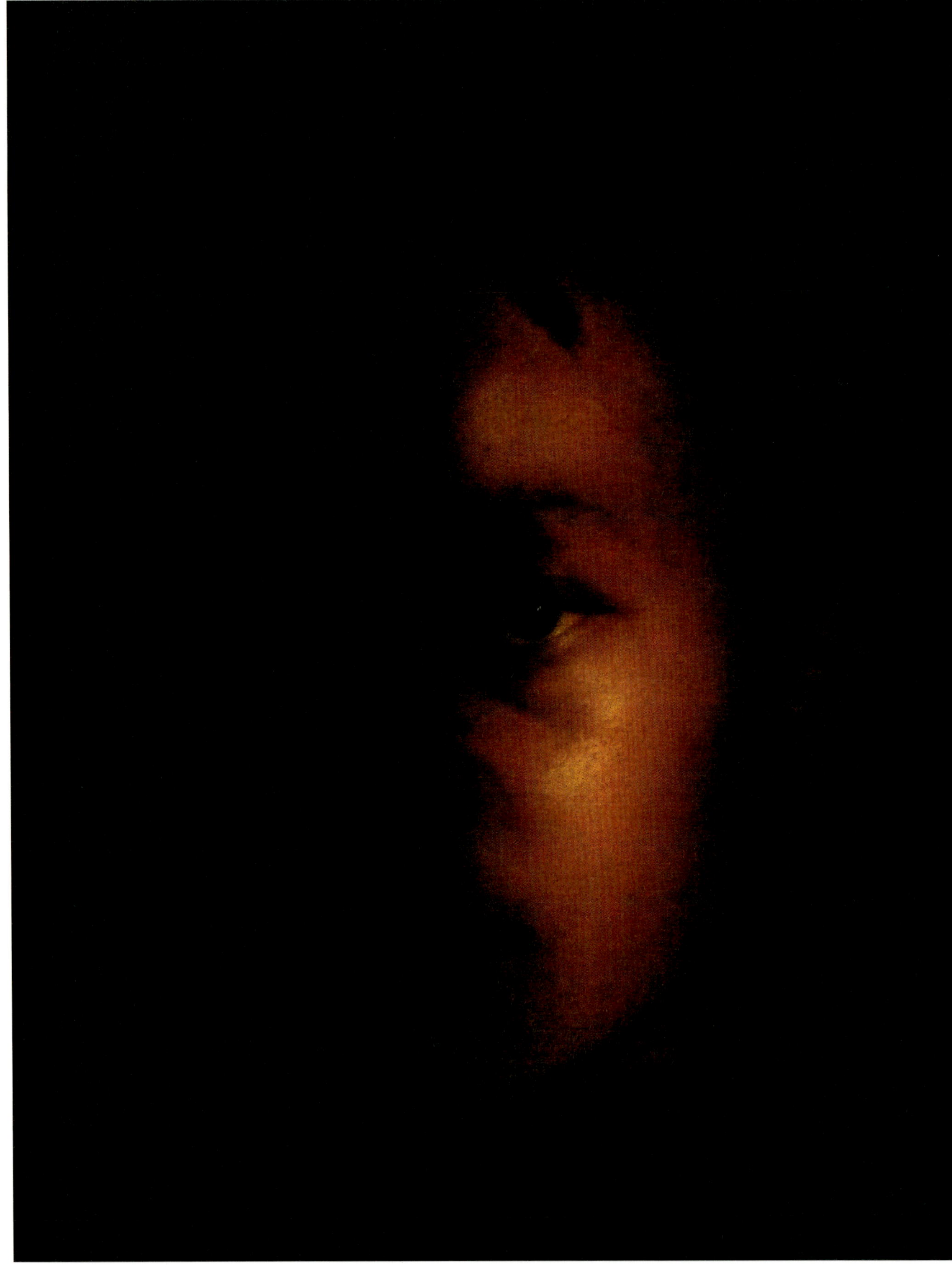

Zandile

I want to preserve my health so that I can see my son grow, even to get married, and I want to see my grandchildren. He's so handsome, my son.

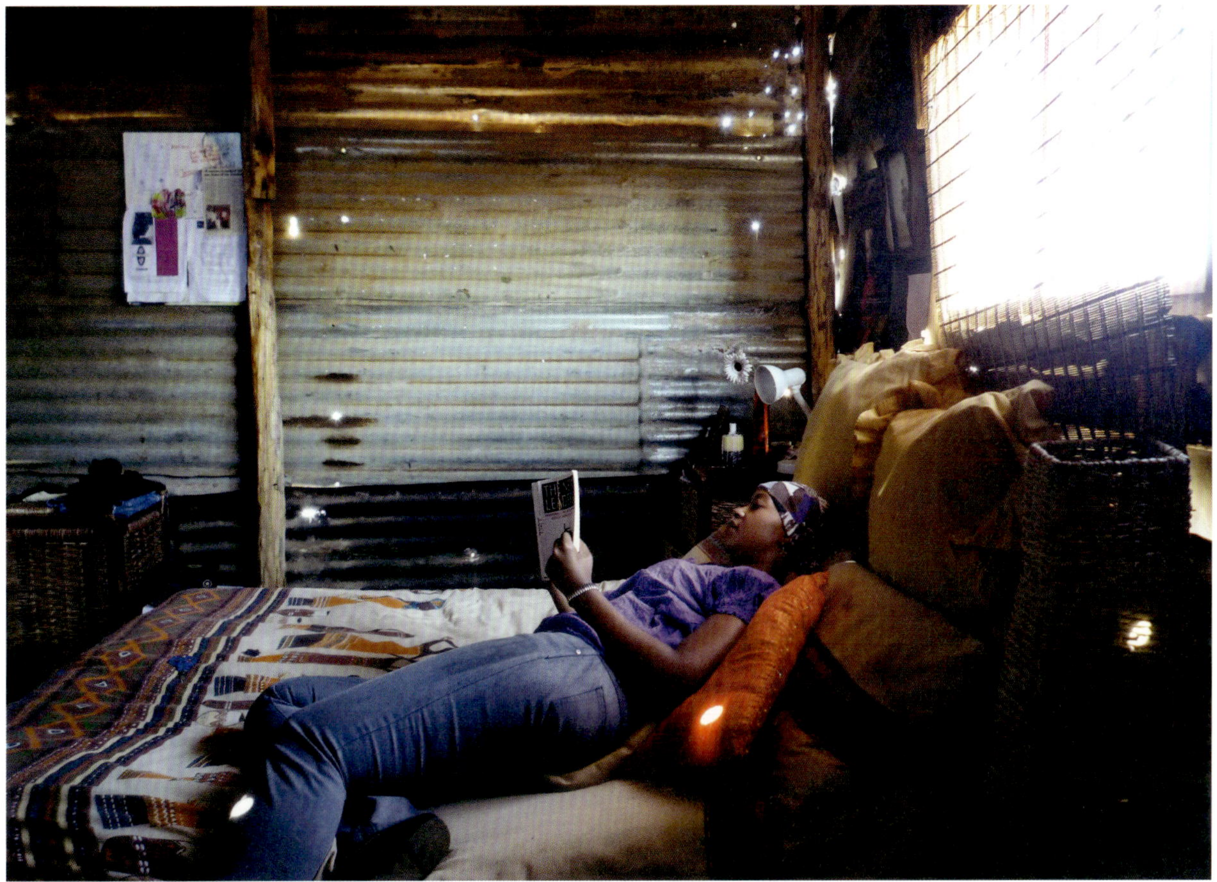

My story begins when I met my baby's father. We were longtime friends, we dated for a short time and, before I knew it, I was pregnant. It wasn't planned. And then he left me for his ex-girlfriend. When I found out I was pregnant, the doctor advised me to do the tests that all pregnant women do. Everything was negative except for HIV. I was twenty-three.

My son is HIV-negative. His name is Loyiso, which means "victory." Honestly, when I gave him the name I never thought of this, but now it has a significant meaning for me, because he's a victor. He conquered HIV. I love him, because if I wasn't pregnant, I wouldn't have gotten tested. If not for him, I wouldn't be alive, because I wouldn't know my status. I've been on treatment for almost four years now. And I'm healthy. Though I'm HIV-positive, I'm healthier than most other people who are HIV-negative. I never even get sick.

I want to preserve my health so that I can see my son grow, even get married, and I want to see my grandchildren. He's so handsome, my son.

I had a very tough childhood. My parents never knew, but as a child I was molested by one of my father's workers. So I've always had this fear that something bad would happen to me. The dark place in my photos represents the child in me who's very scared. Then I look at my son and thank him for bringing such light into my life.

Lindiwe

What often happens is that when you tell your husband you're diagnosed with HIV, he will leave you, or divorce you, or chase you away from home.

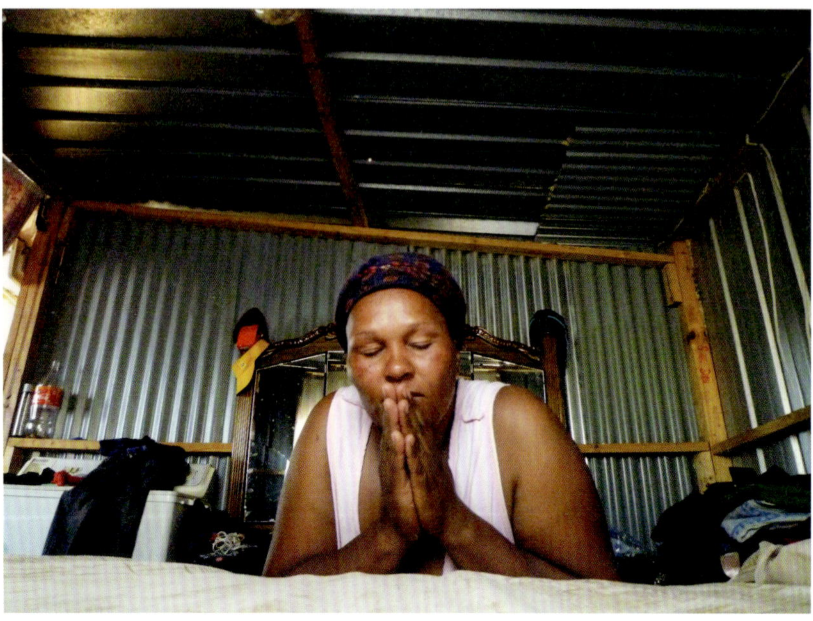

I disclosed to my family after an uncle of mine died of AIDS. They believed he was bewitched. But I told them, "No, HIV is real. I'm living with HIV, and there's nothing wrong with having it."

At first, my grandmother said to me, "You know what, don't tell other people that you have HIV." I said, "Why not, Granny? If I don't talk about this thing, it's eating me up inside. If I do talk about it, I'm feeling free and I'm able to live with this virus." So after a few months she understood what I meant and supported me a lot. Now the whole family knows about my status. My community knows too. And I'm prepared to go on national TV to talk about it. I'm not scared.

I started a support group for women who didn't have any support from their families. What often happens is that when you tell your husband you're diagnosed with HIV, he will leave you, or divorce you, or chase you away from home. If we are alone in a room and we are only women, we can talk about everything. We are free to be open about our status, to share our emotions and our difficulties.

It's better now. Gone are the days when people living with HIV were not allowed to be included in the community, in ceremonies. They would stigmatize you, discriminate against you, and be scared of you. But nowadays there are campaigns that show that a person living with HIV is a normal person. He's your brother, your sister, your lover. Now my community doesn't have a problem with me cooking for them, even for big ceremonies like weddings and funerals. They love me a lot. Some even tell me that I inspire them.

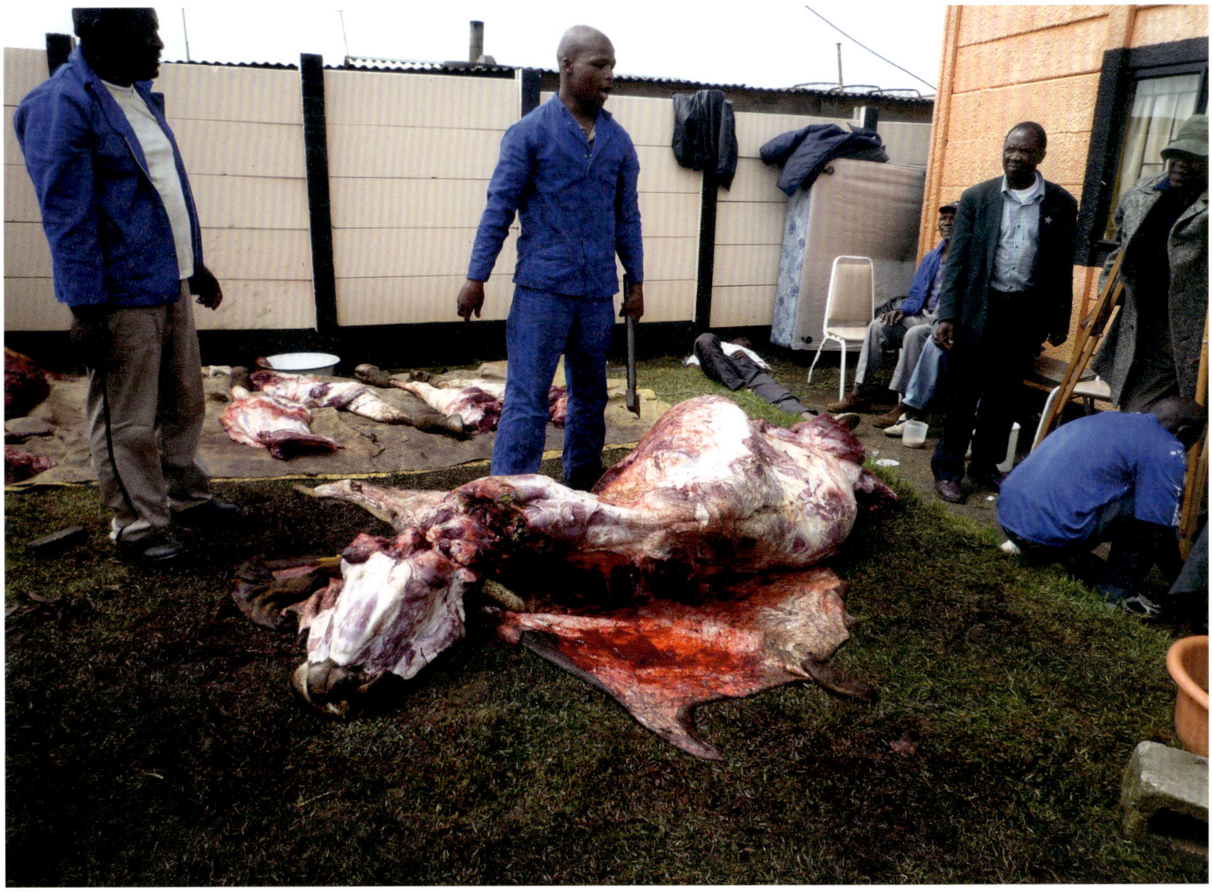

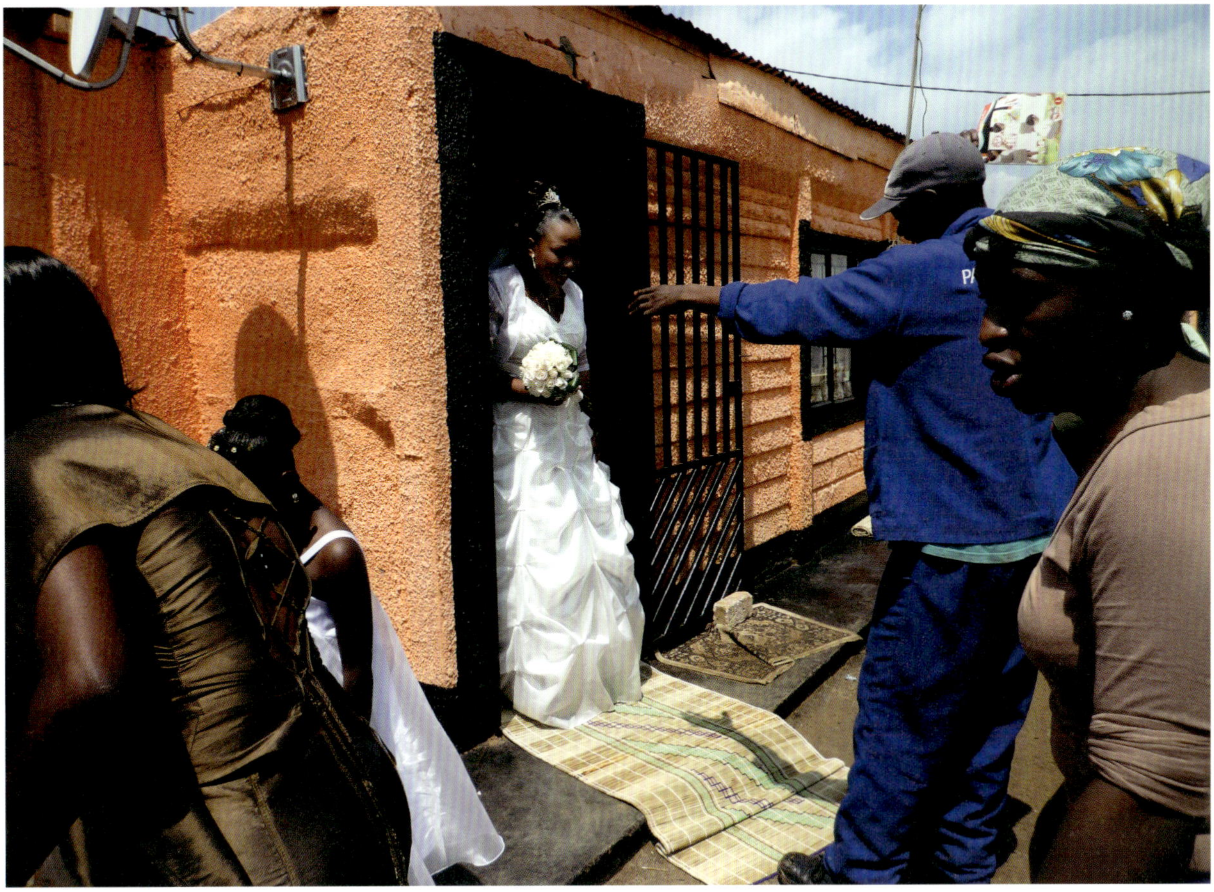

Bhekisisa

As a father, I see that it's important to take care of my children. My father didn't take care of me because of his many wives. I realize that I used to be like him.

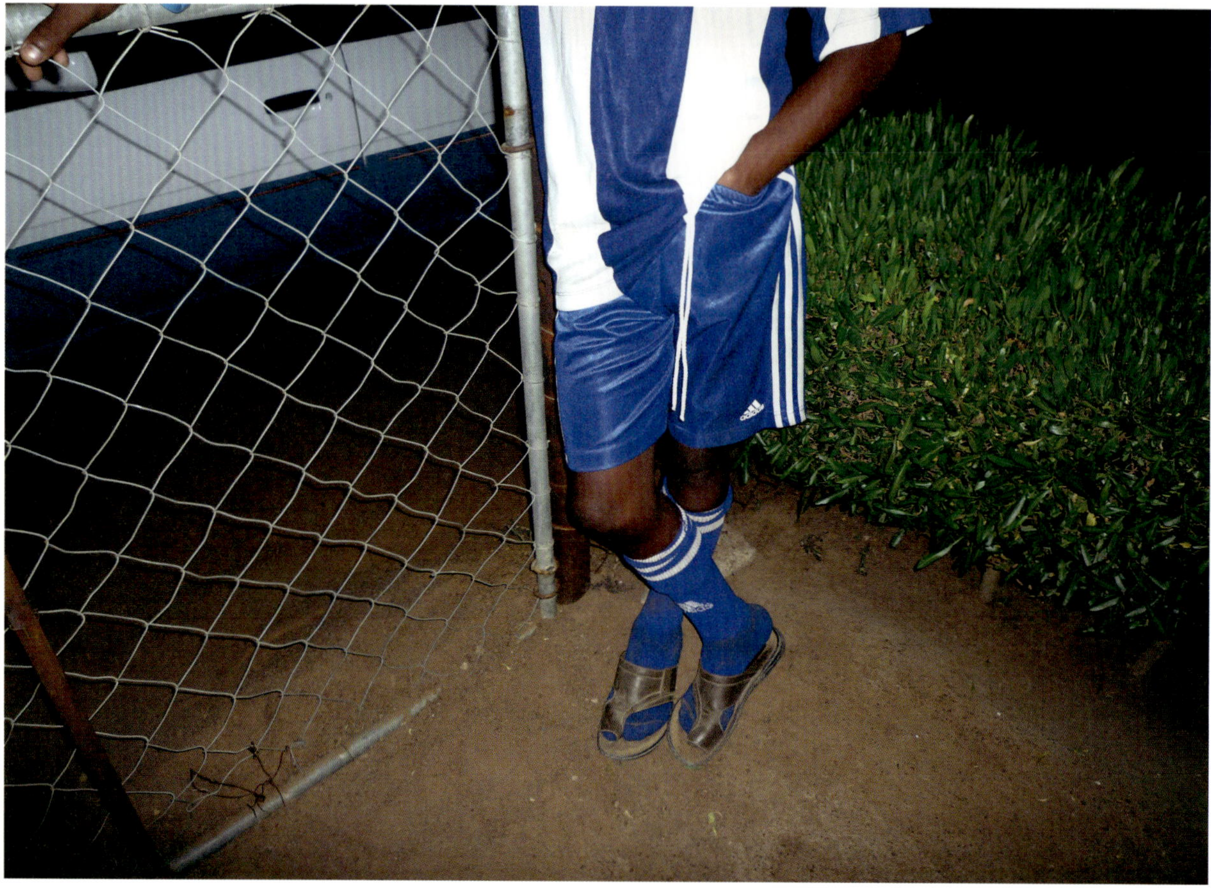

When they told me that I was positive, I was not shocked at all. I knew my behavior had been bad. I had many girlfriends. I was a playboy. You can see how handsome I am. But I was destroying my life. So I told myself that it was time for me to change. I really wanted to live. I really love life.

The same day I found out my HIV status, I went straight to my mother's house and told her. She didn't want to show me that she was very sad, so she said, "You are positive? So what?" I realized that she was trying to uplift me, to tell me I didn't have to give up. So I started to think positively, to take medication, and to pick up my life.

I've got two children in my current relationship, and I'm living with three others. Their mothers just said, "You know what? Take care of these children." I'm so happy that they are part of my life.

As a father, I see that it's important to take care of my children. My father didn't take care of me because of his many wives. I realize that I used to be like him. Then I saw that it was important to change my life completely, to think positively, to take care of everything, to rectify all the mistakes that I had made in my life.

I always want to be happy, because it motivates me and makes me strong. When I become sad, I can feel it in my body—it's not good for me. That's why I've changed.

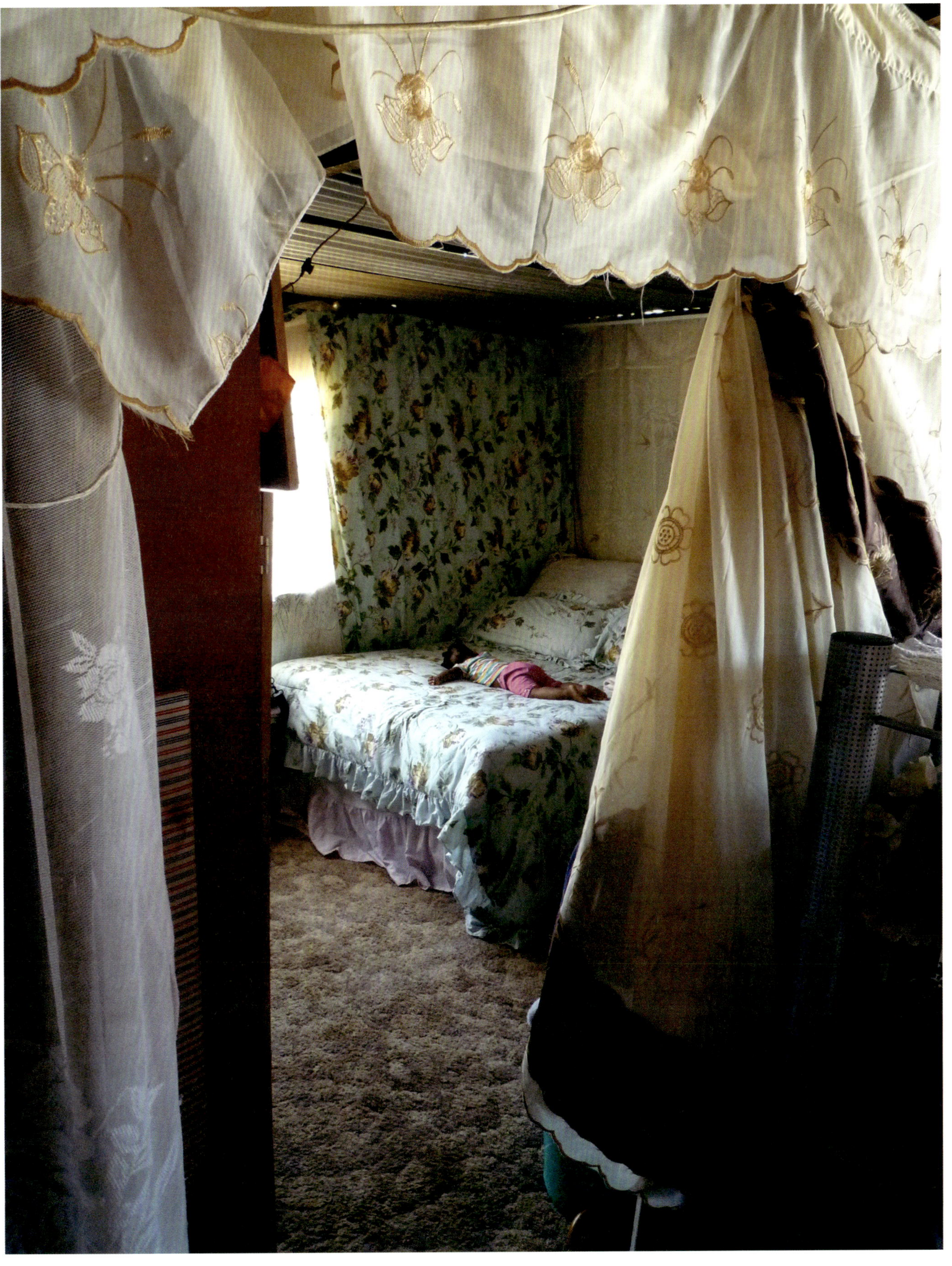

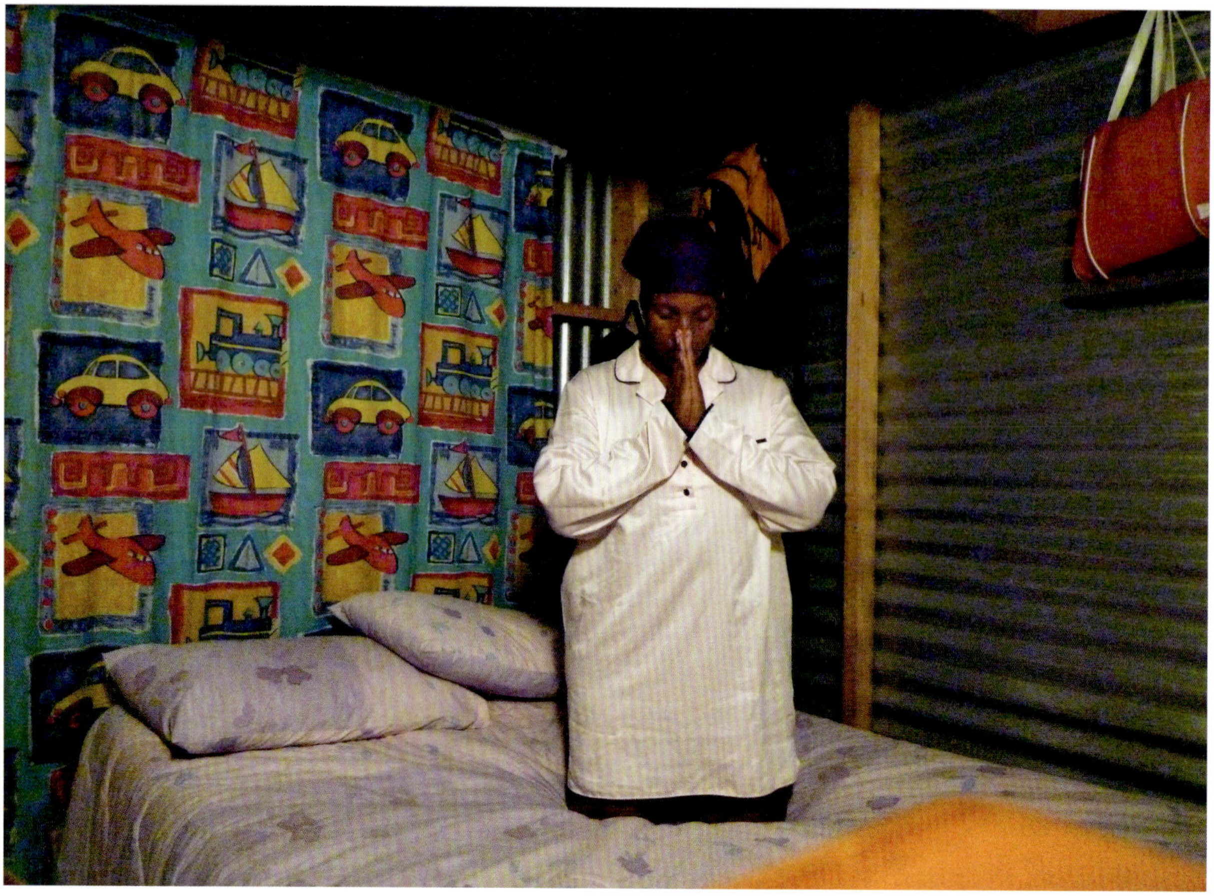

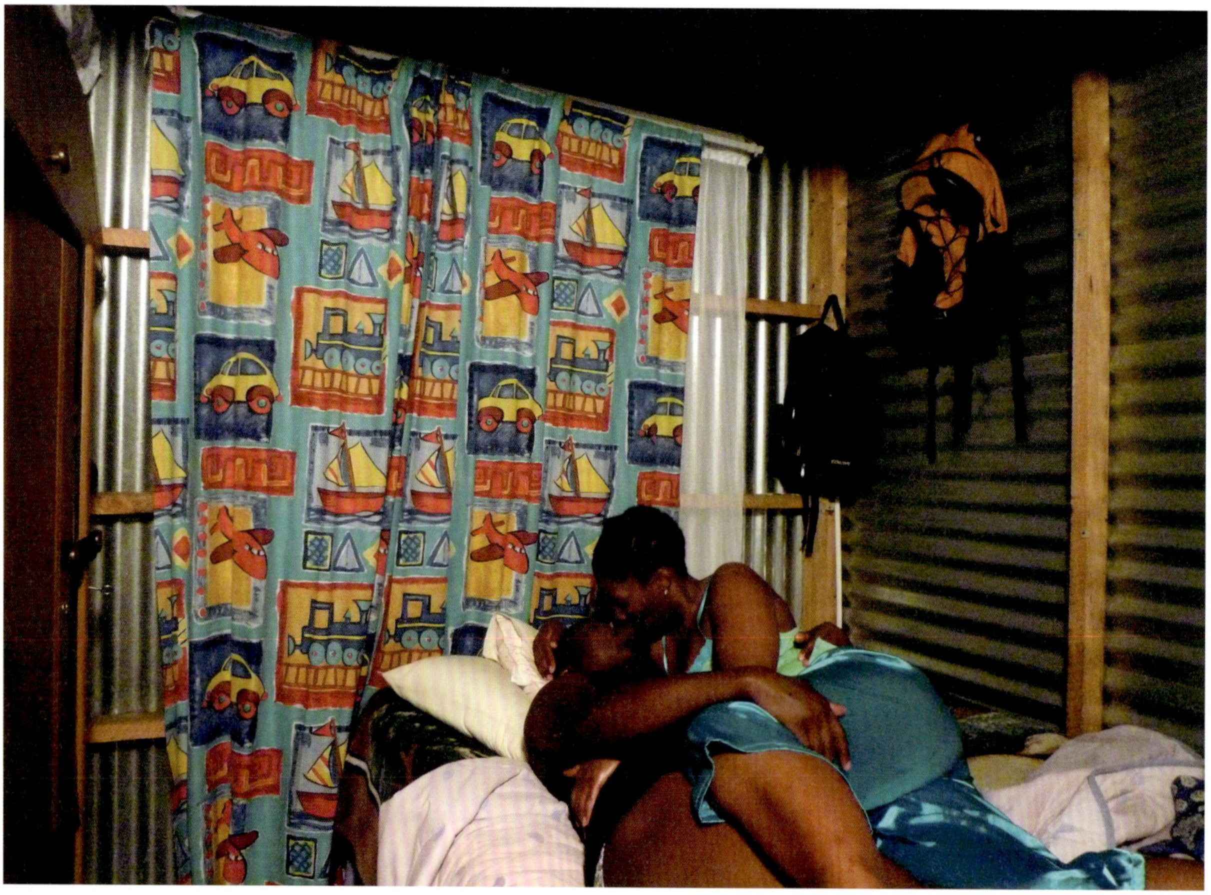

Phindile

She said to me, "Why did you keep it a secret for so long?" And I said, "I was afraid you were going to chase me away from your house. I wanted to tell you, but I didn't know how."

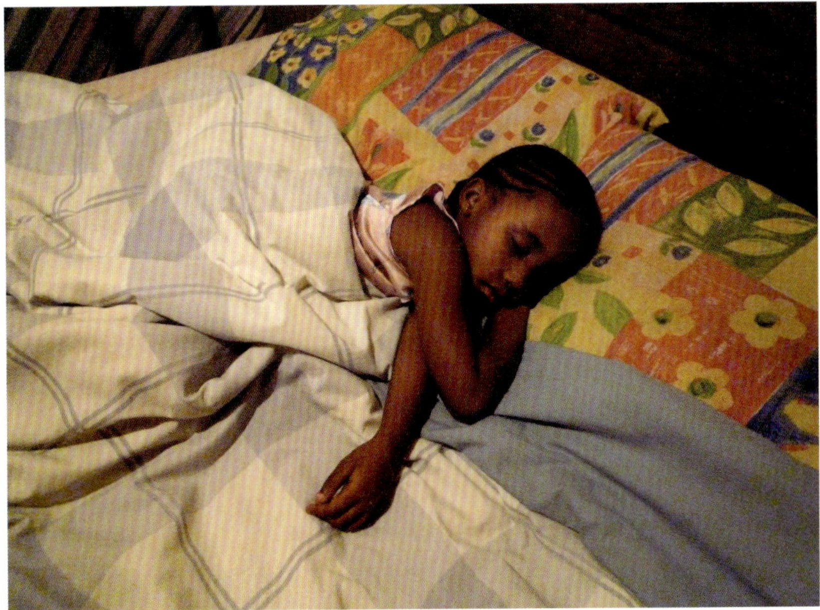

I kept my status a secret for four years. No one knew. A friend of mine used to ask, "Why are you involved in all these organizations dealing with AIDS?" One day I said, "Because I've got HIV," jokingly, not knowing that she would take it seriously.

Then she told one of the ladies, "You know, Phindi has got AIDS." On that very day, I decided to tell my mom. I said to her, "You know what? I'm going to sue my friend." My mom said, "For what?" I said, "She's busy telling people that I've got AIDS, and I don't. I have HIV." My mom cried. I said to her, "You know what, Mom, you don't have to cry. I've been living with this disease for four years now, and look at me, I'm healthy."

Then she said to me, "Why did you keep it a secret for so long?" And I said, "I was afraid you were going to chase me away from your house. I wanted to tell you, but I didn't know how." Then she hugged me and said, "I love you. You are still my daughter." You see?

I was raped when I was sixteen, by somebody I knew. I had kept this secret for twenty years. After both the rape and the HIV, I wanted to start a new life, to do something challenging. I wanted to heal. I thought, "I want to climb Kilimanjaro." So I went to one of the churches and told them, "If I can climb Kilimanjaro, even if I die after that, it will be OK with me." That was December. In January I got a call that the church had raised 15,000 rand for me to fulfill my dream.

When I reached the top, oh, I cried—tears of joy. I'm here, in Tanzania, and I've reached the peak. And I am healed. When I came back, I went straight to the guy who raped me and forgave him. After that, my mom read the story in the newspapers, including about the rape. Even today we haven't spoken about it.

Gugu

"There is something I need to tell you," I said. "I need you then to support me, and I will support you." I told her everything. "Don't feel ashamed," I said. "Don't be afraid. Be proud."

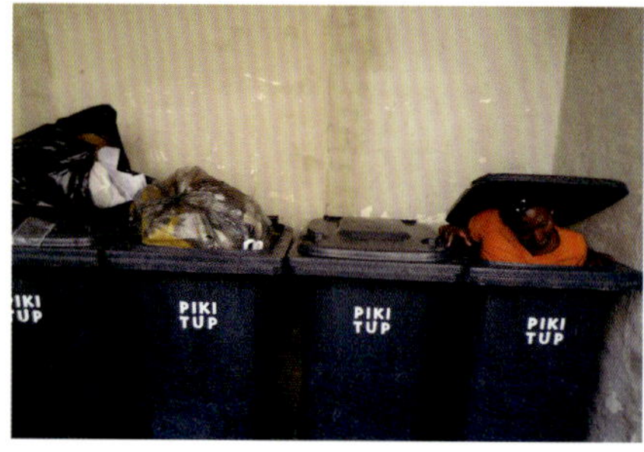

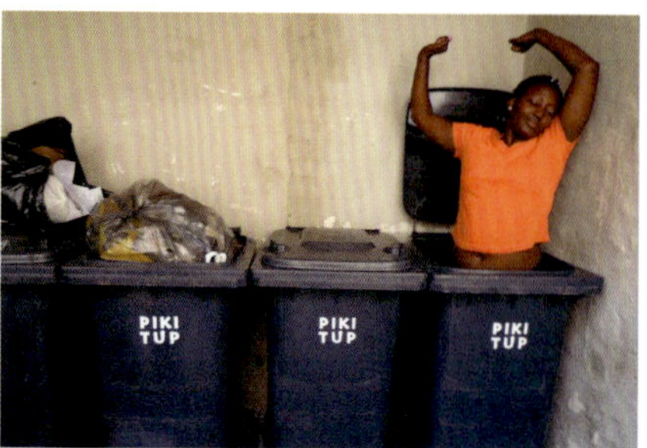

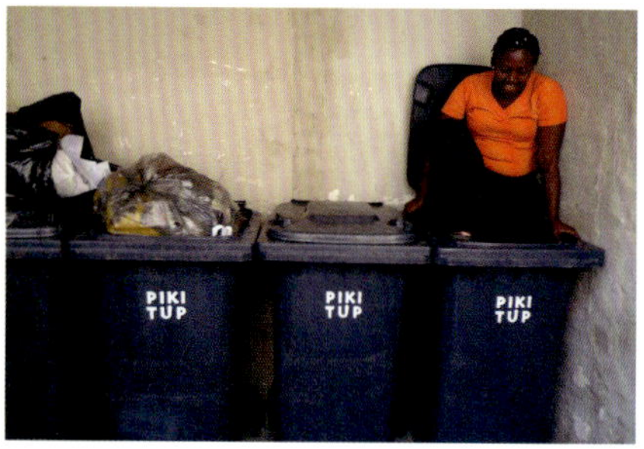

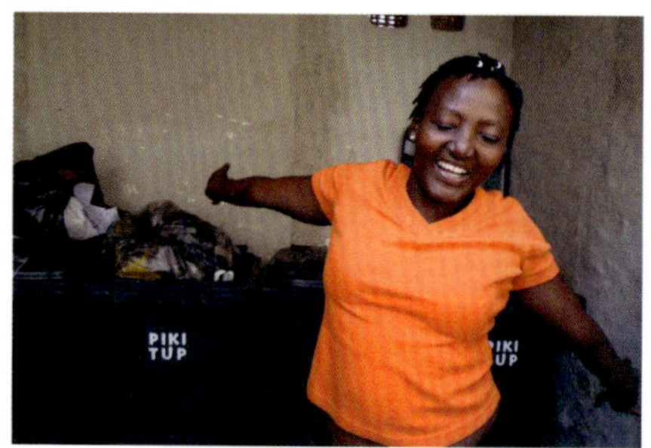

I am a victim of rape. After I was raped, they shot me and left me for dead. I lay in the hospital for three months in a coma. When I woke up, the doctor discovered I was pregnant and told me I had AIDS. My mom did not allow the doctor to do an abortion because it was late already. I was fourteen at the time.

I have experienced a lot of stigma, including from my own family—though not from my mom. When I was not at home they would say to my child, who tested HIV-negative when she was nine, "You and your mom, you're going to die, because you have this disease." Or "Don't disclose, because you are destroying the name of the family." Was I supposed to be quiet then? That's why I decided to disclose my status.

I want to tell other people who are HIV-positive to live their lives openly. Don't care about anybody else. Just live your positive life. You will become stronger, and stronger, and stronger again.

Telling my daughter about my HIV status, and about her past, was hard for me. I said, "There is something I need to tell you. I need you then to support me, and I will support you." I told her everything. "Don't feel ashamed," I said. "Don't be afraid. Be proud."

At school one day, the teachers set the children an assignment, "Who is your hero?" When I was checking my daughter's books, I saw that she had written about me. I said, "Why did you write that I'm a hero, not Nelson Mandela or Jacob Zuma?" She said, "No. They are not my heroes. My hero is you. Whatever difficulty I have in my life, you are always there for me." That's why I love her so much.

Sometimes I tell my daughter, "I will not die until you finish your school and your university." In the meantime, I will stay strong. I'm not the dying type.

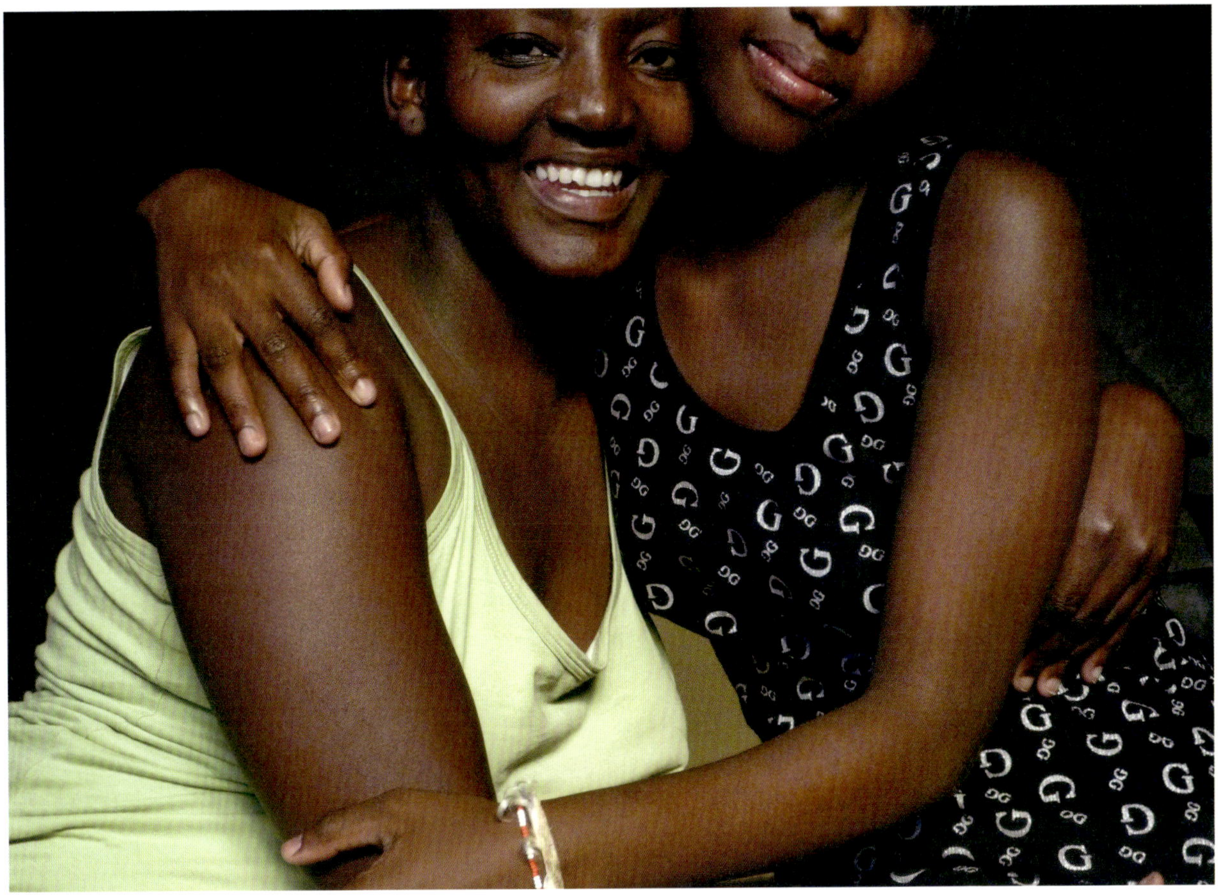

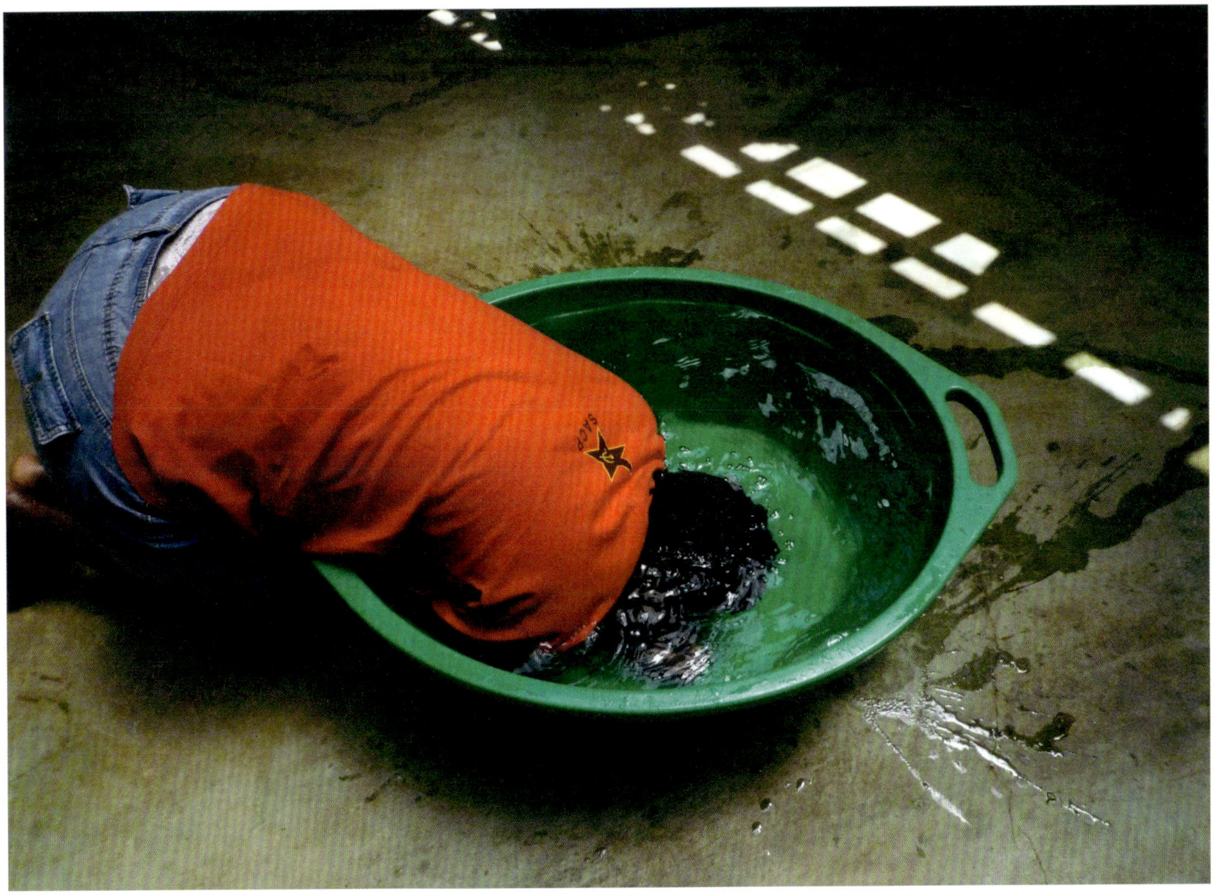

Annah

My baby's name was Tshegofatso. The day we came back from the hospital, he was very big, a healthy baby. He grew nicely and was fat. He looked like his father. He was always laughing. When he became ill he was always frowning, and he didn't laugh anymore.

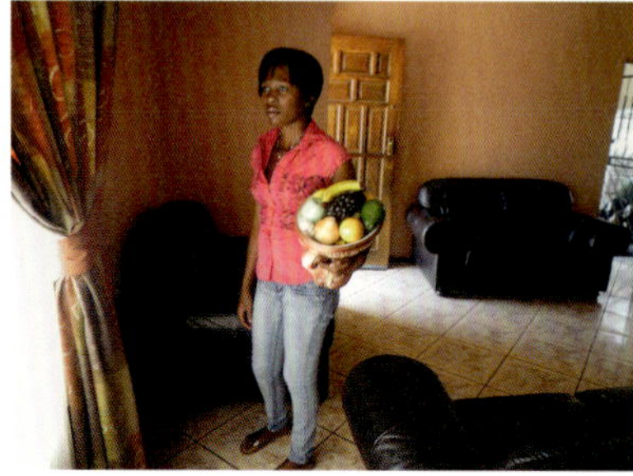

After breastfeeding him one day, he looked at me and then he started making a weird sound. He just died in my hands. I didn't even cry. I just went like, "No. No! This is not happening." But it was too late. I couldn't stop his soul from leaving his body.

We tend to remember God when days are dark. But in the happy days we forget Him. When my baby was very ill, I asked God, "Please help me. If I've done anything wrong, please forgive me. Don't hurt my baby for my sins." But I also said, "Thank you, Lord, for everything you've given me. I know you'll never give me a challenge I can't handle."

I keep a room for disappointment in my heart, so I can accept all the hurts. When it's time, I cry. I allow my emotions to take their place in my body. But I can't turn back the hands of time. I just have to carry on.

Bongi

I first realized I was gay when I was doing my grade ten at school. It was really difficult for me to accept this about myself. I tried to commit suicide. Then my mother and my stepfather took me to a pastor at church. I had to go through counseling sessions with him. He helped me understand and accept myself the way I am.

Five years later, I found out that I was HIV-positive. I told myself that maybe God had punished me because I'm gay. But then, after attending counseling sessions, I accepted my status. The support that I've gotten from my church has been really important. We even have a support group at church for people who are living with HIV.

Even though my family and church are there for me, support from the community is really hard to get. People will insult you, saying disgusting words: "Look at this gay person who has AIDS. We are going to change you and make you a straight guy. But you mustn't infect our girlfriends."

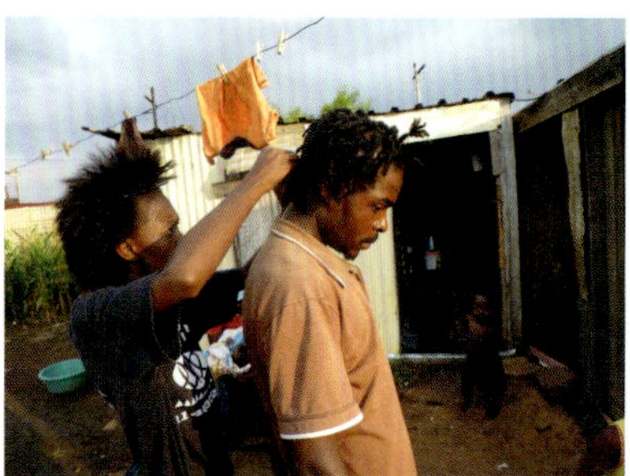

I met my partner last year, and we have been together ever since. He's HIV-negative and he supports me. He loves me and I love him. We live a normal life as heterosexual couples do—we even hold each other's hands when we walk in the street. We are just two guys in love.

Chris

I joined the Zimbabwean Army in 1995 and served in the Congo, where there were a lot of things happening, like beer drinking. Sometimes there were ladies to entertain us. Some guys were not using condoms, or sometimes a condom burst. When we withdrew from the Congo, the situation back home in Zimbabwe was not right at all. The money we were getting was not enough for us to survive. There was no food. We soldiers were sent at night to beat people for no apparent reason, even older people. So I decided to leave, to come and support my wife and daughter in South Africa.

Today, when I disclose my status, some of my friends don't take me seriously. "Ah, you think I was joking when I was telling you I'm HIV-positive? You have to go and test, my friend." To me, disclosure is a way of showing people that having HIV does not mean you are already dead. People should say, "Ah, Chris is living. Let me also go and test."

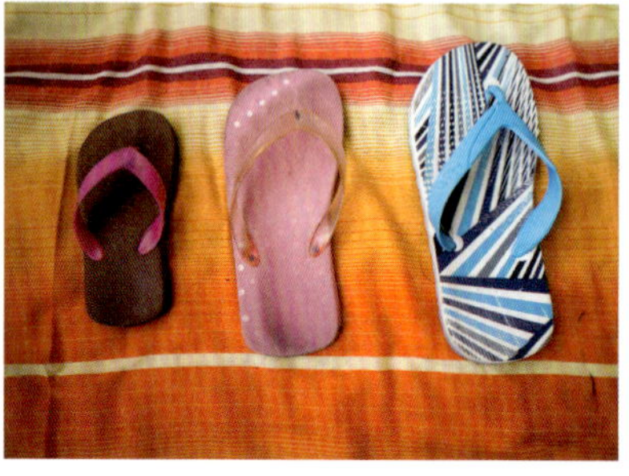

The way we live in Hillbrow now is terrible. In a single flat there will be four or five families—these are not healthy conditions. But I try to sacrifice for my family, because I am much happier to be with them, especially my daughter. We always play and joke together, running up and down, jumping on the bed. Even people who are HIV-negative have to admire me.

Gladys

At the clinic, my husband came in and was told that I was positive. He said, "Not my wife! Maybe there's a mistake somewhere." But when I tested again, it still came back positive. I did the test seven times with different labs. "Where did I get it from? I've never cheated. Why me?" I could not understand.

I wasn't thinking of myself. I was thinking of the baby that was inside of me. I was sure my baby was going to die. I was very scared. Now the girl is very big. She's OK. She's perfect. And this woman has picked up the pieces of her life.

I used to be heartbroken. But now I call myself "the chosen one."

I know I am positive, and I'm going to live positively.

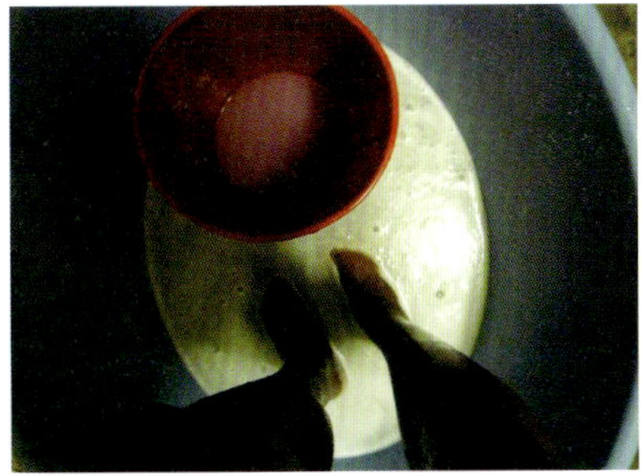

When I separated from my husband I said, "I'm going to change everything about myself." I had loved Reggae ever since I was a small child. I loved Bob Marley. I loved his music. His words always comforted me very much. I'm a new person now. I am proud to wear my colors. I love being a Rastafarian because, even if I'm positive, my fellow brothers and sisters love me and I love them.

Kau

I'm going to be honest. At twenty-five, I knew how to prevent HIV. But coming from a remote rural village and being in Johannesburg where everything is new, everything is at your fingertips—it's difficult to control yourself.

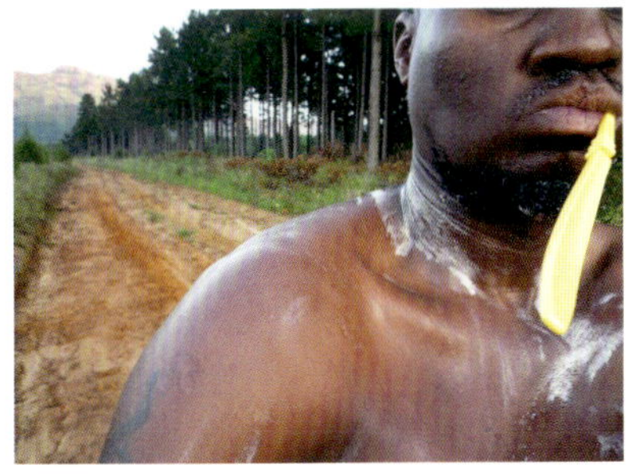

I knew I was doing some things sexually that I was not supposed to, but there was this idea in my mind that the people most likely to be infected were the uneducated, or prostitutes, those kinds of people. I had a good job as an aircraft technician. I didn't imagine I would get HIV from someone who looks nice.

I actually waited until I turned twenty-one to engage in sexual activities. And then for me to get infected at twenty-five, I felt really ripped off. If I were to go back and do it all over again, I wouldn't abstain, but I would condomize.

Nowadays, relationships are a challenge for me, because you meet a person, you like her very much, but then you need to disclose your status to her. I always prefer to disclose before I get too attached, to protect myself. Based on my experience there will be some rejection, either indirect or direct. People who like you initially might just go away.

I decided I needed to meet more HIV-positive people, so I started volunteering. Eventually I resigned from my job and became a treatment literacy practitioner. For me, being HIV-positive and being in a position where I can empower other people is great.

Ludick

I found out about my HIV status while I was in maximum security prison for committing murder. I saw that most of the inmates living with HIV in prison were dying there. So I thought, I'm going to die in prison too.

I was fortunate, though. Because I was a teacher and one of the most active inmate representatives, the wardens arranged that I be placed on medical parole.

My physical condition at that time was extremely bad. Instead of going on medication, I started to consult traditional healers. But I felt steadily worse. I was looking death in the eye. Finally, my eldest brother took me to a private doctor who arranged for me to get Western medication.

Before I went to prison I had been a member of SAPS, the South African Police Service. We used to say that the police uniform got us many girls. I never used protection. Deep down in my heart I knew that my past was not right. Still, it was hard for me to understand that I had to live with HIV.

Some people say, "Ludick, you are thirty-five years old. By the time you become a completely free man, you'll be fifty-four. Do you really think you are going to survive until your parole is finished?" I say, "I hope that you will be around so I can show you that I am here, living my life."

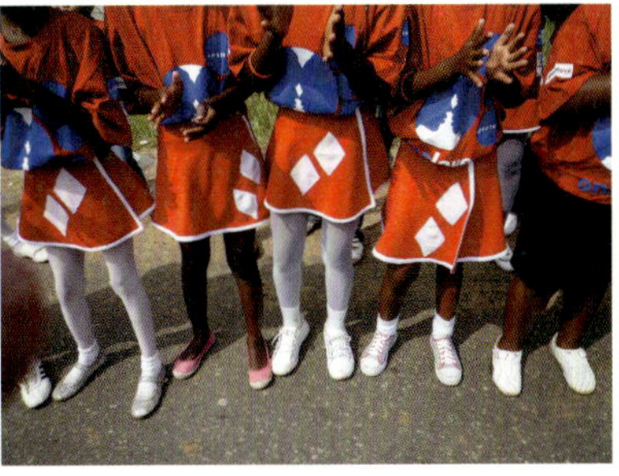

Mlungisi

There was nothing wrong with me, just a small swollen lymph node at the back of my ear. The nurse asked if she could give me an HIV test. "Let's do it," I said.

At that time there was no proper counseling. The fact that I was still alive and feeling OK was confusing to me. I went straight home and told everyone about my status. My brother was shocked. "We'll support you," he told me, "but don't go around telling people you are HIV-positive, OK?" As time went by I realized that it's me who's got HIV. If I want to tell someone that I am HIV-positive, I'm going to.

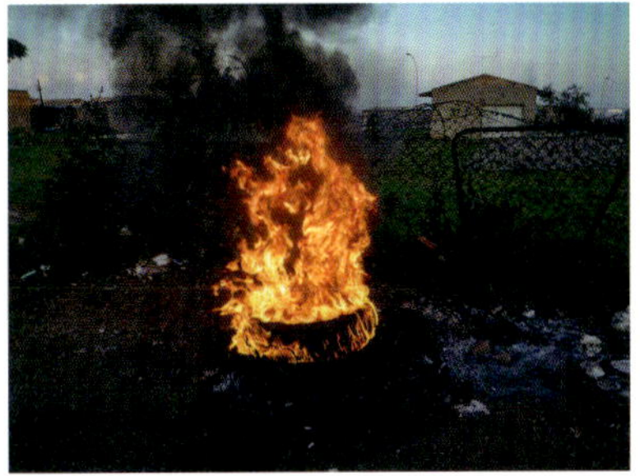

I grew up using traditional medicine. If I needed something for my stomach, I wouldn't just go to the shop and buy some medicine. Granny would prepare it. If I were not HIV- positive, I believe I would still be using traditional medicine. But after studying HIV, the science of medication, and virology, I came to understand why I have to take antiretrovirals.

I am especially fascinated by fire, which is important in traditional medicine ceremonies. There is a lot of good that comes from fire and a lot of sadness too. In that way, fire is like sex. People glorify sex as a sacred thing, because it creates life. But some people become HIV-positive from sex, like me. It's both.

Nomsa

I disclosed to my family the same day I got my results. Now they refer their HIV-positive friends to me when they need information. "My cousin is also positive, and she's living openly with her status. She can help you."

When my son was seven years old, I told him too. We are very open with one another. On Saturday mornings, we have our time where we sit in bed together and reflect on the whole week. We laugh together. We cry together. Still, at times, I feel like there's too much on his shoulders because of HIV.

After I learned about my status, I went to church and found my true identity, that I am made in the image of God. But my church doesn't address HIV, although I have fought for years that they need to do something. It's a no-go zone. Even the Bible says, "My people are perishing because of lack of knowledge."

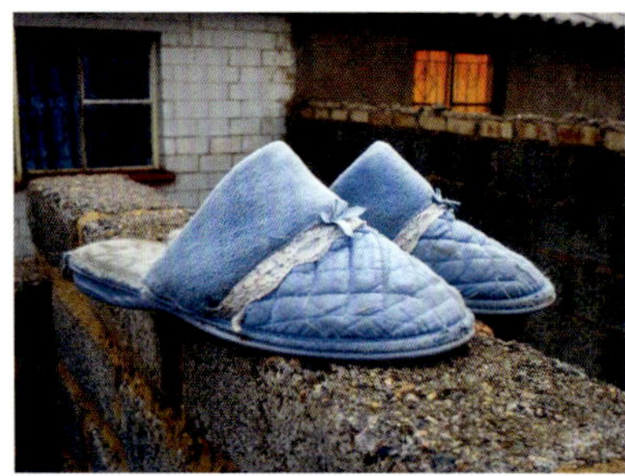

A part of me died when I became HIV-positive. That's the part about being a woman, about being able to have a husband and a fully functional family. But I always remember my aunt who said, "When you feel like crying, cry until you don't have tears anymore. Then just look at yourself in the mirror, wipe those tears, and move on." That's how I cope at times. I cry the pain out and then I wipe my tears and I'm myself again.

Nontyatyambo

One day I had a dream. I saw myself disclosing in front of a stadium full of people. When I woke up in the morning, I told my mom that I had dreamed this, and she said, "We are going to support you as a family. Definitel can do it."

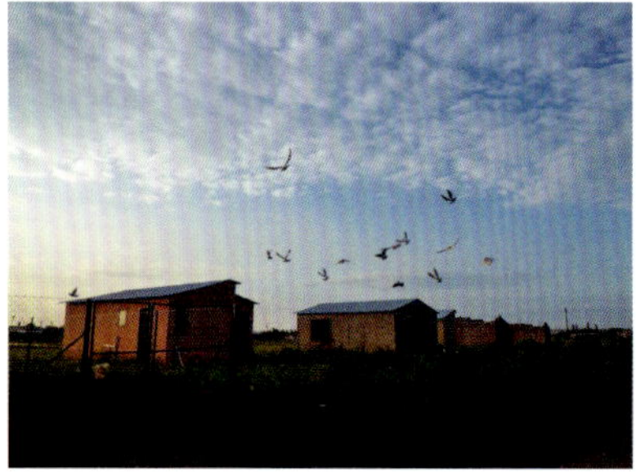

That's the day I started to accept my status, which was the first healing for me. You can take medication, but if you don't accept your HIV status, you are not going anywhere. I looked in the mirror and I asked myself, "Nontyatyambo, do you want to die or do you want to live?" Something told me, "I want to live."

Now, when someone approaches me and wants to have a relationship, the first thing I do is explain that I am living with HIV: "I've got this little friend in my blood." I'm in a relationship now and my partner is HIV-negative. Fortunately, she is very supportive and we are so happy.

My step-kids and I have a good relationship. There are three boys. The two older ones know about my HIV status. They are comfortable telling me anything, even things they don't tell their biological mom.

I want to see them grow. I want to see them experiencing life—without being infected. I'm already talking with the two older ones about sex and sexual intercourse. They must start taking care of themselves now.

Pleasure

After the diagnosis, I went to my boss to explain. My coworkers started distancing themselves from me and, eventually, my employer asked me to leave. The news spread that I had AIDS and my friends started to run away. I didn't have support from my family. I was chased away from my two children. I had to start another life. I lived alone, without friends.

At that time, around the 1980s through the late 1990s, AIDS was so scary. No one wanted to associate themselves with AIDS. Even me. I could not accept myself as a person living with AIDS.

In the early 2000s you started to see education programs—I think these assisted a lot. Through treatment literacy programs, I learned about the life cycle of the virus, how the virus operates in your system, how to control it.

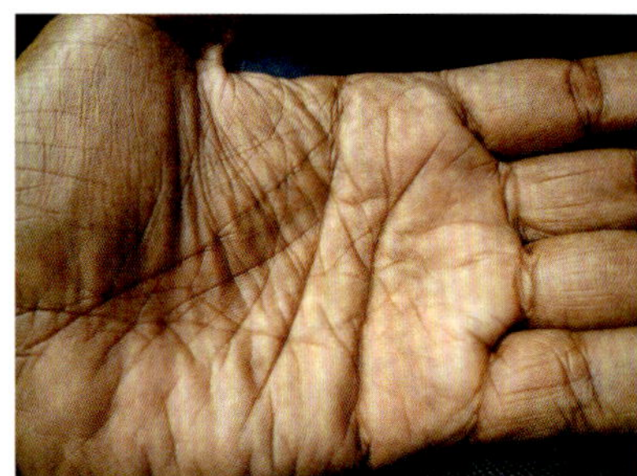

Eventually my children said, "We want our father." As they grew up, they started to realize how life works. Now they visit me whenever they wish. I tell them, "Any time you want me, just call me. Daddy will be there for you." So the relationship with them is OK. And with the mother, I told her that I forgive her. I just moved on.

Me and the virus, we need to have a clear understanding. If the virus kills me today, the virus is going to die. I've made a bond with the virus to say, "Spare my life and I'll spare yours."

Los Angeles

The Los Angeles *Through Positive Eyes* workshop, held in April 2011, highlighted the experience of long-term survivors, those who have lived with HIV for more than twenty or thirty years, some from the very first years of the epidemic. The early availability of medications in the global North has made survival possible, even as it has reduced or even eliminated one of the greatest causes of HIV stigma: physical disfigurement. Many people living with HIV no longer appear sick, while others report suffering from the long-term side effects of medication.

United States' AIDS epidemic, as of 2011

Number of people living with HIV:	1.2 million

Transmission category (numbers)

Men who have sex with men:	548,000
Injection drug use:	139,700
Heterosexual contact:	273,500

Treatment

Antiretroviral therapy has been available since 1996 but despite state-aided programs, low-income and uninsured Americans have less access than others.

Percent diagnosed:	86%
Percent in HIV care:	40%
Percent on antiretroviral treatment:	37%
Percent undetectable virus:	30%

Key events

1992 *AIDS is the number one cause of death for American men aged 25–44.*

1998 *Centers for Disease Control issues the first national treatment guidelines for the use of antiretroviral therapy.*

2006 *Bush administration strengthens federal funding for abstinence-only sex education programs.*

2008 *Same-sex marriage legalized in California.*

2010 *The Obama administration releases the first comprehensive national HIV strategy.*

Update 2019

In 2017, 1.1 million Americans were living with HIV. 56% of new infections were occurring in black and Latino men who have sex with men (1% of the population). The percentage of Americans diagnosed with HIV who were in care increased to 63% and those who were virally suppressed increased to 51%.

Since 2014 there has been a significant expansion of pre-exposure prophylaxis (PrEP), but the program still reaches less than 20% of those who would benefit from it.

Through Positive Eyes in Los Angeles was organized in partnership with the HIV/AIDS Prevention Unit of the Los Angeles Unified School District. Major funding was provided by The Herb Ritts Foundation, with additional support from the City of Los Angeles AIDS Coordinator's Office and UCLA .

Lynnea

After being diagnosed as a child, I grew up thinking that it was impossible for me to have a child of my own. I failed to plan for my future because I honestly couldn't imagine having one.

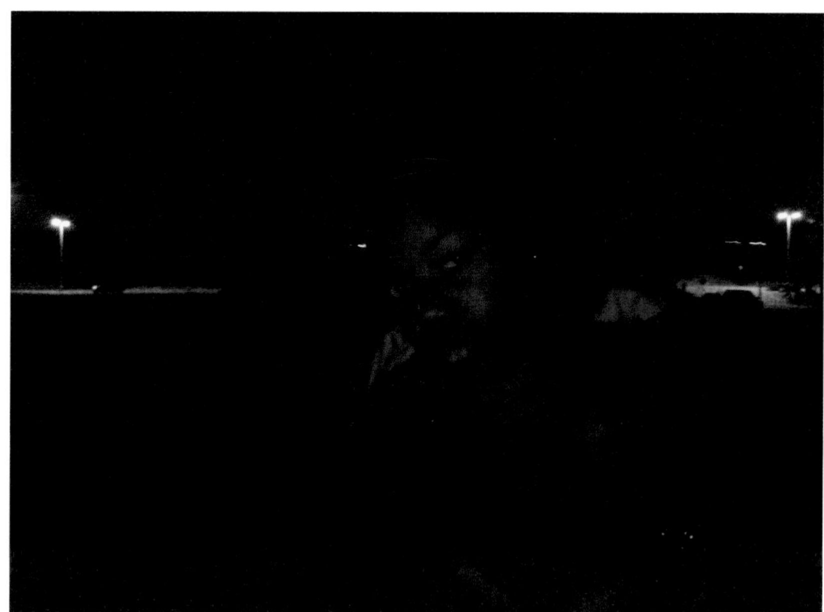

When you're a person living with HIV, you need your friends, to get past the stigma and also to share moments of genuine love. I think I was born with HIV. My mother has it, and one of the ways it can be passed is from mother to child in the womb.

A lot of times people give me more sympathy than they give someone who has contracted HIV through drug use or sexual activities. They say it's not my fault and I didn't ask for it. But who asks for HIV? The only difference between me and other HIV-positive people is that I don't know life without it.

After being diagnosed as a child, I grew up thinking that it was impossible for me to have a child of my own. I failed to plan for my future because I honestly couldn't imagine having one.

As an adult, I began hearing about a decrease in mother-to-child HIV transmission, using a new treatment regimen. After consulting with my doctor, I made the decision to try. With the currently available medications, HIV is no longer terminal. It's a chronic treatable disease, like diabetes. So my doctor gave me the green light.

In the past, doctors preferred a Cesarean birth, to minimize blood sharing, but, following the medical instructions, I was able to have a natural birth. Doctors recommend that the mother be on an IV drip of AZT for at least four hours before birth. After birth, the baby receives a low dose of AZT for the first six weeks. I did everything as prescribed. Despite all the negative things I had learned in the past, I wanted my child to have the best possible outcome. And that's how it turned out. I had prayed for a girl. I dreamed of a girl. The ultrasound confirmed I was having a girl. She would be the remixed version of myself, so I scrambled the letters of my own name, Lynnea, and created the most beautiful name I could imagine: Nae'Lyn.

These days, Nae'Lyn is my life. She's a happy, healthy, HIV-negative little girl. She's sassy, spunky, and very opinionated. She is quite the opposite of me, not shy at all. She sings in church. She remembers everything. She is very loving, the sweetest little girl I've ever met. And she wants everything her way. She's a handful.

And here I am, looking forward to being an old woman, decades from now.

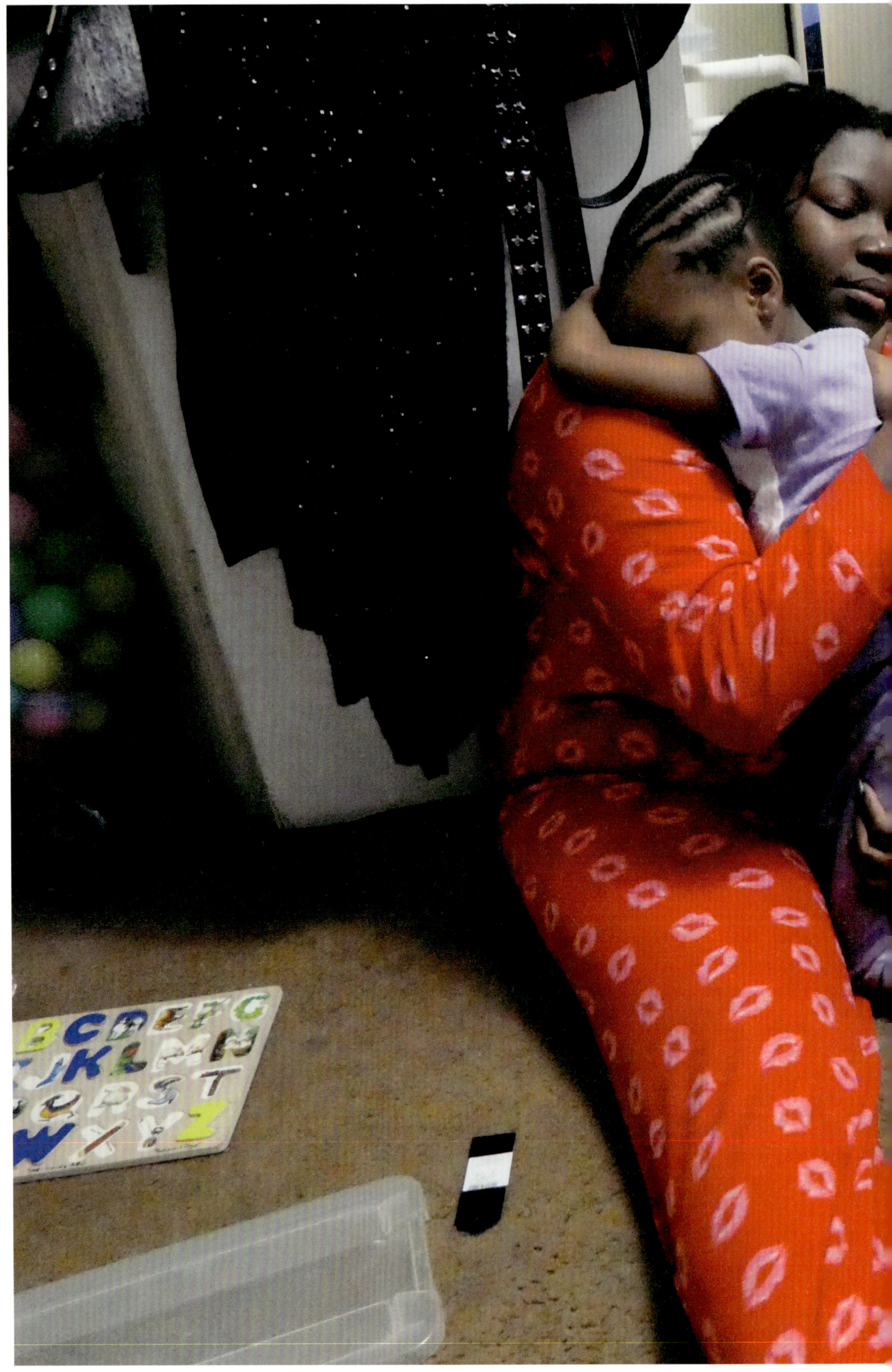

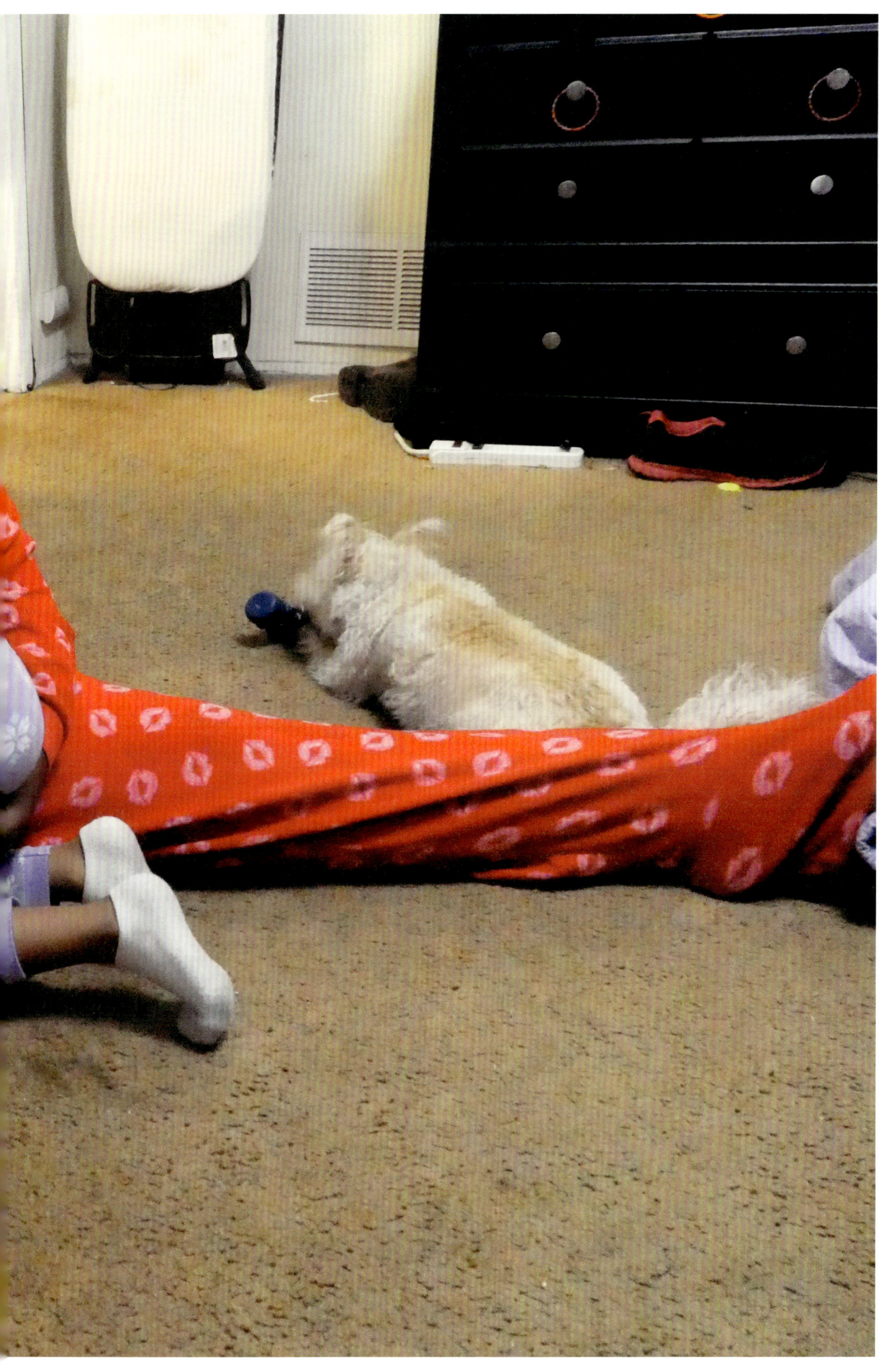

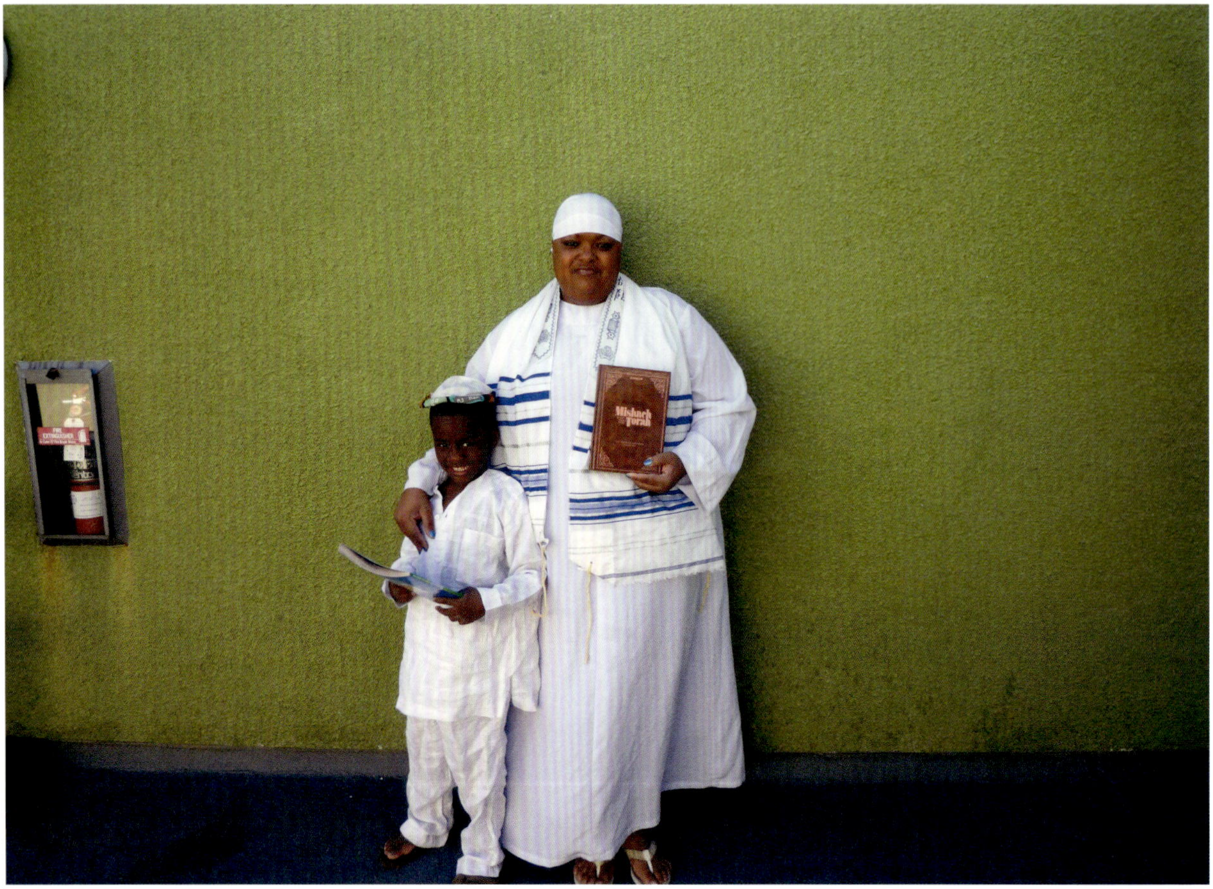

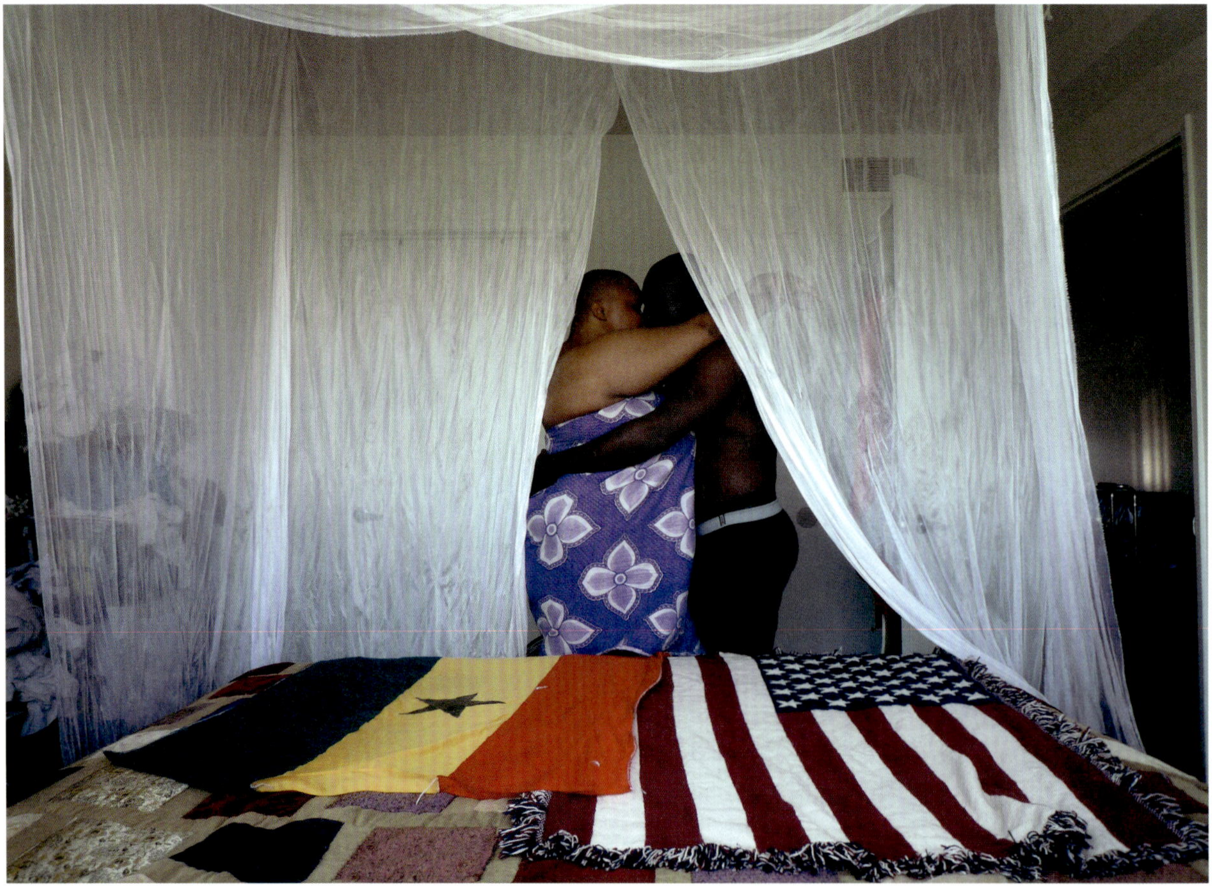

LaVera

Guess what? I may be in a monogamous relationship with my partner, but that doesn't mean my partner is in a monogamous relationship with me.

When I found out I was HIV-positive, I had just re-entered the United States after a trip to Nigeria, and I was having some pregnancy-related complications. When the doctor told me, I broke down and started crying. I was scared. I felt like I knew absolutely nothing about the illness, and on top of that I was looking at, "Wow, I'm pregnant." I was already in my second trimester.

My husband is negative, and we use condoms every time so that he stays that way. At the time I found out, he was living in Nigeria. I didn't tell him I was HIV-positive. He comes from Ghana, where, if the community finds out that you have HIV, you could be ostracized. For him, coming to terms with the fact that his wife is HIV-positive is a big deal. It's been a journey.

I know I got it sexually, from the man I had been engaged to before my husband. There was nothing that said, "Oh this guy may be sick." Nothing. But I started experiencing allergies, repeat sinus infections, a fungal yeast infection under my breasts that would not go away, and a swelling of the lymph nodes behind my ears. I was running back and forth to the community health clinic. No one thought to ask me to get tested for HIV.

If you say you're in a monogamous relationship, they don't think to ask you to get tested. But guess what? I may be in a monogamous relationship with my partner, but that doesn't mean my partner is in a monogamous relationship with me.

My son saved my life. The doctor explained to me that with intervention there was less than a 2% chance of passing the virus on to my baby. Moreover, if I had not gotten pregnant with him at the time I did, I wouldn't have been tested. He put me on track.

Now I'm in school for my master's in counseling. I'm the first person in my family to earn an undergraduate degree. I still shake my head like, "I'm in school for my master's. Wow!" I've gone to Washington to speak with legislators, I speak to classrooms, I've joined community outreach efforts. None of this was in my life before HIV.

And my HIV-negative son has been there pushing me the whole time. He's happy, he's vibrant, he's very energetic. He lets me know that there's hope.

Jazmine

I got a tattoo of the word *Love* where the L is an HIV ribbon. I got it because I think I'm still lovable, even having HIV.

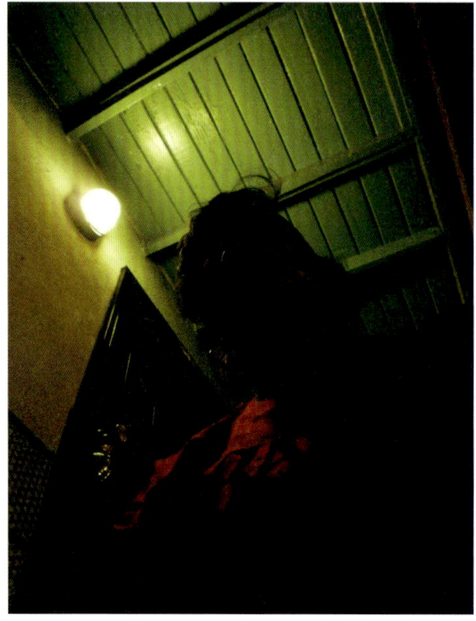

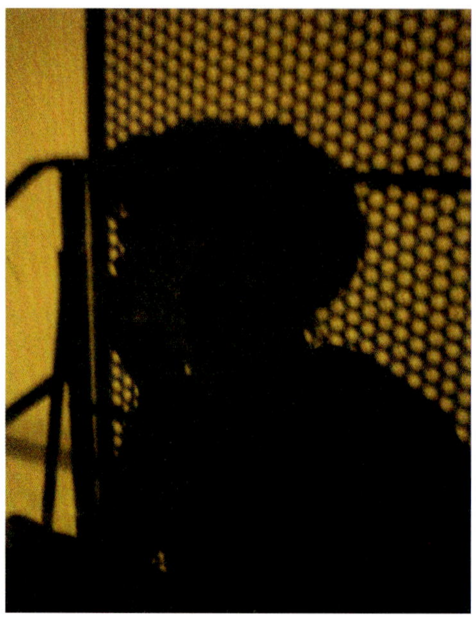

Back in 2008, when I was sixteen, I was having stomach problems. I went to the hospital and the doctor said I had a cyst on my ovary and he was going to remove it. When he did the surgery, he found an infection in my womb, so he ran more tests. After a week of being there, some doctor came and told me, "Oh, you're HIV-positive," and walked out the door. I didn't even know I was being tested for HIV.

I was heartbroken. It was about to be my senior year, I was playing varsity basketball. I decided to be home-schooled instead of finishing and going to prom and doing all the fun stuff you do in senior year. I missed my senior year, but I'll get over it.

I got HIV through unprotected sex with my ex-boyfriend. I told him, "If I have it, I believe you do, because you're the one I lost my virginity to." And he's like, "Don't talk to me anymore." I was trying to make sure we were both on medicine, that we were both OK. But he doesn't want to come to terms with it. It bothers me still.

The house where I stay, everyone there is HIV-positive. At first, I didn't want to talk to anybody. But then I had a horrible break-up and the people I live with were very supportive. They're like my aunties and big sisters.

I got a tattoo of the word *Love* where the L is an HIV ribbon. I got it because I think I'm still lovable, even having HIV. I still go out to parties. I put my freak 'em dress on. People think that people with HIV are dirty. I remember telling this boy and he was like, "What! You can't have HIV. You don't even look sick." I don't have to look sick to have HIV. I'm straight, I had sex, I got HIV. It can happen to anybody.

A few of my coworkers at Home Depot know that I'm HIV-positive, and they've all been supportive. But it's not like you just go up and say, "Oh, you know, I'm HIV-positive," and keep walking. After doing this photography project, I want to go out and make people more aware of HIV. We're not different. We're not this weird group of people. We're just like you.

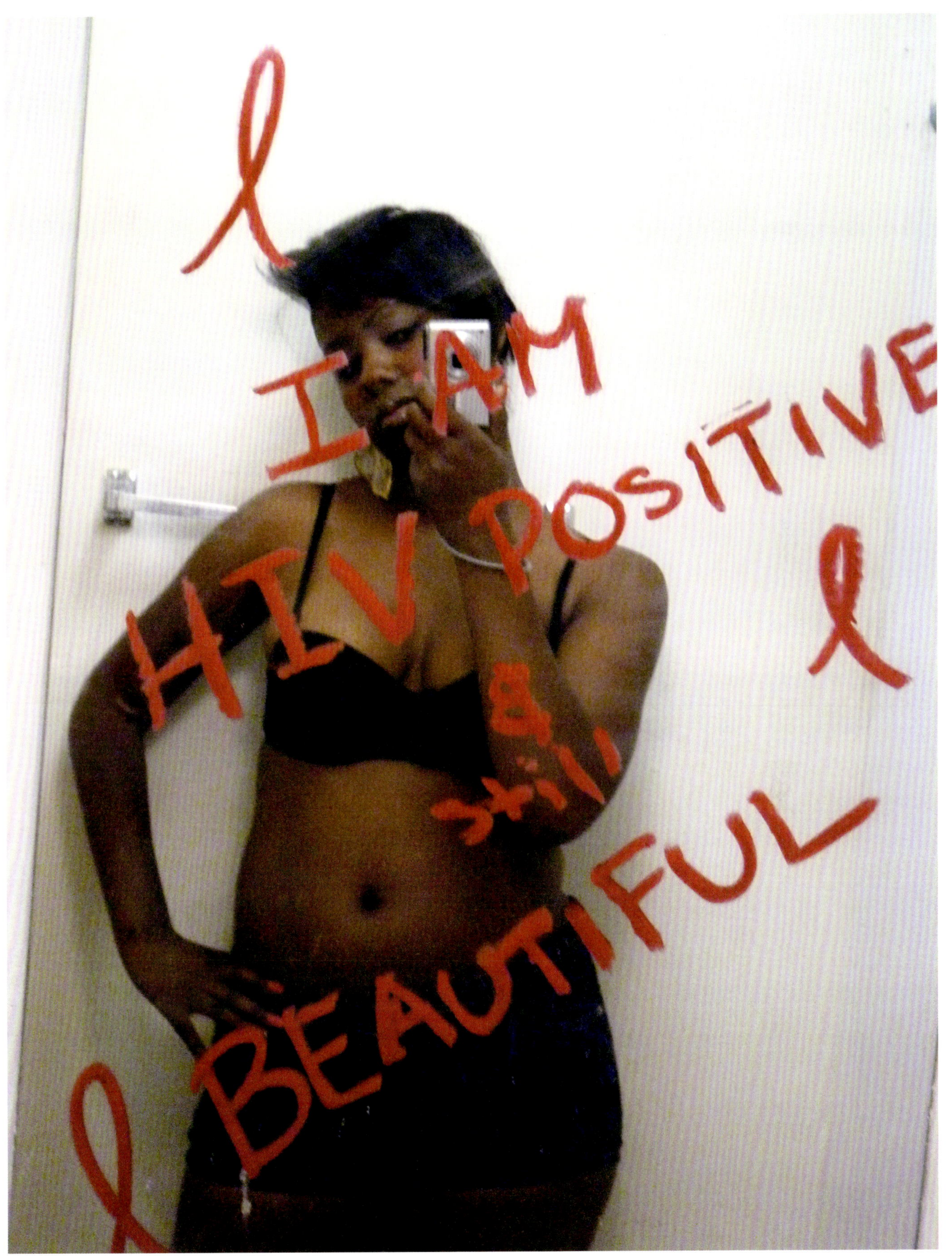
I AM
HIV POSITIVE
& still
BEAUTIFUL

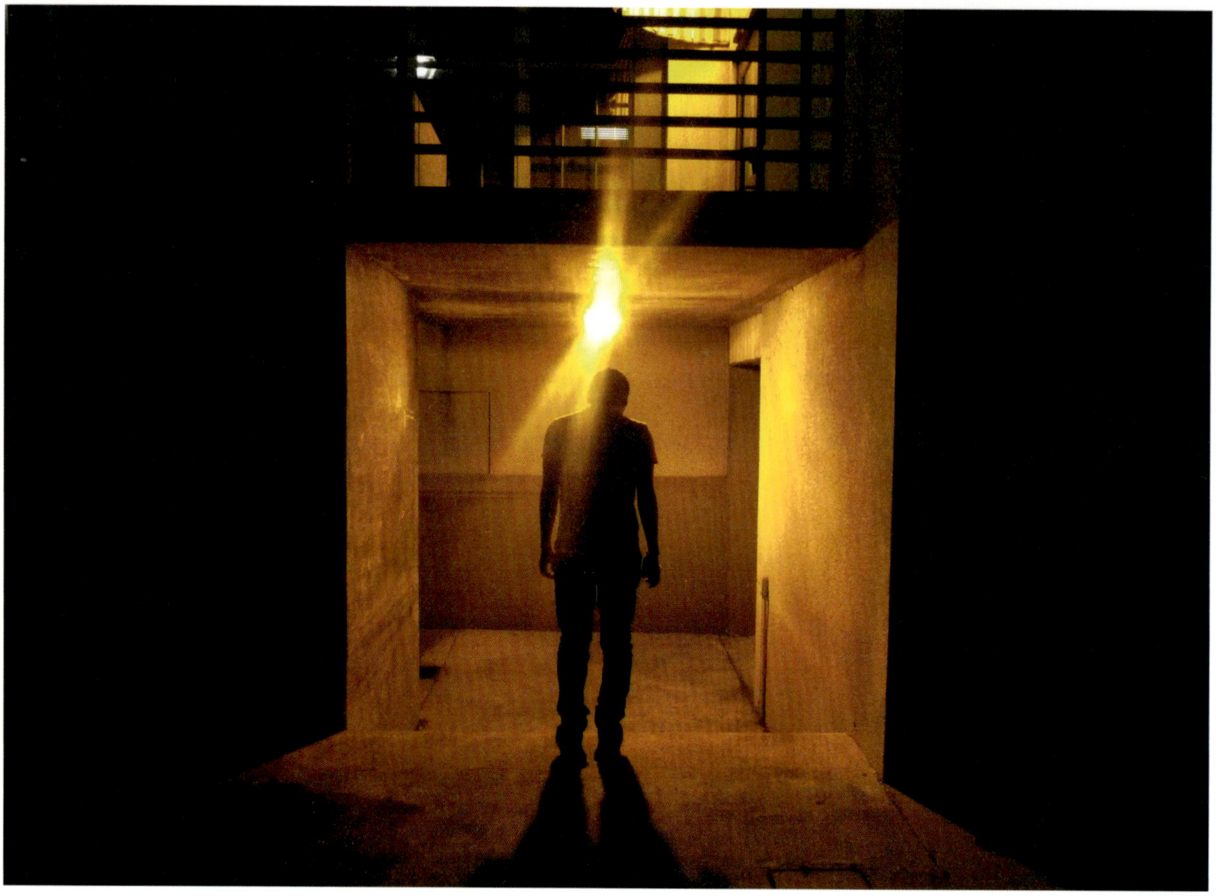

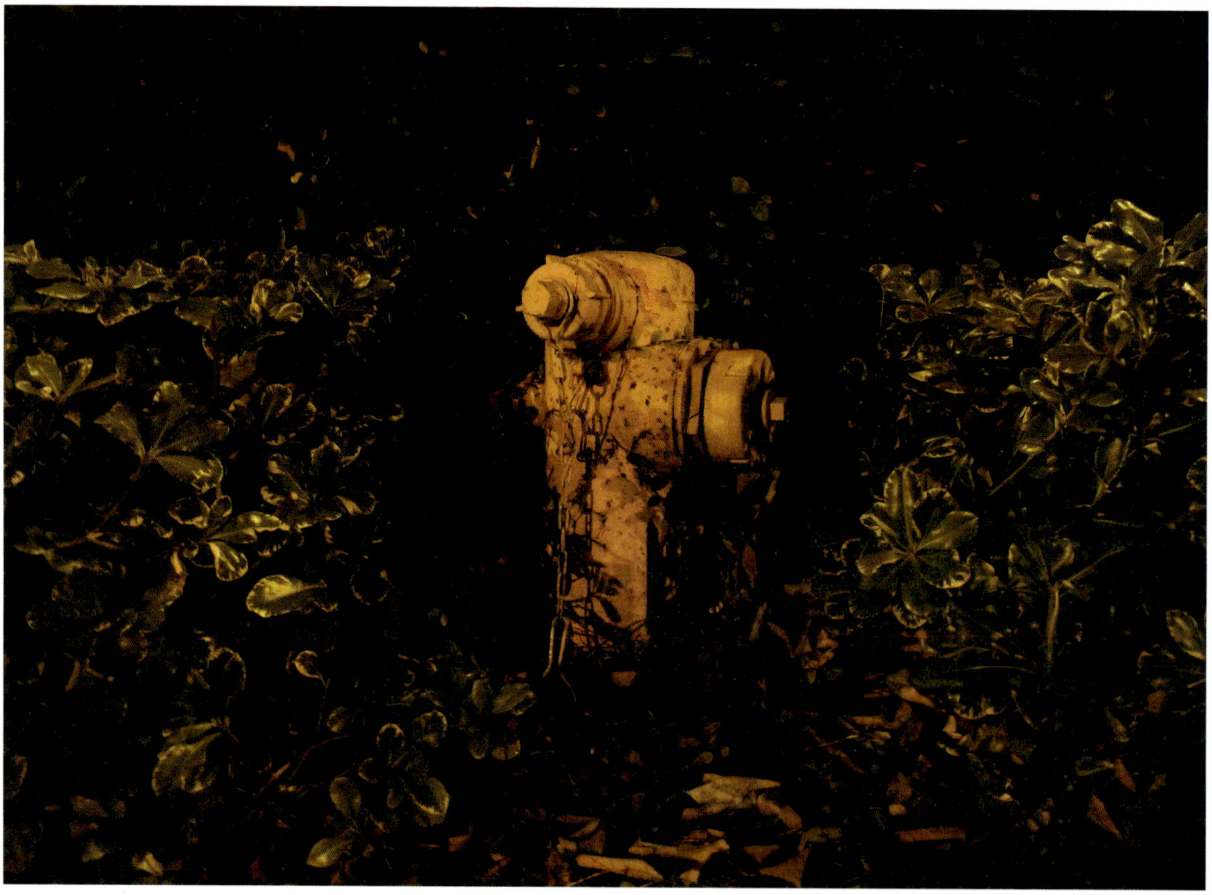

Jose

At school, it was really therapeutic to tell people that I was positive and see that nothing had changed. They would still shake my hand after class, and a lot of them sent me cool letters.

How HIV entered my life is pretty simple. I had unprotected sex with someone who was infected, and he didn't know. He was arrested for something minor and when he was in jail they tested him and they gave him his results that same evening. After he came out of jail, he suggested that we go get tested. I found out two weeks later that I was positive. It was the worst moment of my life.

I grew up in a very loving, caring family, the youngest of five kids. My mom would talk to us ever so slightly about sex. "Te cuidas." Take care of yourself. My sister would bring home condoms. I grew up in the social justice movement, I learned how to discuss healthy sexual lifestyles, and how to feel comfortable saying no. I was like, "How could I be so stupid?"

Self-stigma made me go into a hole. I didn't tell my family. I went into a really negative drinking binge. I knew people with AIDS were wonderful people, but I still felt really bad and shameful.

One day, I realized I wasn't dying, and that something needed to change in me. All those negative feelings started disappearing. I decided I had to forgive myself and love myself, my surroundings, my family, my partner.

It was such a relief to finally tell somebody. After I told some friends and they were OK with it, I felt brave enough to tell other people. At school, it was really therapeutic to tell people that I was positive and see that nothing had changed. They would still shake my hand after class, and a lot of them sent me cool letters. A couple of girls said that I was cute—"Too bad!" they said.

A year later I told my mom. She cried because she thought it was a sad thing. She said what any Mexican mother would say, "Te dije que te cuidaras." She had told me to be careful. "But you're my son and I love you." Once I'd told her and she was OK, I told the rest of my family. They were all very supportive of me, not just about being gay but being positive too.

At this point, I don't care who knows. I would get on top of the biggest mountain and scream, "Jose is HIV-positive." Because it doesn't matter.

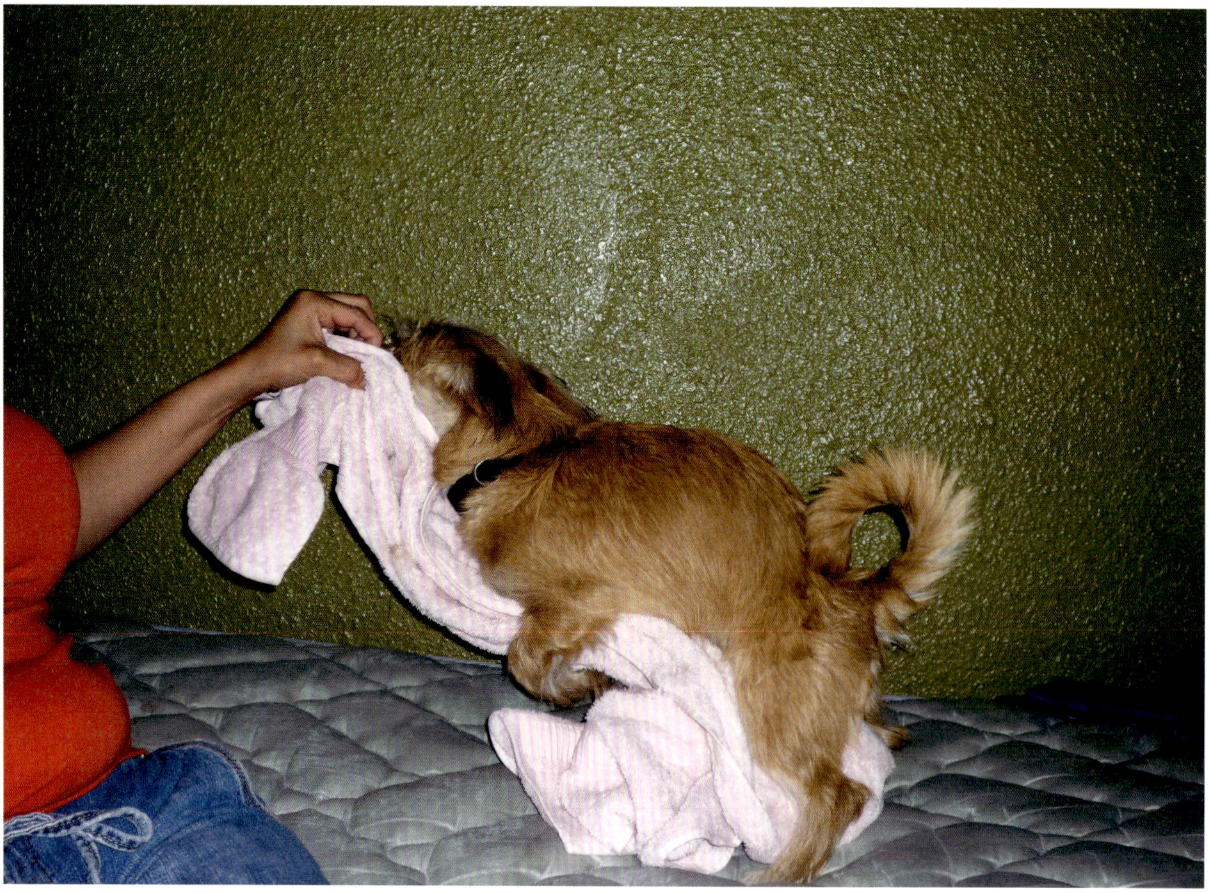

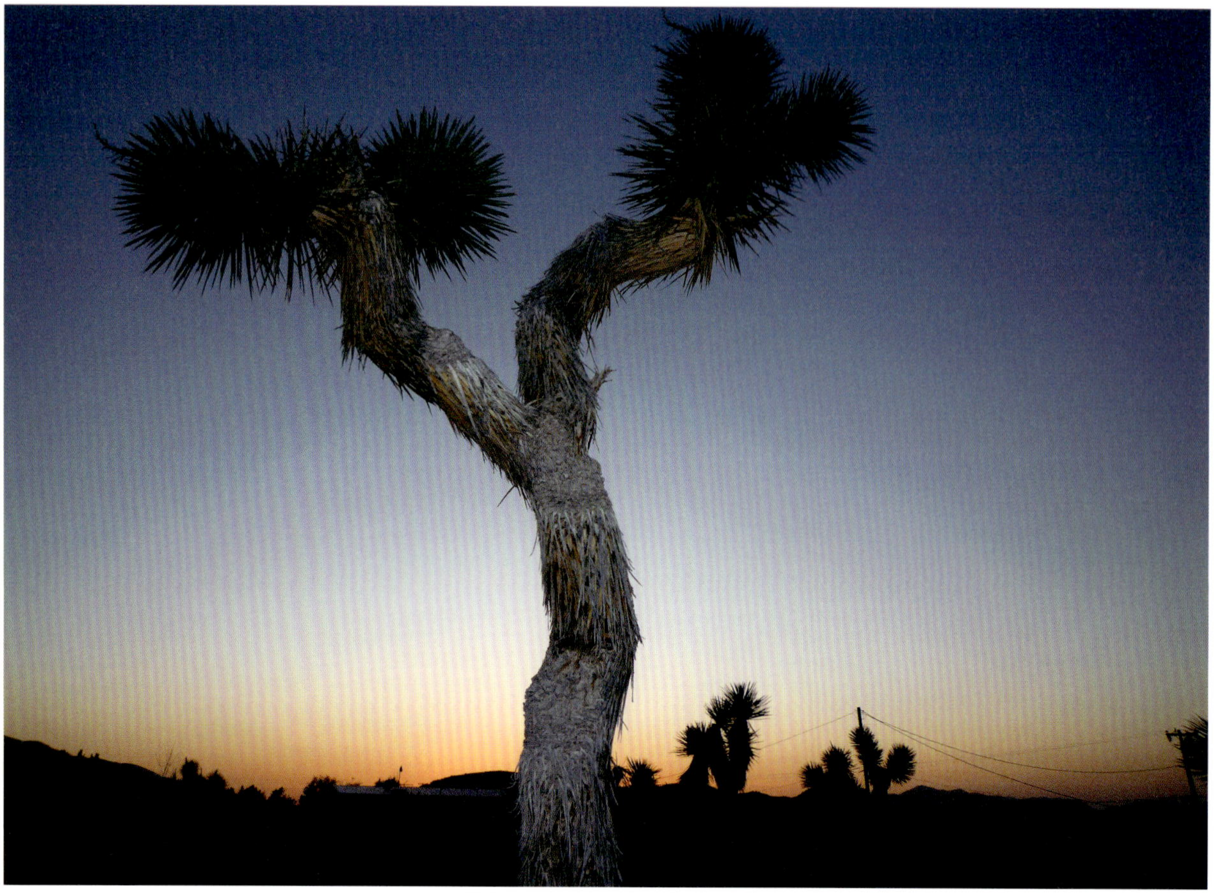

Ralph

I prayed to the great artist up in the sky that if he let those women be healthy and safe, that I would give him ten years of celibacy. They all came back negative. I kept my promise.

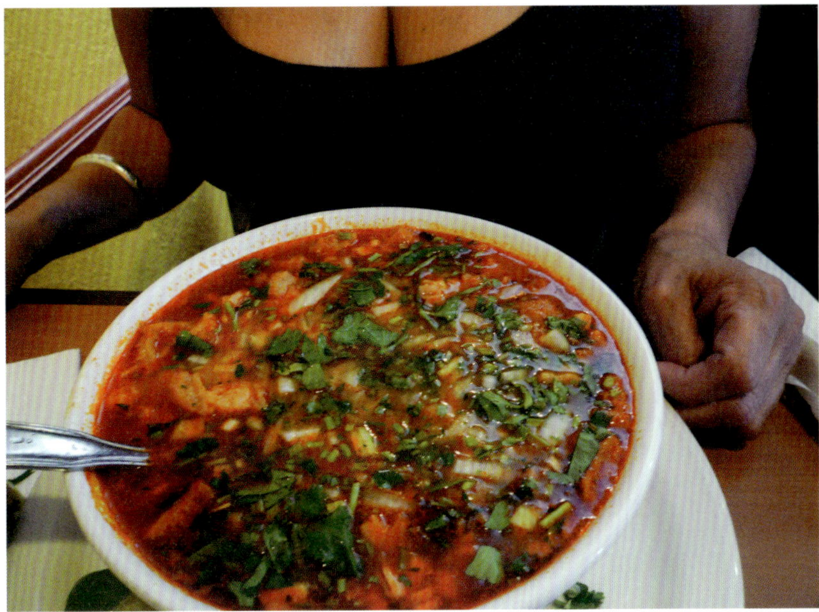

Everybody always goes, "Why do you walk with a cane?" I've been known to say, "Oh, I have a slight case of AIDS."

I got my test results on April Fools' Day, one month before my twenty-fifth birthday. Back then, I was a mohawked punk rocker. And I was a fighter. I had been fighting since I was eight years old. When your dad kills your mother, it makes you pissed off.

Those first two years of being HIV-positive were mad years. I had unprotected sex with several different women, and I didn't tell them. I figured, I was damned by somebody, so I was going to damn the world. After that I came to my senses and realized I was wrong and I had to tell those girls. Of course I got smacked. I got told I was going to be killed. I just told those girls, "You know this shit's out there. Go get tested. If you feel the same way after you test, then do what you got to do."

I prayed to the great artist up in the sky that if he let those women be healthy and safe, that I would give him ten years of celibacy. They all came back negative. I kept my promise. In those ten years I educated a lot of women. I called it "working the bar circuit." I'd go out and meet women who were ready to go home and get busy, and I'd tell them I was HIV-positive.

I have a hard time walking now, because it has crippled me. I'll never have kids, I'll probably never have a wife. But I love women. Everybody thinks Ralph likes big boobs, but Ralph likes all kinds. Whatever clicks. They come and they go, though. Maybe one will come and stay. If I get that lucky.

I live in the high desert now, to breathe some fresh air and exercise. I'm trying to get my lower end to come back to life. I woke up one day, went to turn on the stereo, and I collapsed. Turns out I had developed a neurological disorder on account of my HIV. When they told me I was going to be in a wheelchair, I was like, "Cut my legs off if they ain't going to work." They said, "No no. We don't have to do that." Good thing, because I got myself out of the wheelchair. I'll run again.

In the game of life, you need to follow the instructions. Eventually we all have got to die. Nobody gets out of here alive.

Rodney

"Be here now." That could be the best mantra ever. It keeps me from worrying about the future or feeling shameful about the past.

I found out that my partner had been layering crack in our pot. He would put it in without me knowing it. One day I reached into his pocket and I found this little white square. And then I started smoking crack, just straight out. We got evicted five times in a seven-year period. Sleeping on the streets, drinking huge amounts. Just lost.

I remember at one point thinking, "The fly on that piece of shit is better than me." My partner would beat me down a lot, tell me how ugly I was, how skinny I was, how stupid I was. And I started believing it.

My T-cells dropped to one. I was down to 120 pounds, wasting, having diarrhea like thirty times a day. I had a staph infection on my back. I threw my meds out the window. I could see them on the roof of the building next to us. I just figured, if I stop taking my meds, I will die and then I won't have to commit suicide. But I kept not dying. And those meds sat out there.

I had a sore on my hand and it was really hurting badly, so I decided I had to go to the doctor, because I still wasn't dying. The hospital put me in the Carl Bean House, an AIDS hospice, and that's where everything changed. I started going to Alcoholics Anonymous meetings twice a day.

I was kind of broken when I started doing yoga. I was in a lot of pain after all those years of drug and alcohol abuse. But I found a great sense of calm, of serenity and peace. "Be here now." That could be the best mantra ever. It keeps me from worrying about the future or feeling shameful about the past.

I fall out of poses, but I've learned how to fall gracefully. I've learned how to get up and laugh about it and dust myself off and keep going.

I once took a yoga class and the guy would have us sit for twenty minutes in meditation at the beginning of class, and I would be screaming in my head like, "Oh my God! Get out! Run!" Now I meditate for ten to fifteen minutes every day, and that's amazing.

Life is interesting. It's crazy and fun and hard and depressing. But it's certainly a lot better than it was.

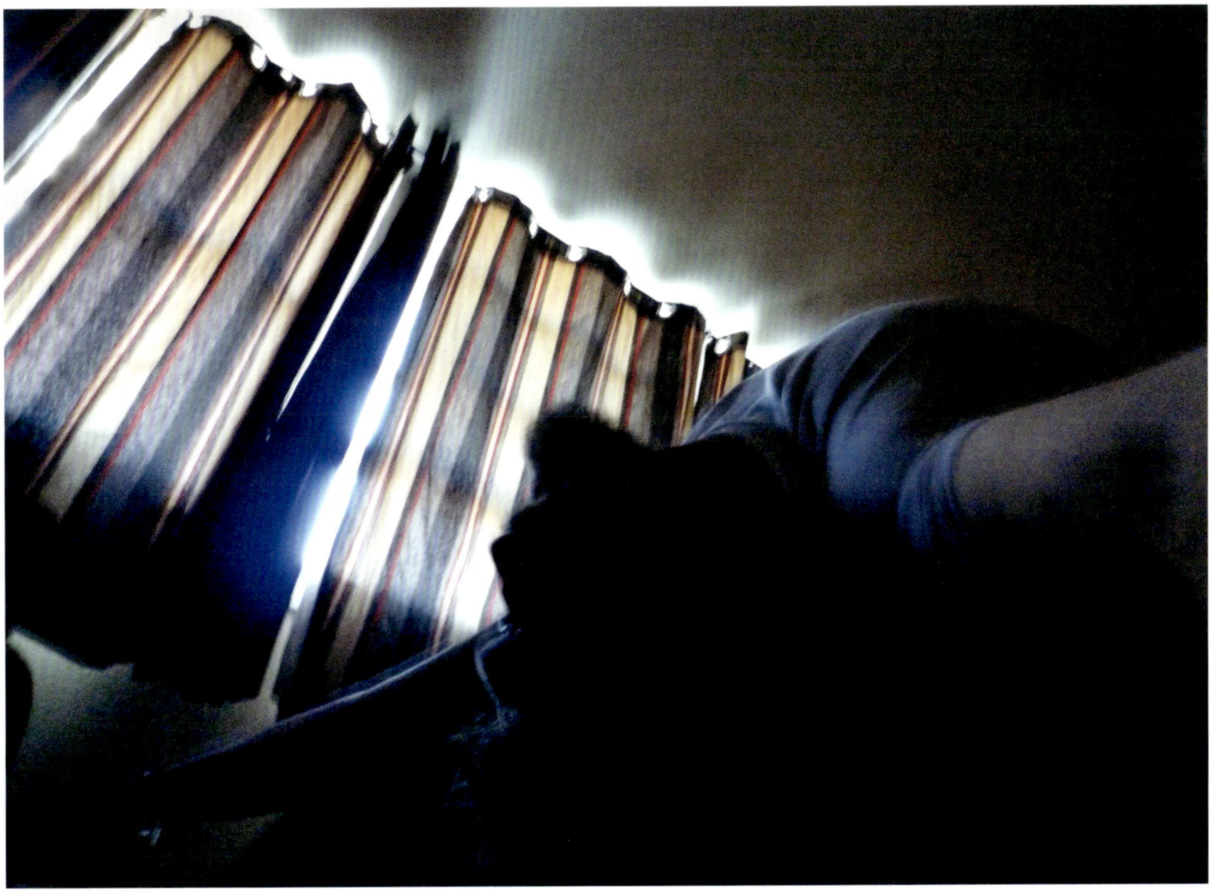

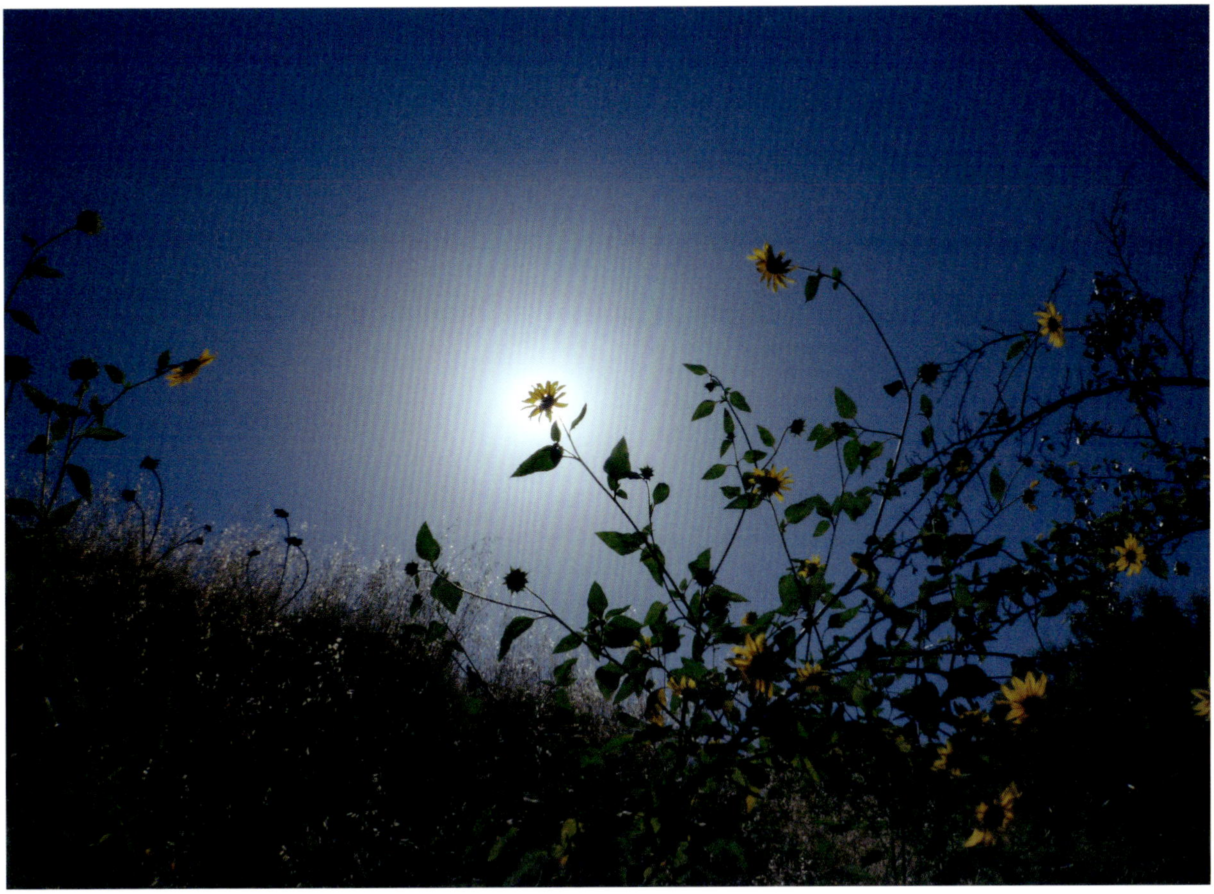

Nancy

I was supposed to die young. I always said I would die beautiful, on the pillow with my Mexican hair, just like Cinderella or Sleeping Beauty.

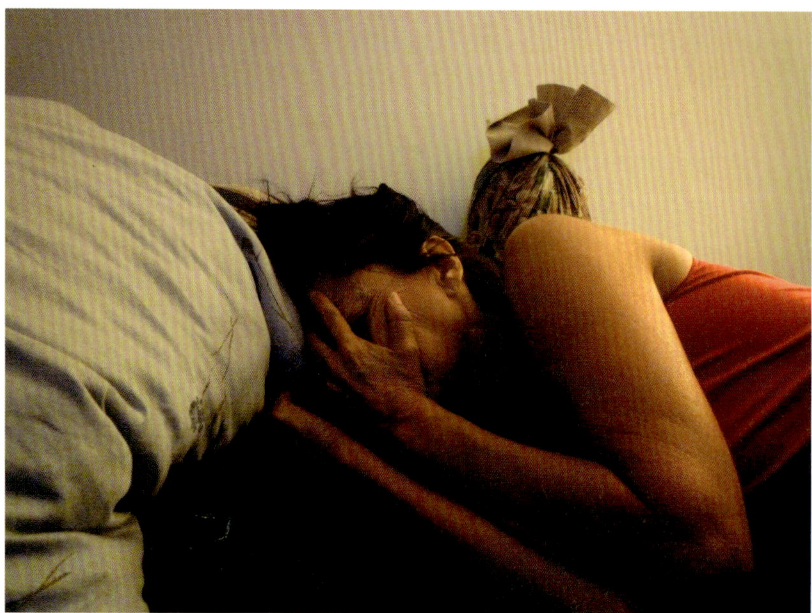

When I was a young child I had polio. I grew up with a brace on my right foot, I had a limp. With all that, and being skinny and awkward, I was laughed at. But being stigmatized for having HIV is different. You don't grow out of HIV.

I first found out I was HIV-positive when I was pregnant with my son. I was listening to a radio station and they were doing a special on HIV and AIDS—I didn't know that a mother could transmit HIV to her baby through breastfeeding. I decided right then that I had to get tested, because I also knew a person could get HIV from having unprotected sex.

My behavior wasn't that wild, but I did have sex before I got married, and I had sex after I was married, and not with my husband. Being Catholic, there was a lot of guilt and shame about that. Then, my partner, Ray, developed an AIDS-related illness. He died when my son was about eight months old. It wasn't until I became more HIV-educated that I realized I didn't give him HIV, that he gave it to me.

As Ray was dying, I realized I had to tell my family, because there was nobody else there for me. But first, I had to tell my older child, my daughter. This was around 1993. She was only twelve and she was scared out of her mind. She'd seen Ray die and she thought I was going to be next—we all did. I had to reassure her that I would outlive everybody, though I had no idea what was going to happen.

I was supposed to die young. I always said I would die beautiful, on the pillow with my Mexican hair, just like Cinderella or Sleeping Beauty. I wasn't supposed to be with my son when he was sixteen and rebelling. I didn't want wrinkles, saggy skin, everything falling. I wasn't going to see my daughter get married, or see my grandchildren.

My son, Raymond, always said when he turned eighteen he was going to get a tattoo. He came home one night, and he said, "Wake up!" He turned on the light, put his arm up, and showed me my name: "Nancy" across his whole forearm. He said that he always wants me close to him, and he doesn't want to lose me. No shame, no embarrassment. That's a huge honor—even though I'm still not that happy about the tattoo.

Cesar

I was born in East L.A. and started being sexually active when I was thirteen. I was really curious and experimented a lot.

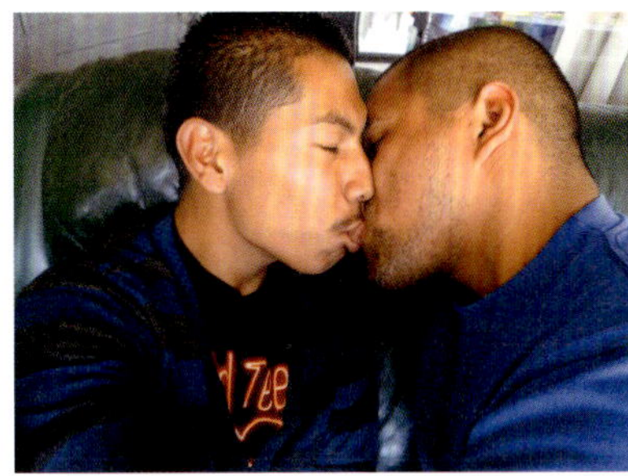

When I was in high school, I wanted to know my HIV status, because I had many partners in the past. So I took a test. I went to the clinic with my mom. The doctor told me that I was HIV-positive and I was shocked. I didn't cry or anything, I just couldn't believe it. I never knew anybody who was HIV-positive. I was in denial. The doctor told me that I needed to see a therapist, to get help.

I was diagnosed when I was seventeen. I'm nineteen now. I haven't finished high school yet. I was going to drop out because I was depressed, but I decided to go back to school so I could have a career. I want to study ultrasound tech for pregnant women. I think it's interesting—babies, and being born. I think it's really cool.

I have a big Mexican family. I love spending time with them, especially my cousins. We're really close. My family knows that I'm gay. But they don't all know that I'm HIV-positive because I don't want to freak them out. My mom knows, but my dad doesn't. He's not really involved in my life. He just works. And drinks, every weekend. That's pretty much it.

I'm not really a sexual person. Maybe before, but I look at it differently now that I'm positive. Before, I would have sex with friends, guys I knew, and now I'm HIV-positive. So it didn't go that well. But now it's different. I'm in a relationship and sex is not the major thing.

Jose and I met in an HIV group. We're both HIV-positive. We come from the same background. We're Mexicans and we have the same last name. He's taking meds. I used to take meds, but I stopped. I want to start again. It's just a little problem with my medical insurance.

Jose is really kind. He likes to eat a lot! As soon as I saw him, he caught my attention. He was really loud. He asked me for my number and after a few weeks he called me, because he didn't want to sound too desperate. We've been together one year and four months. It's my longest relationship. We've been talking about having kids, about the future. It's great to have someone in my life.

Dwayne

I was in Atlanta, Georgia, and I was working with this very professional corporate company, traveling all over the country to motivate people to be amazing in their work and help them make money. I was feeling run down, so I went and saw my doctor. He said, "You know, I think we need to test you for HIV."

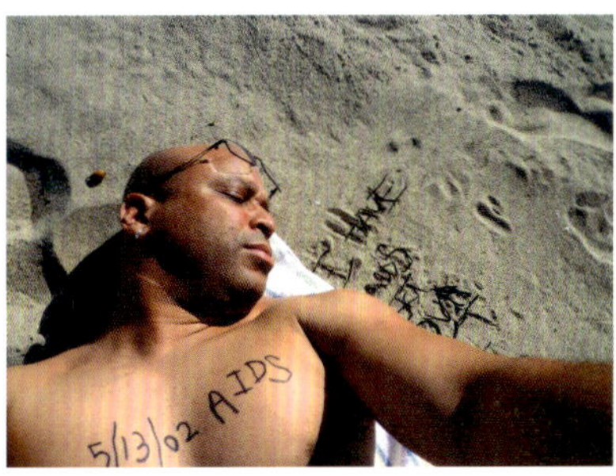

I learned I had 8 T-cells, a viral load of over 200,000, pneumocystis pneumonia, thrush, wasting, lesions on my body—which obviously should have been a telltale sign—gastrointestinal infection, MAC (Mycobacterium avium complex), and a cranial bleed. Wow, I mean, where do I go from here?

I was out of the workforce for about six years. It took a long time to get back to where I am now. I went through seven different drug therapies that had an adverse effect on my system and made me very ill. It's like poison in your system. And then some of the horrible things that were said to me by people finding out, like that this was God's punishment for being gay.

I've learned that people can be cruel.

I was invited to a Christmas party. The person who invited me loves me dearly, but her relatives couldn't deal with me having AIDS, so then she had to call me, crying and sobbing, to disinvite me. I spent Christmas alone.

You'd think that gay men would be more accepting. But there is still stigma within the gay community about HIV and AIDS. I've gone on dates and the guys start talking: "Oh that's just gross, I would never date a guy with HIV." I went through my first two or three years after being diagnosed alone in my apartment in Atlanta.

But I've also learned that there are some angels out there. Like the friends of mine who paid my rent. Project Open Hand brought me food. I had a bill collector call me and I disclosed to her that I have AIDS. And she said, "Listen, you're going to make it. My brother has AIDS, and he made it. He's doing just fine." And do you know what that woman did for me? She paid my bill.

Eventually I rejoined the workforce, but I was let go when I disclosed my status. I fought back and prevailed. I see this as a victory for people with HIV/AIDS who have had to face any type of injustice in the work place.

Guillermo

A few years ago there was a fire in Griffith Park and the area where I normally hike was destroyed. I felt devastated—it was a blackened atmosphere, with gnarled trees. But then I stepped back and realized that even in the most adverse circumstances you can find beauty. After that, every time I walked through that area, I saw new life starting to spring up. I saw green come back, the trees blossoming, flowers growing, the animals coming back. I said, "It's just like my body. My body is healing, but at its own pace because that's nature."

I became infected in 1989. I had been working as a prevention worker at the AIDS Foundation of Hawaii. I counseled transgender people and prostitutes in the red light districts of Honolulu. I feel a lot of guilt about my HIV, because I knew better.

When I became HIV-positive, my partner, Juan, could have left me. But he made the decision not to. We are going to be celebrating our thirty-fifth anniversary soon. Ten years ago we officially became domestic partners. I don't know how we made it this far.

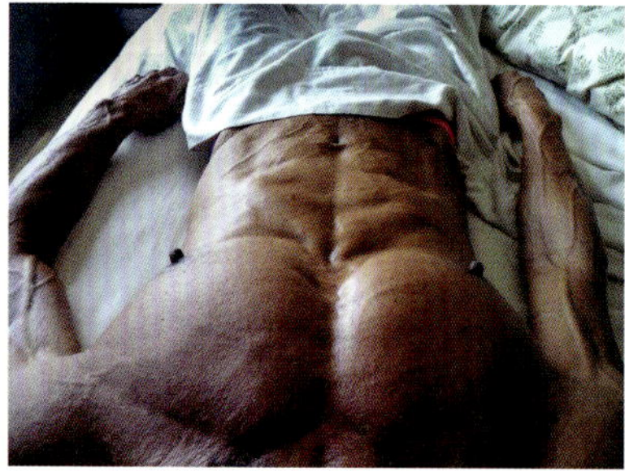

I was diagnosed with Kaposi's sarcoma, an AIDS-related cancer, in 2006. It was on a large portion of my body, so I was forced into early retirement. It has been resolved except for one location, on my penis. It's bad enough just to have KS, but at that particular location, for a gay man, it's just so traumatizing. It's taken me five years to learn to accept what I have. It's not growing, it's not shrinking, and I can live with that. It's not about beauty anymore.

I've always been told I have a remarkable body. Now I have lipodystrophy, the absence of body fat. It's a side effect of my AIDS drugs. In my photographs, I tried to capture some of my body topography, and to show that I'm resisting, I'm fighting against what binds me. It's there, I can't change it, but I'm not defined by HIV. I don't consider myself a victim. I consider myself very much alive and resilient.

I have a favorite phrase, from the Indian poet and playwright Rabindranath Tagore: "The butterfly counts not months but moments, and has time enough." I understand the butterflies because they're beautiful, but they have such a fleeting moment of life. I've learned that if there's an opportunity in front of you, just jump on it. Don't even think.

Mark

In 1981, I moved from Minneapolis to New York City and partied on Fire Island all summer.

That was the summer that HIV arrived. The gentleman I was dating then died in early 1983. He was probably one of the very first AIDS deaths. I realized at that point what my status was, though there was no test yet. I got verification in May 1984. It destroyed a perfectly lovely vacation in the Bahamas.

My partner of seventeen years, Rick, died two weeks before protease inhibitors were approved. I got protease inhibitors, the first effective treatment, immediately after his death. It was just the timing. I was down to twenty-eight T-cells, but the new drugs immediately stopped the progression.

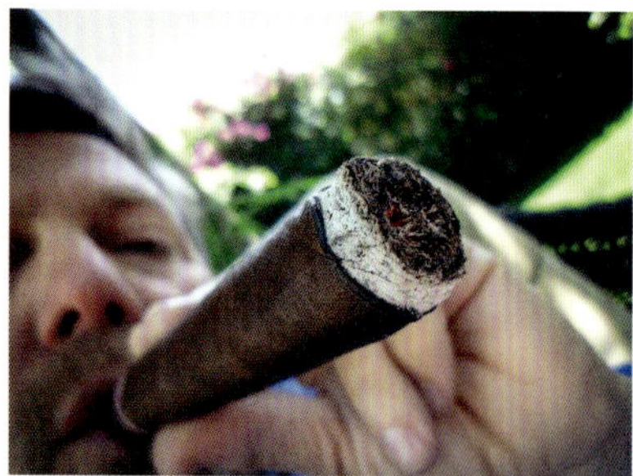

I didn't know how to react—whether to be grateful and happy, or depressed and guilty, for surviving when nobody else was. Sometimes I feel like a war survivor. I can relate to these kids who are coming back from Afghanistan, like, "Why aren't I dead?"

I get every new drug that's developed, early. The most arduous was called T20. You needed to inject it twice a day. The thought of injecting myself like that was harrowing, but diabetics do it, so I just got down to it. Now I take six different antiretrovirals, plus vitamins and elite suppressors and whatever else we all take.

Along the way, I discovered I was losing some of my color perception. I'm an interior designer, so my eyes are the only tools I really have. An eye clinic discovered that the virus is thinning the walls of a nerve. How to fix it, how to change it, they don't have a clue.

Because I've been living with HIV for so long—thirty years—my whole life is a reaction to health issues. This has completely altered my viewpoint, from being a very casual, happy-go-lucky, try-anything kind of a personality, to a very careful personality. Surviving HIV requires that kind of focus.

I joined the Los Angeles Gay Men's Chorus in 1994. You've never seen such a wild group as the boys in the chorus. The range is dramatic, from very conservative older gentlemen—in their seventies and eighties— who've been there since the beginning, all the way to the young kids—I call them "bug chasers." In the early days there were multiple deaths every week. There was a lot of singing at memorials, a lot of "Gaelic Blessing." It's only poetic justice that the next man I fell in love with was a chorus member.

Washington, D.C.

In the United States, communities of color experience the highest rates of HIV infection. Racial and ethnic disparities reveal themselves most strongly when it comes to basic access to care. Notably, the Washington, D.C., workshop, held in July 2012, included many participants who shared stories of drug use and addiction, a prominent feature of the AIDS epidemic in the nation's capital. The inequities built into the judicial system in the U.S. can be overwhelming and are magnified for people living with HIV. The urgency of the participants' stories was further amplified by the fact that the workshop took place shortly before the XIX International AIDS Conference in Washington, D.C. Drawing attention to the need for compassionate addiction treatment and needle exchange programs.

Washington, D.C.'s epidemic, as of 2012

Number of people living with HIV:	16,072
New infections:	680
AIDS-related deaths:	221

Treatment

Antiretroviral therapy provided to all diagnosed HIV-positive:	8,449
% linked to care within 3 months of diagnosis:	87%
% viral load undetectable:	61%

Washington, a model local response

The XIX International AIDS Conference, held in Washington D.C., turned the spotlight on the epidemic in that city, which emerged as a model local response. New infections and AIDS-related deaths had declined by 42% and 36% respectively since 2008. D.C.'s successful needle exchange programs had cut new diagnoses among injecting drug users in half since they began in 2007. By 2012 everyone in the city had access to antiretrovirals, regardless of ability to pay or immigration status.

Through Positive Eyes in Washington, D.C., was organized in partnership with ARTLAB+ at the Hirshhorn Museum and the Smithsonian Folklife Festival. A coalition of sponsoring organizations included: La Clínica del Pueblo, Community Education Group, HIPS, Metro TeenAIDS, National Council of Negro Women, SMYAL, Us Helping Us, Whitman-Walker Health, and The Women's Collective. Major funding was provided by The Herb Ritts Foundation, with additional funding from The Ford Foundation, The Andy Warhol Foundation for the Visual Arts, International AIDS Society, and UCLA.

Christian

Soon after I was diagnosed, my mom told me she and my stepdad had been diagnosed positive three months before. She just didn't know how to tell anybody. We went through it together, until she passed.

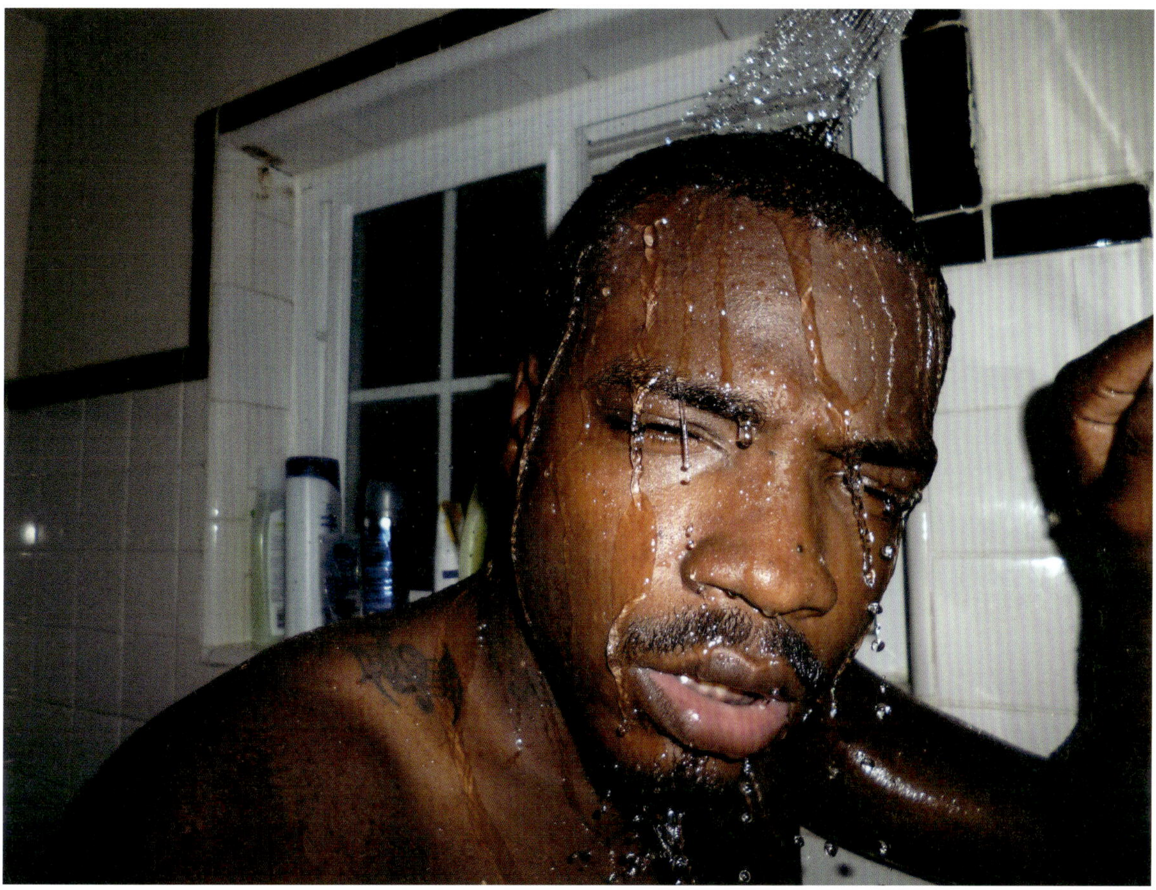

When I came out of the closet at sixteen, it was hurtful to my family. They're devout Baptists, in North Carolina, and to be gay—and then to be black, and then to be in a small town—was kind of embarrassing. When I turned eighteen, I moved out and I became homeless. I was living in my car and going to school in Fairview, North Carolina. I didn't have anybody to connect with. So one day I just called my mom and I talked to her. This was before I was diagnosed. And we started bonding then.

I think my story is different from others. I contracted HIV through a rape situation when I was eighteen, with somebody who I was dating at the time. I just wasn't ready and I guess he was. And it seems weird to say this, but, after the rape, we were still friends. Later on I found out I was positive and that was a dramatic moment, because, where I'm from, they don't talk about this stuff.

Soon after I was diagnosed, my mom told me she and my stepdad had been diagnosed positive three months before. She just didn't know how to tell anybody. We became really good friends. We went through it together, until she passed. I wish we had bonded earlier in life, so I could have enjoyed that family relationship, but it was so good to have it at that time.

Now I am thirty-one years old with three stepchildren and grandkids. My husband is forty-two. He is HIV-negative. I never knew that someone could love me as much as he does. And I never thought that I would love someone as much as I love him.

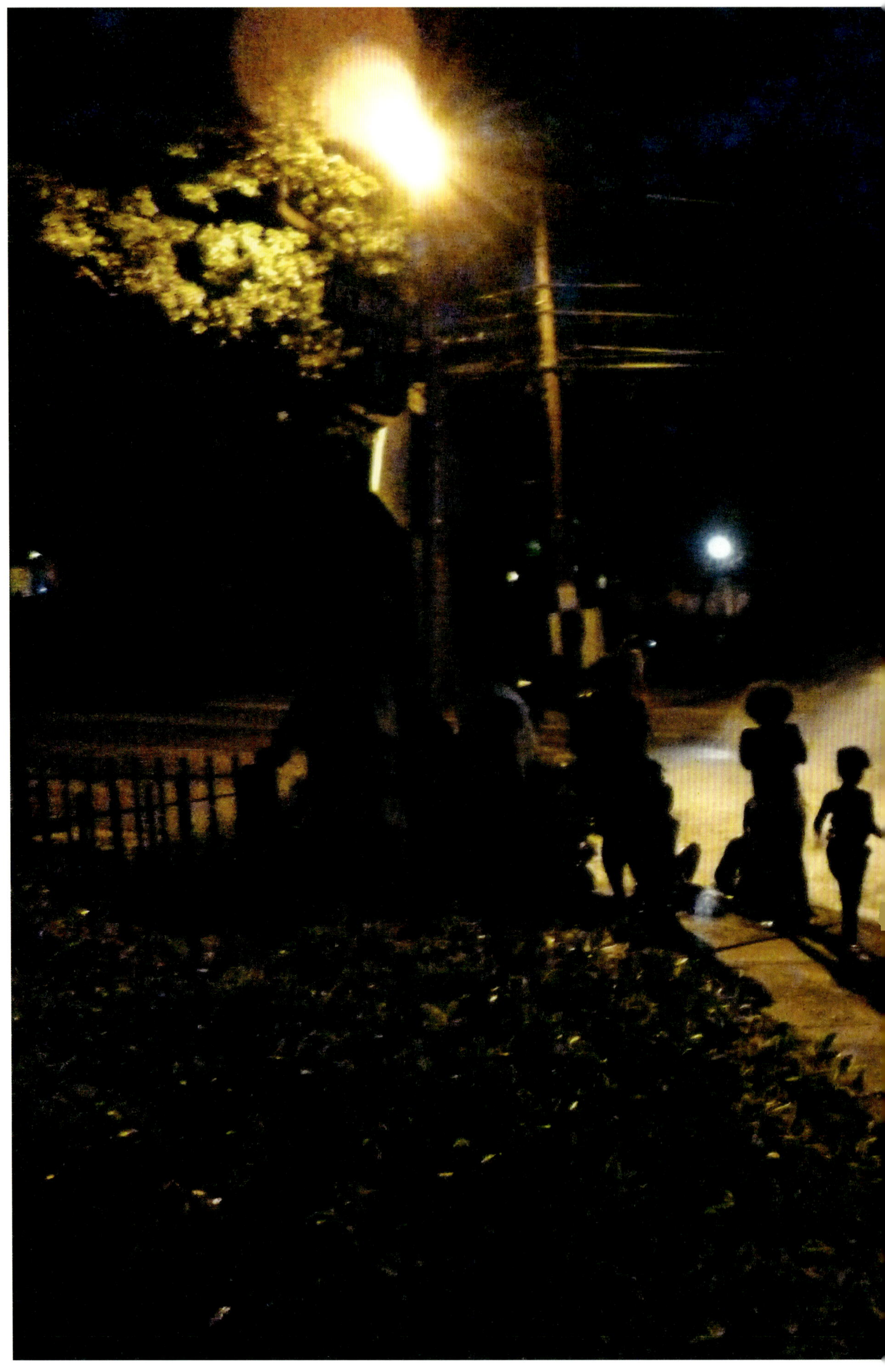

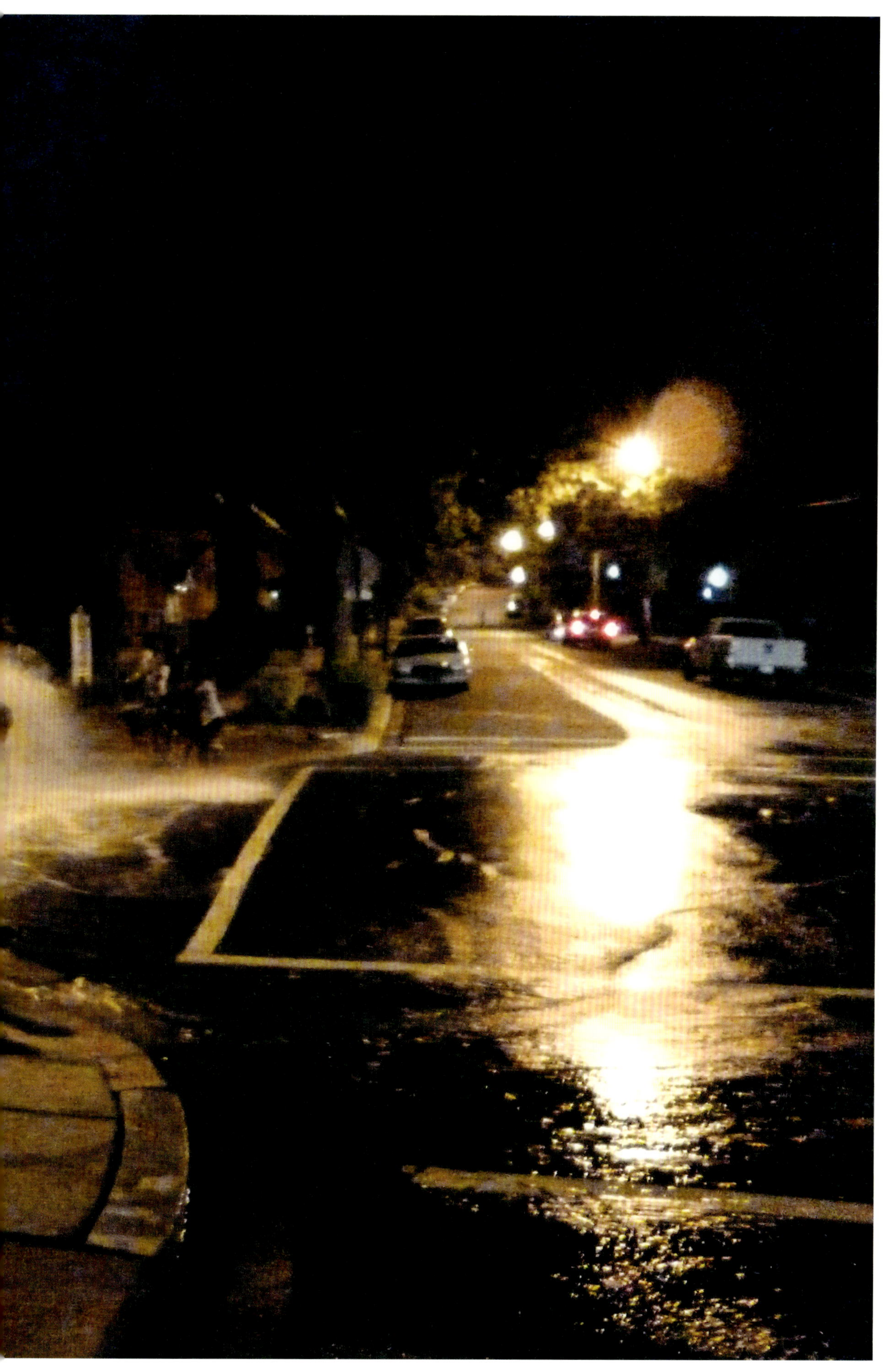

Mary

Every time I get to that point in the poem, where I disclose, I get this rush of nerves, like, "Oh my God, I'm going to tell them I'm HIV-positive." It just feels good to tell my story.

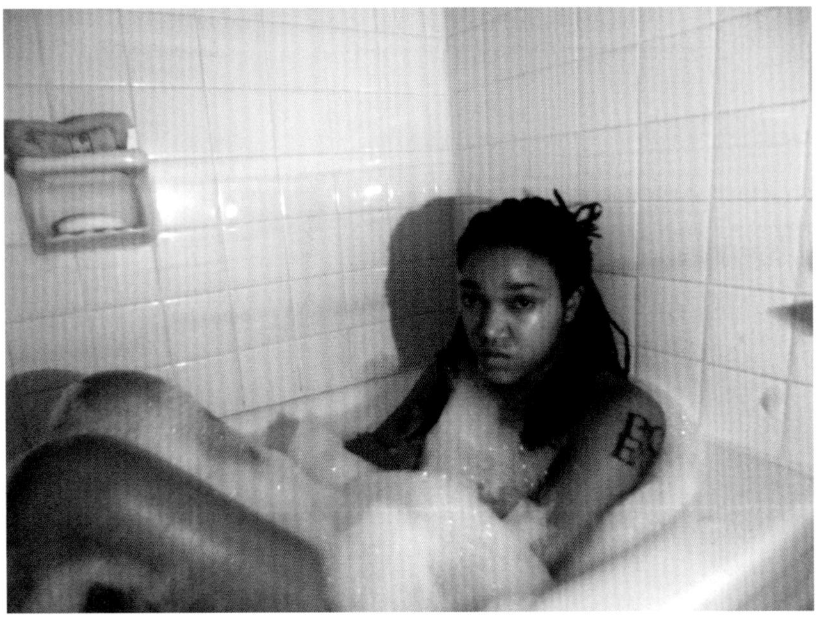

I'm twenty-three years old, and I'm bringing swag to HIV awareness. I'm swagtastic.

I was born HIV-positive. My biological mother passed away of complications from AIDS. I really felt abandoned. I went through a period where I hated my birth mother, because I felt like, "You just going to leave me here with HIV?" But I loved her at the same time. It was very confusing.

A lot of my poetry has to do with my mom and her absence in my life. One of my first poems was about my father being a drug dealer and my biological mother being his customer and sexual partner—that whole enmeshed relationship that they had. At first, in my poems, I spoke about my mother having AIDS, but I didn't share my stories of living with HIV. In high school, I stayed quiet because I didn't want people to be like, "Well how do you know all this stuff about HIV?" It would blow my cover. Then, I was inspired to write "Dandelions," my first poem exposing my status. "The sickness she denied lies in my blood with a lesser value." Every time I get to that point in the poem, where I disclose, I get this rush of nerves, like, "Oh my God, I'm going to tell them I'm HIV-positive." It just feels good to tell my story.

Lately it's been difficult, especially with my mom who raised me. My dad cheated to have me and I think she chose to let me live with her because she wanted my dad around. My mom doesn't want me to be exposed and she doesn't necessarily support me being an advocate for HIV. But this is what I feel I have to do.

I love my camera. I named it Scotty. Scotty has to come everywhere with me because she's my friend. I hope my photographs inspire people who are HIV-positive to tell their own stories. I hope that my photos let someone know that they aren't alone. I really hope my pictures normalize HIV because I think that if people see the relationships between my HIV-negative best friends and me—who don't look at me as being any different from them—they'll realize that we're all human, and that it's OK to love someone who is HIV-positive.

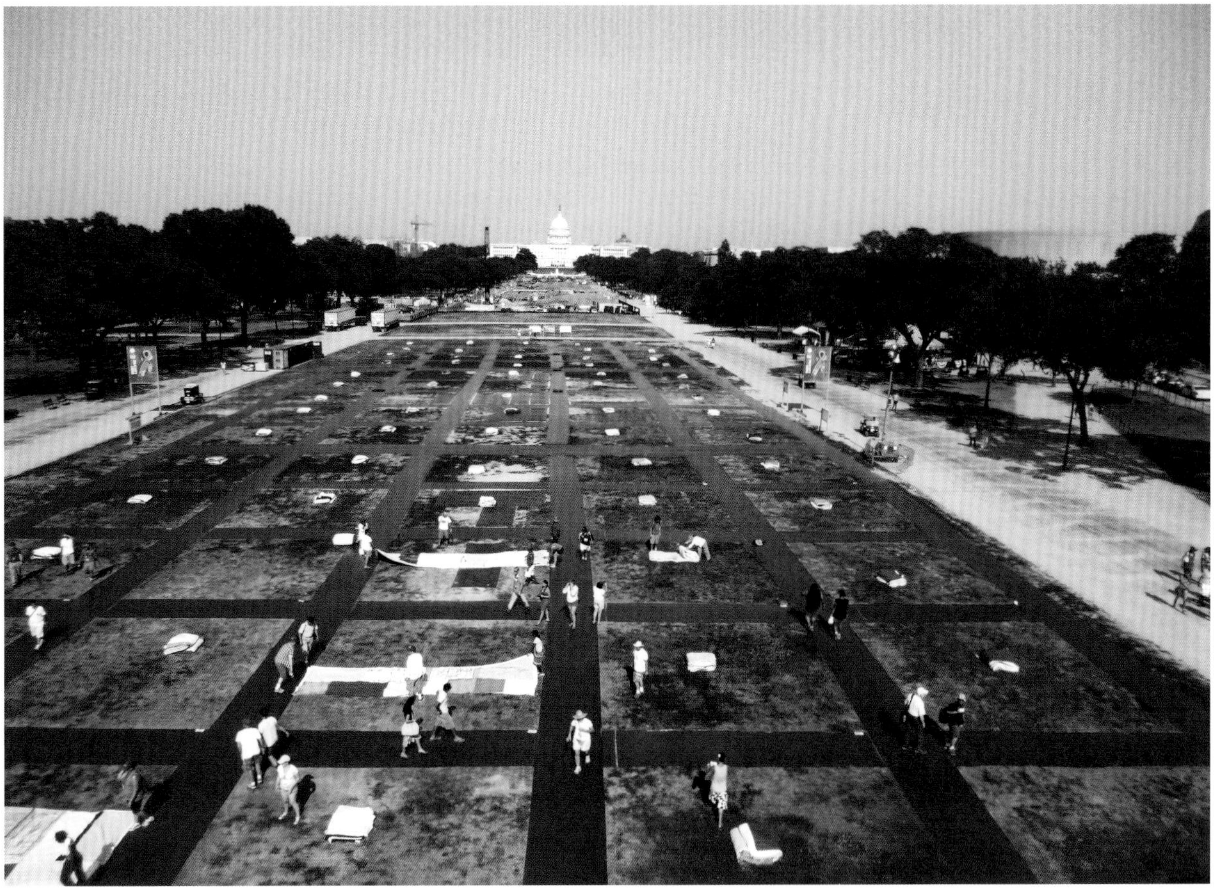

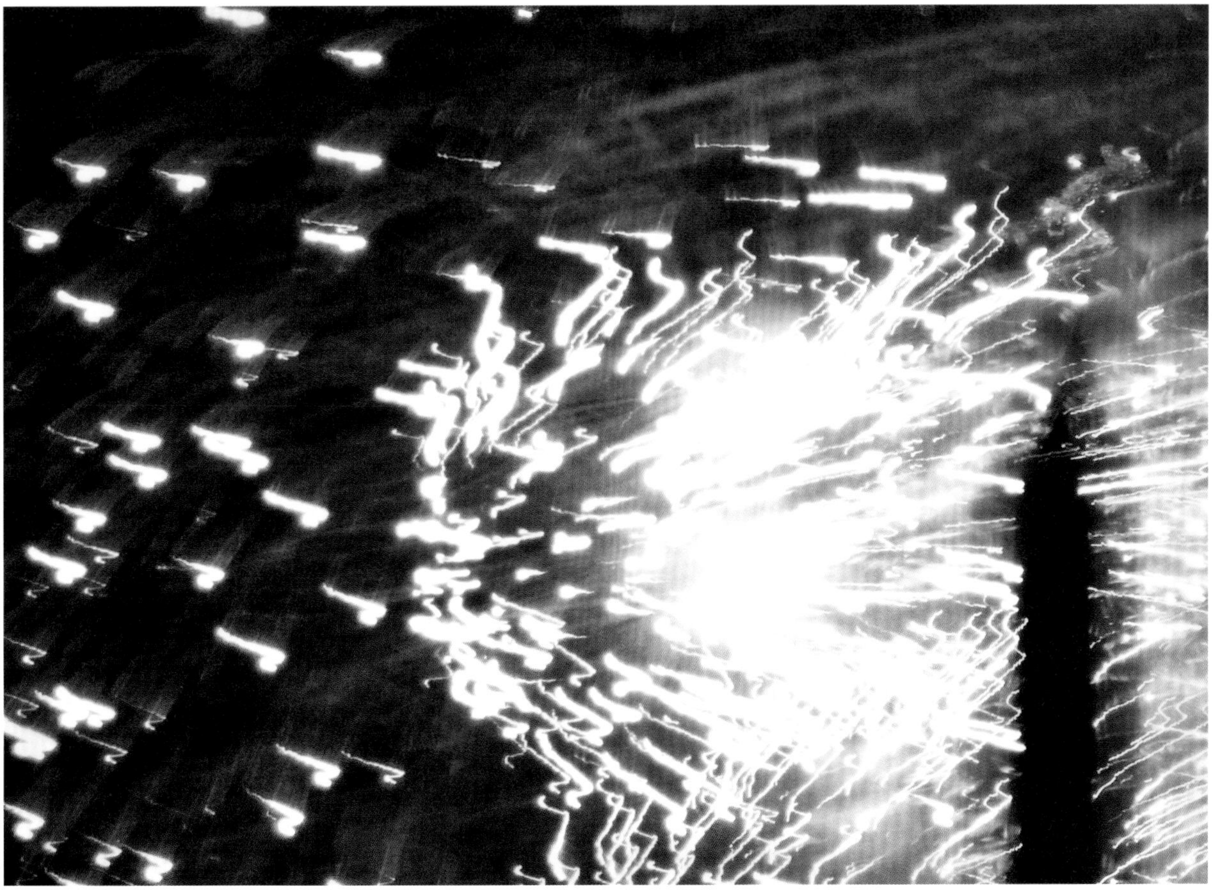

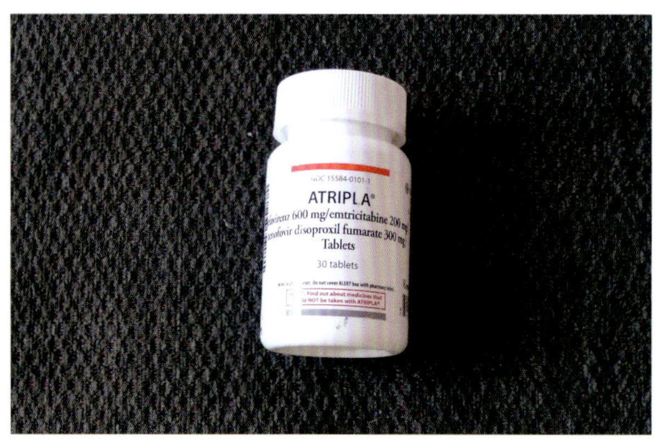
ATRIPLA®
Tablets
30 tablets

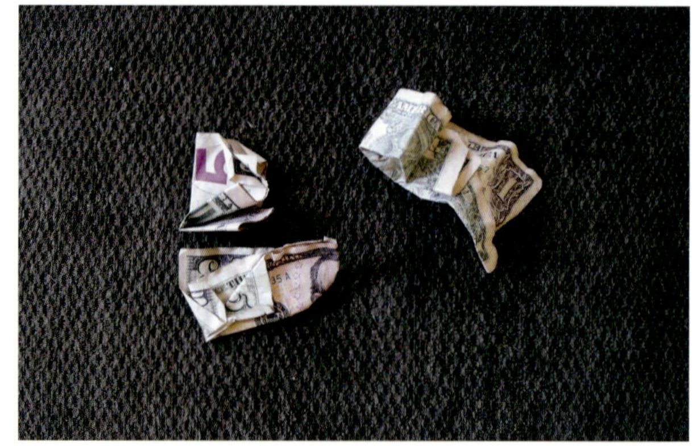

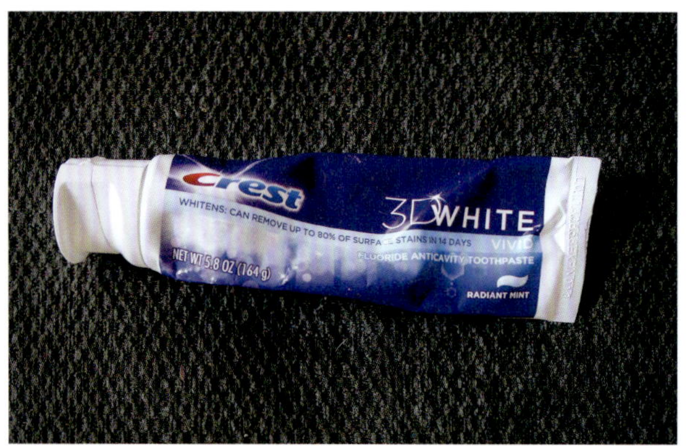
Crest
3D WHITE
VIVID
WHITENS: CAN REMOVE UP TO 80% OF SURFACE STAINS IN 14 DAYS
FLUORIDE ANTICAVITY TOOTHPASTE
NET WT 5.8 OZ (164 g)
RADIANT MINT

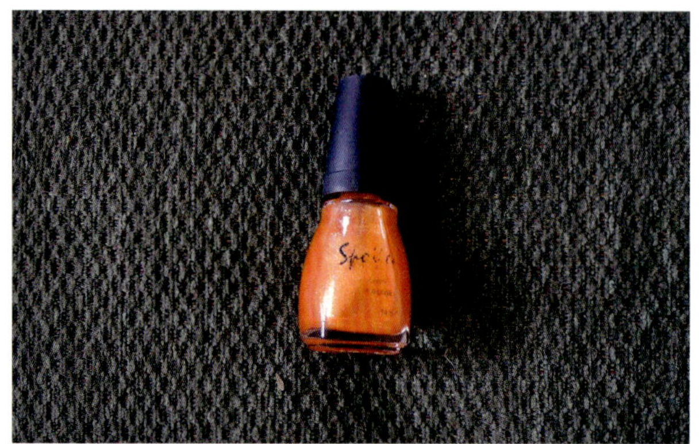

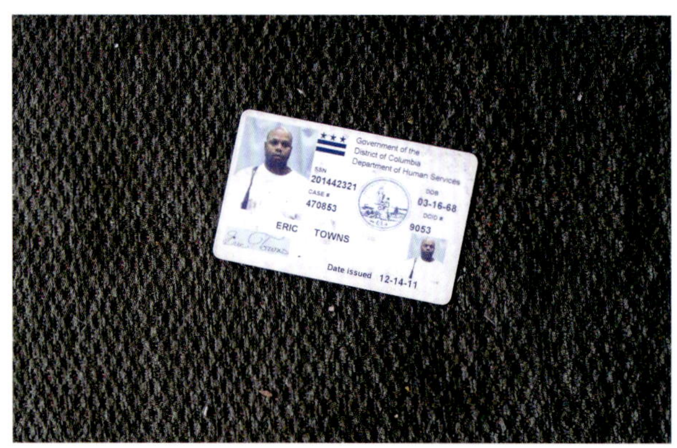
Government of the
District of Columbia
Department of Human Services
201442321
470853
03-16-68
9053
ERIC
TOWNS
Date issued 12-14-11

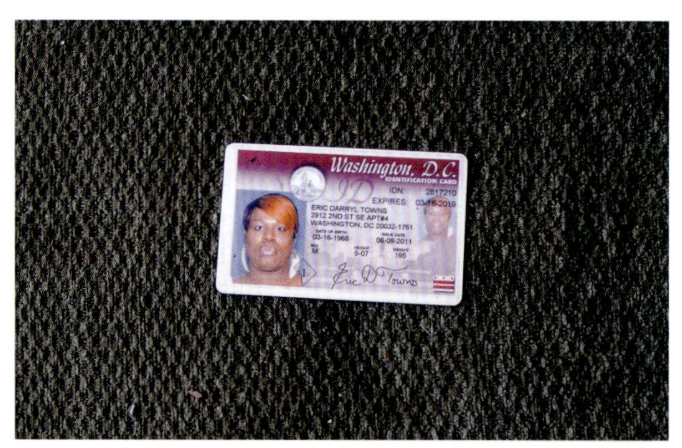
Washington, D.C.
ERIC DARRYL TOWNS
03-16-1968

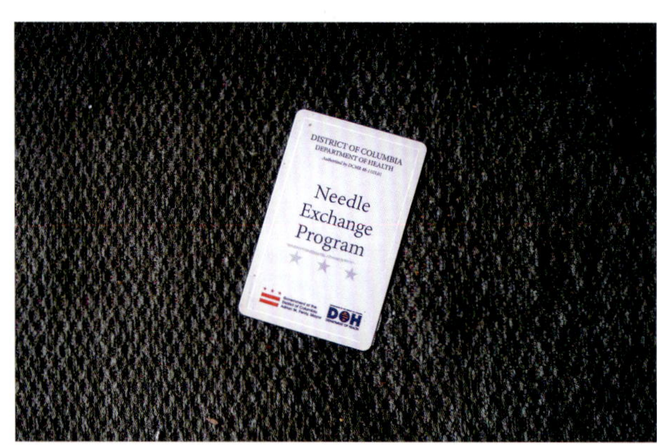
DISTRICT OF COLUMBIA
DEPARTMENT OF HEALTH
Needle
Exchange
Program
DOH

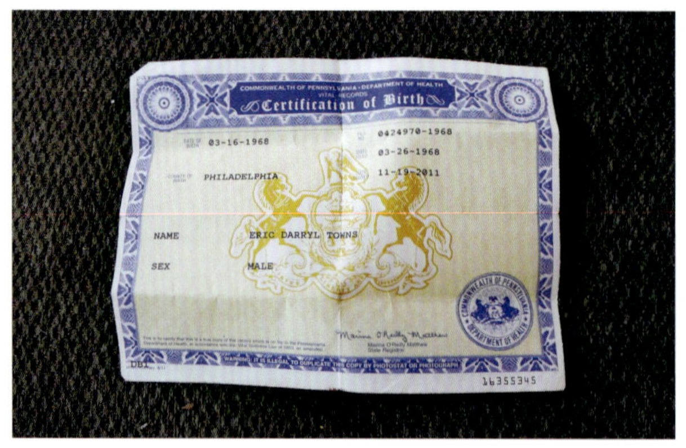
Certification of Birth
03-16-1968
0424970-1968
03-26-1968
PHILADELPHIA
11-19-2011
NAME
ERIC DARRYL TOWNS
SEX
MALE
16355345

Ericka

I don't know how to explain it, but when I see other people who may be struggling with something in life, I feel their pain. I just do.

I was raped in prison. When they told me I had HIV, I was nineteen years old.

From then until I was twenty-five, I prostituted. It was the only way to get more money to supply my habit. I had a really bad drug addiction. I lost my place because I was indulging in drugs. Any drug to alter my mood was my drug of choice. I've dibbled and dabbled with heroin, ecstasy, crack, marijuana, PCP. I'm not proud of it. No one is. I'm learning from the mistakes that I made, and I'm no longer indulging in any drugs. I just want to move forward with my life.

I have been a year clean. I'm working towards getting myself back on the right track, because I know my parents didn't raise me up to be sleeping on someone's couch. I plan to get my General Education Diploma. I plan to have a stable roof over my head. I would like to travel. I really would love to go to Paris, to see the Eiffel Tower. As long as you move forward, HIV doesn't have any control over your life. That's how I view things.

I took photos looking into my bag, showing different parts of my life: my birth certificate, my medicines, my wallet, my diabetic pills, my makeup. These photos show my everyday struggle, what I have to go through in life. I'm diabetic, I have HIV. I've been living as a woman for about five years now. I've been taking hormones and I'm using lasers so hair won't grow on my face.

I never really got teased in school. I never had any problems with kids as far as the stigma that goes along with being transgender and gay. All the kids really liked me. They used to call me Preppy. As I got older, though, I've been beaten up because of my gender. But I never really experienced any true hate, ever. It's always been love. It's always been that way for me.

I have a really strong spiritual connection. It is just really strong. I don't know how but in some way I feel as though my higher power speaks to me and through other people. It just makes me feel calm. I don't know how to explain it, but when I see other people who may be struggling with something in life, I feel their pain. I just do.

John

I spent a lot of time nursing my mother. After she passed away, I was in shock. I picked up a camera and just started shooting. It was definitely a release. It was like my counseling session.

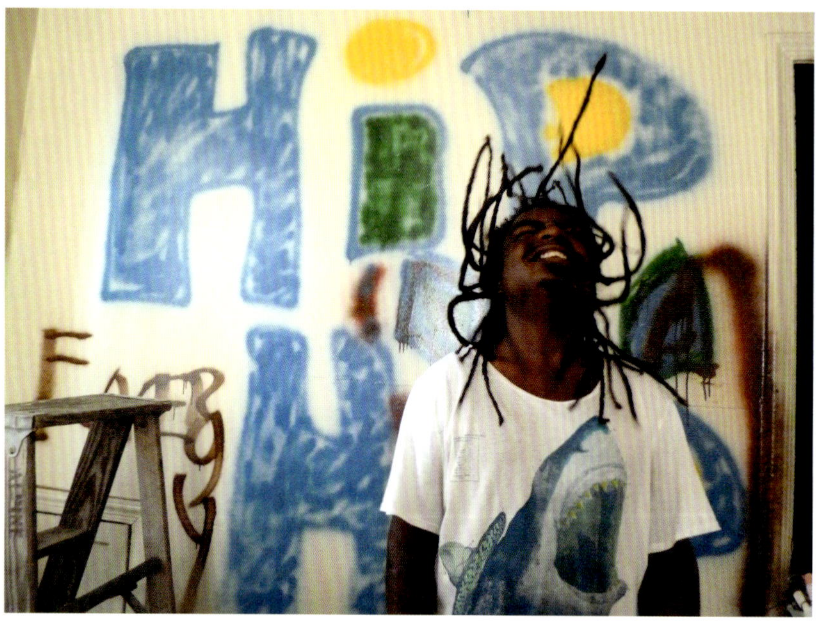

I was born with HIV twenty-three years ago. At the time my mother and father got together, my father was doing drugs. He contracted HIV and I was born with it. So I always knew I was sick. I didn't really know what the sickness was, I just had to live my life and keep taking my medicine. That's how I still see it now.

I was nineteen when my mom died and twenty when my dad died. I have a brother who is twenty-six and another brother who is twenty-five. We actually got closer when my mother passed away. Everybody sits in my room and we chat for a couple of hours, and then everybody goes about their business. That's how it works.

I spent a lot of time nursing my mother. After she passed away, I was in shock. I picked up a camera and just started shooting. It was definitely a release. It was like my counseling session. Capturing beautiful things and moments in time is always priceless.

With my pictures, I am trying to make a statement that everyday life can be beautiful, that the things around you can be awesome. I burn incense to send blessings to my mother and father in heaven. That's part of my Buddhist practice. (I'm a Rastafarian too.) God doesn't give us anything we can't handle, and I feel like God knew that I could handle it. I know He knows that my parents made a mistake and my father made the mistake of doing what he did, and I know that He forgave him for that. Having me gave my father an opportunity to do something good.

I want to photograph people and things that are unknown or unspoken. I want to get to those people whether they are in the United States or on the other side of the world.

When I was in school, I didn't speak much. I didn't really talk at all. I was so into the whole "being sick" thing, and not into living. I was just surviving. I feel like it's time to live now.

Hopefully it takes me somewhere—I don't know where—because only God, or Jah, as Rastafarians call Him, can decide that.

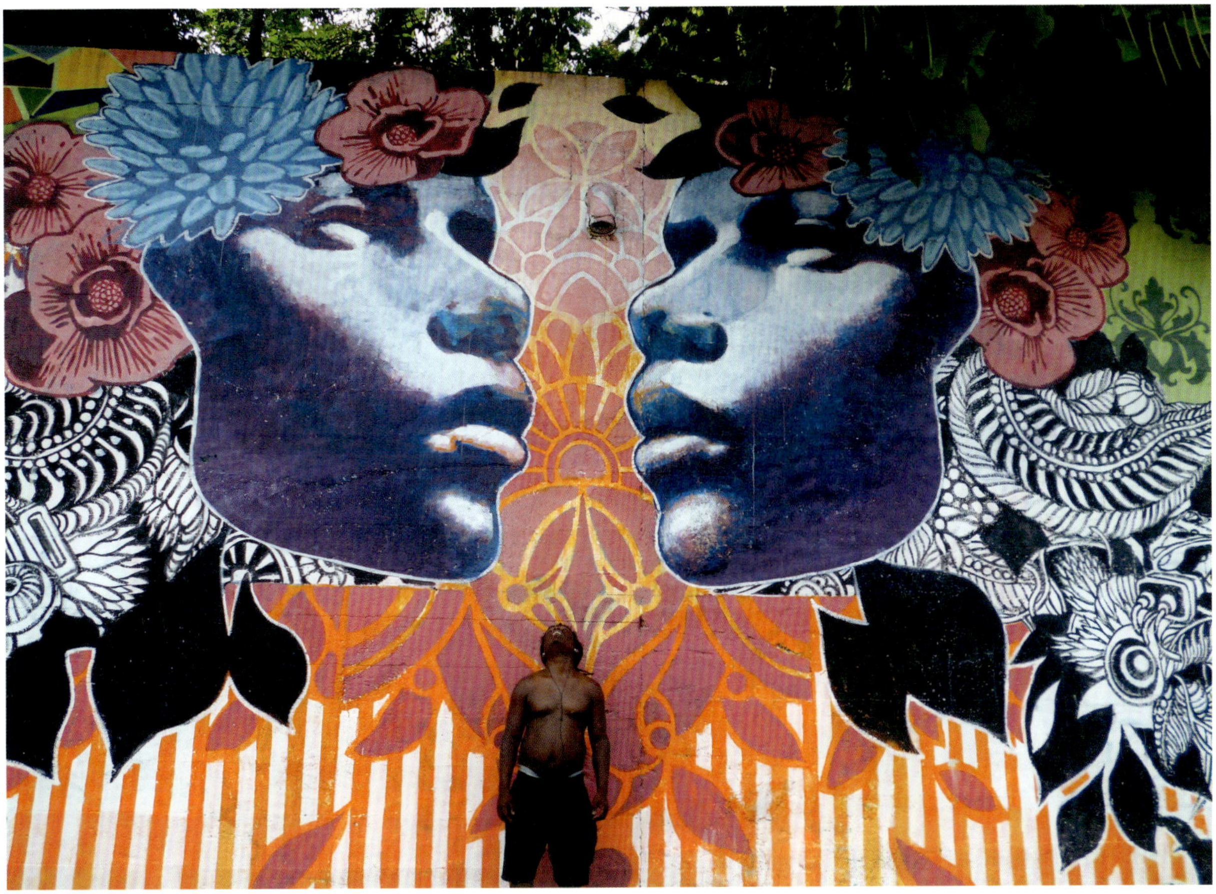

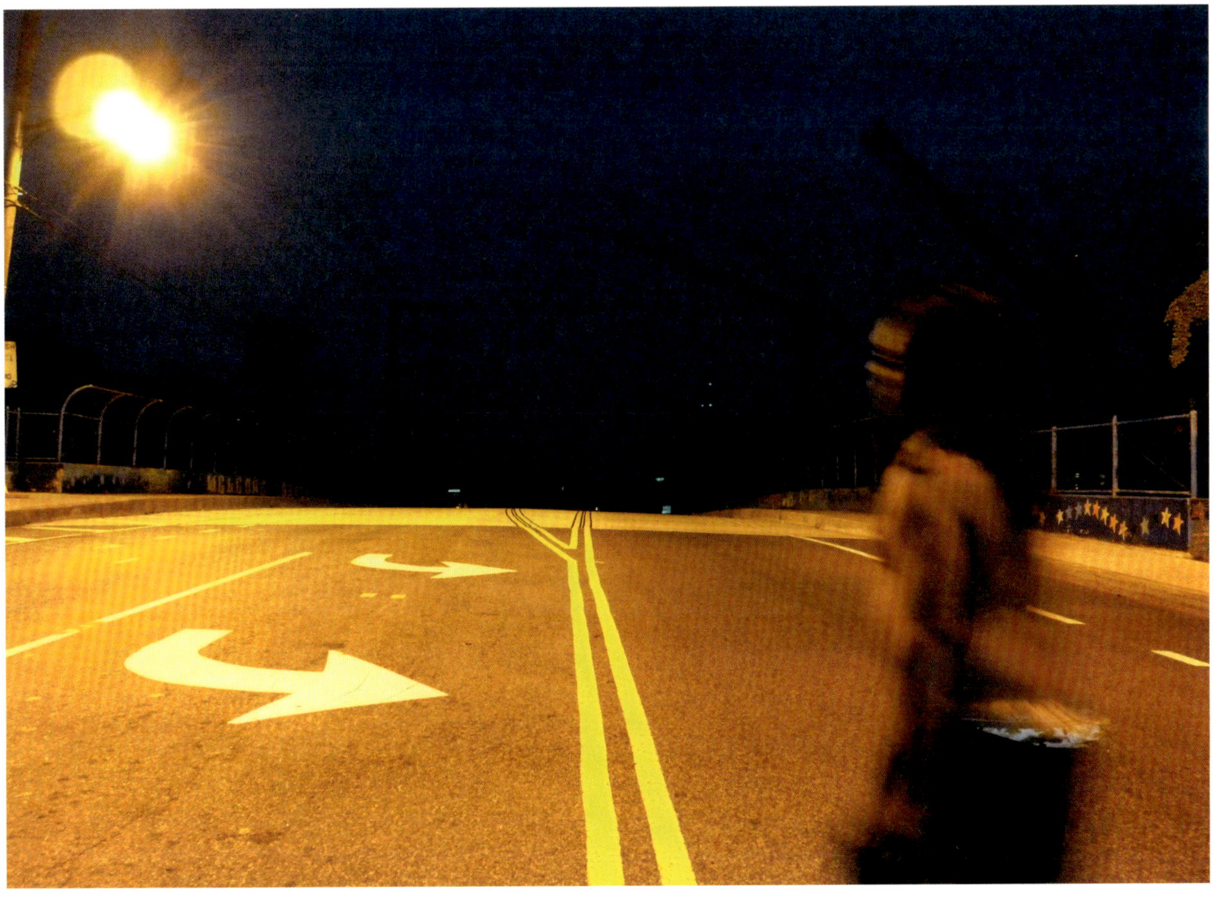

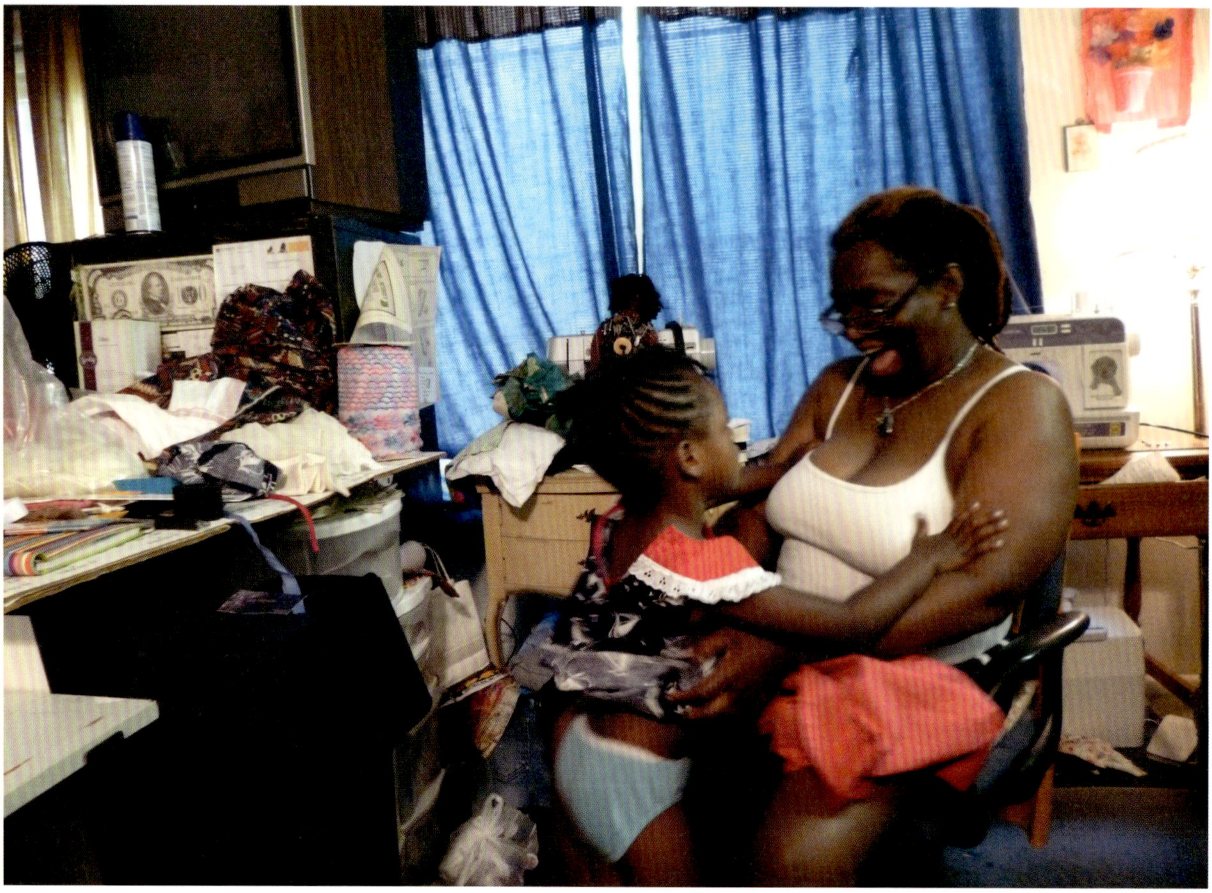

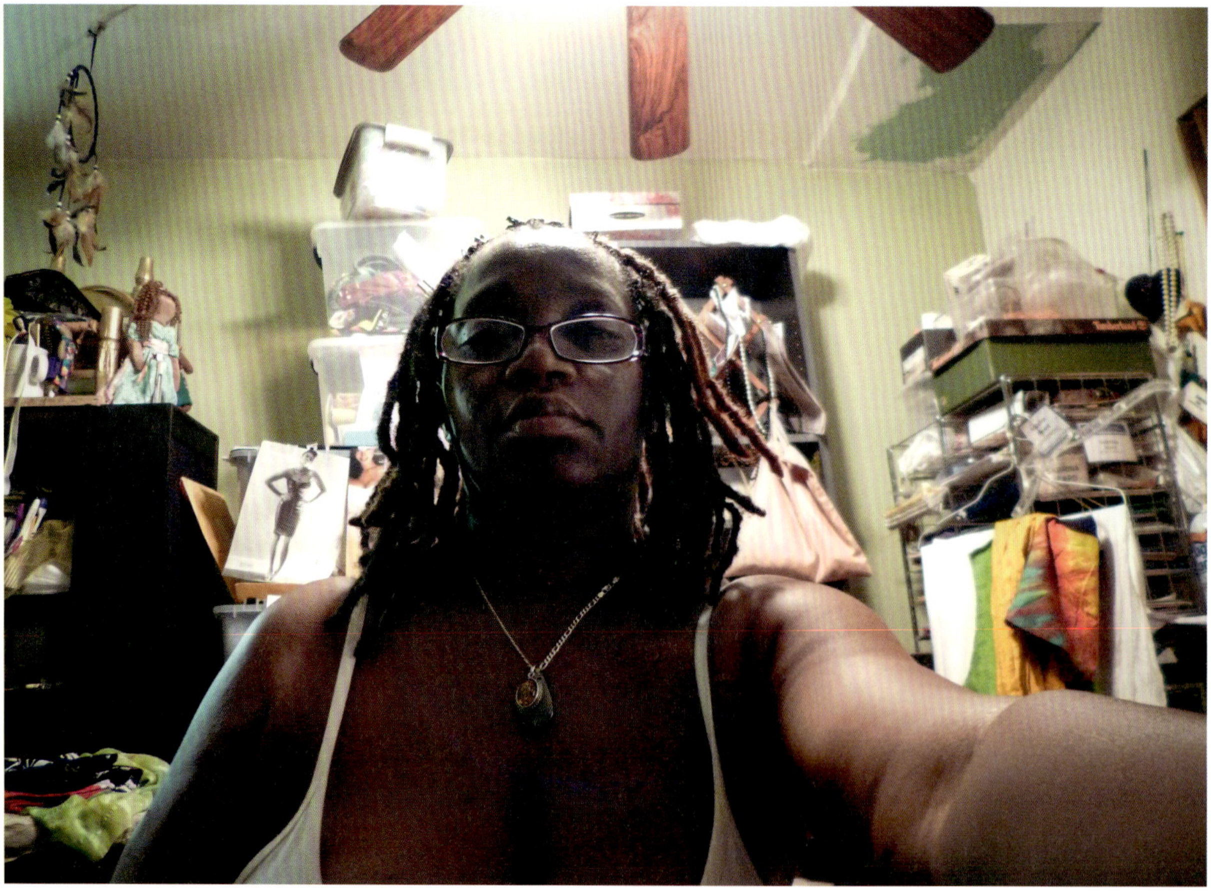

Sabrina

When I was taking my babies to get them their shots, those nurse ladies would look at me so mean. "Why you do this to these kids?" You know, just making me feel like a horrible little mother.

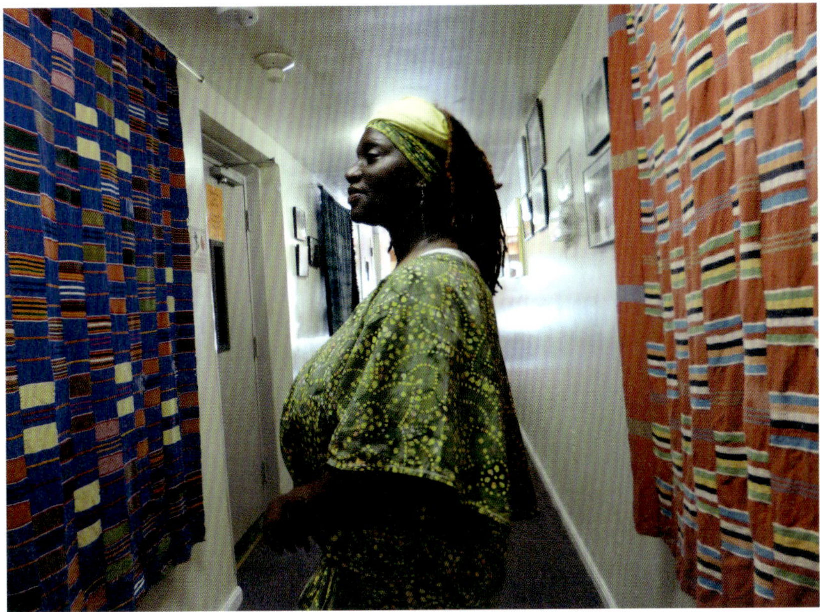

I was diagnosed twenty-three years ago, when I was thirty-three and pregnant with my daughter. I was still using. I smoked crack cocaine and drank alcohol and smoked cigarettes and marijuana, in different combinations, through all those years, as we transitioned from public housing to subsidized housing.

When they were still young, my children were taken away from me. The Court stipulated that I go into treatment in order to get them back. That was the turning point for me, especially the part where you have to have supervised visitation with your children, I just couldn't take it. So I entered rehab. At that time I wasn't open to anyone knowing that I was HIV-positive. I was terrified.

But in the hospitals, those nurse ladies—oh! I'm just smiling about it now. They allowed me to hear them debating over who was going to draw my blood, and how many gloves they was going to put on. When I was taking my babies to get them their shots, those ladies would look at me so mean. "Why you do this to these kids?" You know, just making me feel like a horrible little mother.

But the hardest thing was the stigma I felt myself, about being HIV-positive.

I now work at an agency called the Women's Collective and I'm a community health worker, so I work directly with clients who find it really hard to stay on their medications, or to make their doctor visits. They have life factors that come up. In the case of someone who has children, they prioritize and put their children's needs in front of their own. In the case of someone who might be challenged with housing, there ain't nobody think about no medicine when you ain't got nowhere to live. Sometimes there are a lot of other factors that stop a person from doing the things that they need to do, and it is my job to find ways to encourage them or find ways to remind them, maybe just by staying in contact with them and giving them support.

Me, I take my medicine every day because I realize that this pill is keeping me alive and healthy. I surround myself with things that I like to do. I have—Lord knows—about four sewing machines. I like to sew! Right now my main focus and my goal is to live.

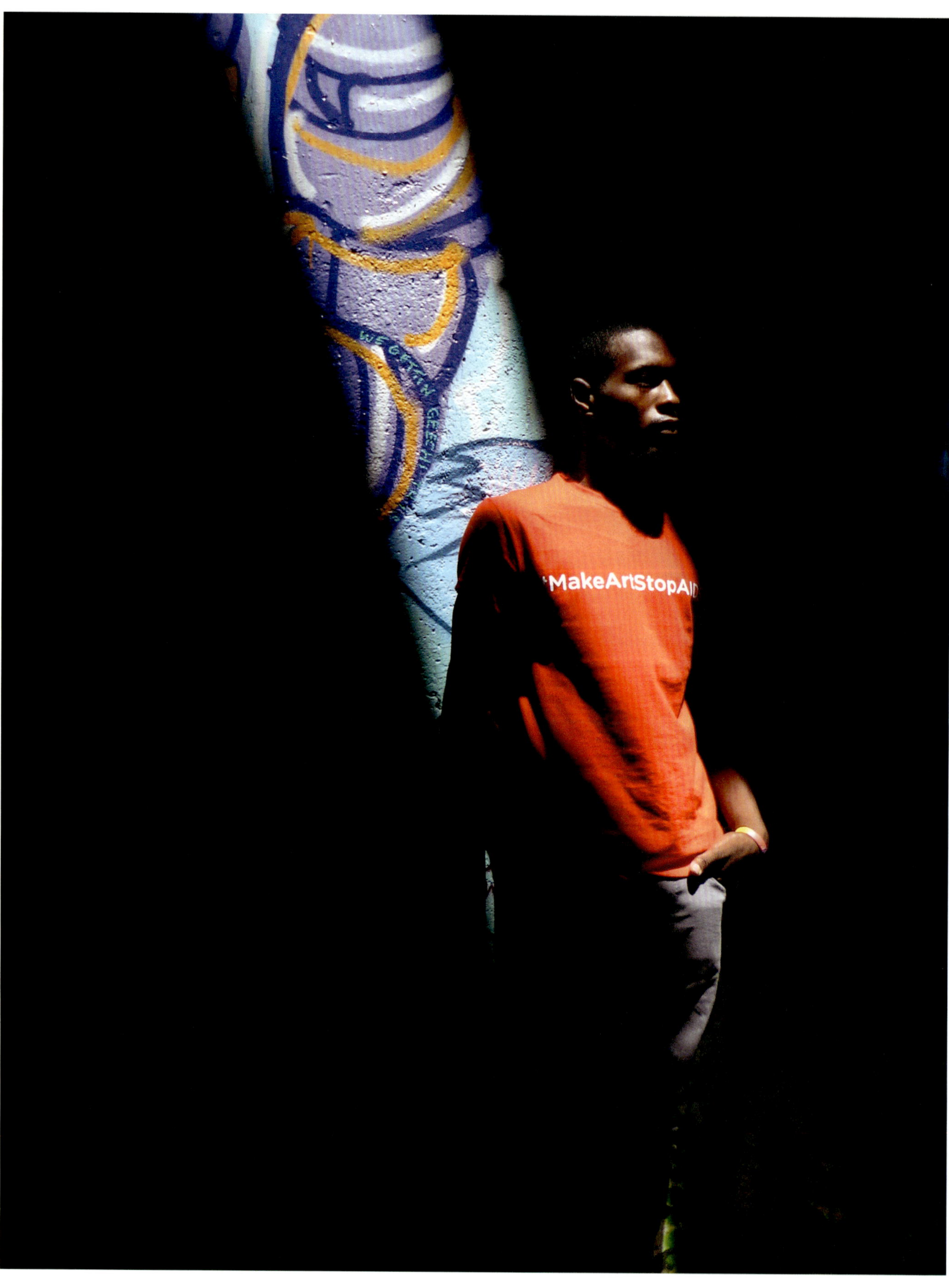
MakeArtStopAI

D'Angelo

I actually knew about safe sex and everything. But, you know, at the time, when you are hungry and you don't have anything to eat or you don't want to be sleeping on the subway... I did what I had to do.

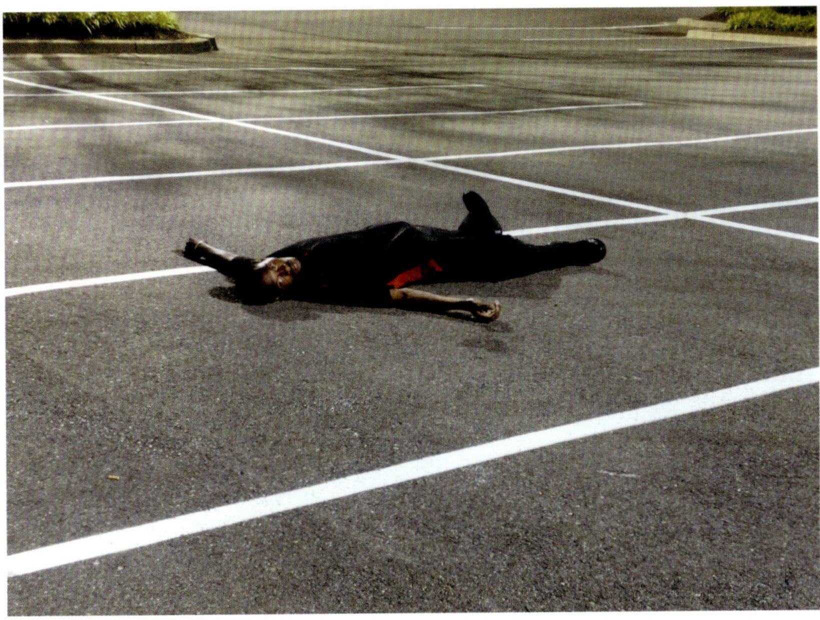

My mother and I used to be very close before she found out that I was gay. We were inseparable. I was fourteen when she found out. Things started going downhill from there. She didn't approve and we fought. I've been kicked out of the house and I have ended up homeless, living on the streets of Atlanta.

I mean, not to blame her, but I don't think I would have HIV if I wasn't kicked out, because I wouldn't have been doing the things that I was doing in Atlanta. You know, there was some sleeping with people for places to stay, and for money. I did things that weren't healthy for me, just to survive. I actually knew about safe sex and everything. But, at the time, when you are hungry and you don't have anything to eat or you don't want to be sleeping on the subway...I did what I had to do.

As far as the photos that I take, if you look at them you'll see that they are pictures of me, a lot of them alone, just somewhere, sitting or standing or walking. And that's because I'm trying to portray someone who is lonely and feels like he doesn't have anyone.

I am twenty-two years old. I'm from Atlanta, but moved to D.C. five years ago. It's tough, I'm back to square one now, out on the street again. I don't like to portray myself as someone who is homeless or doesn't have a place to go, but that is reality at the moment, and I can't depend on my best friend and his family to host me forever.

I want to dedicate my life to advocacy work within the LGBTQI community, particularly for youth, so what's next for me is trying to put my life together and move forward and take care of myself. So I am going to be trying to find new work and continue in my advocacy and doing what I need to do. Just because I'm down-and-out right now doesn't mean I can't still put my best foot forward and go out there and advocate for people. I mean, I've been unhappy before, I've been depressed before, so I know it's nothing I can't defeat.

Edgar

I am from El Salvador. I came here to be reunited with my mother. When I arrived she gave me one hug and one kiss. That was it. I expected more after such a long time. I was eighteen and I hadn't seen her in thirteen years.

My dream was to go to school, but I never got the chance because I needed to make money. I got a job in construction. For six years I worked long days, with no opportunity for anything else.

When I was twenty-four, I felt a curiosity and started a relationship with a man, someone who was not out about being gay. (It's complicated.) We broke up. I got depressed and was getting drunk every day. And then, suddenly, in my mind I said, "OK, I have to start again. I want a new life." So I turned to another guy who was supposed to be a friend. We didn't use condoms. That turned out to be a bad decision.

One month later I got really really sick with all the symptoms of HIV. I realized I needed to get tested. The person who tested me didn't counsel me at all. He just said, "You know you're positive, right?" I cried for three days.

My mother doesn't know about any of this. I'm scared about her reaction. I still have a lot of problems with her.

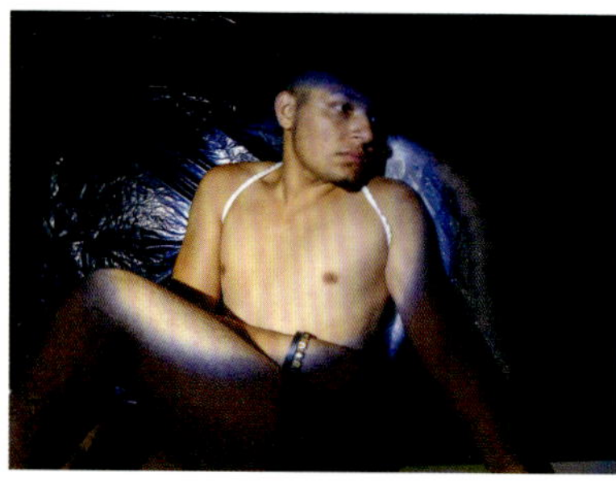

The guy I slept with, when I told him I tested positive, he just said, "We all have to die some day." I said, "OK. Thank you so much."

I know it doesn't make sense, but since this all happened, I feel free. I have a lot of friends who have helped me. I feel so strong now.

I always loved to draw, from the time I was seven years old. Now I paint. At La Clinica del Pueblo, where I volunteer, I painted a mural of condoms and funny cartoon characters, with a positive message. I'm happy. I see light in my life now. I take pictures of lights, like the sun. And I feel it is my light. I feel I am alive. I don't know why, but I feel I can express myself now, how I am.

Gemini

I was diagnosed with HIV when I was sixteen. I didn't cry. All I could think about was my mother because that's what she passed from. She was a prostitute and she used to shoot up intravenous drugs and smoke crack. One time she stabbed her finger with a crochet needle. Me being a mama's boy, I ran upstairs to get a Band-Aid. I tried to put it on her finger and she hit me. She was like, "No! Mommy's sick. Mommy do it myself." I didn't know then, but I know now. The day before Mother's Day she left, and she just never came back.

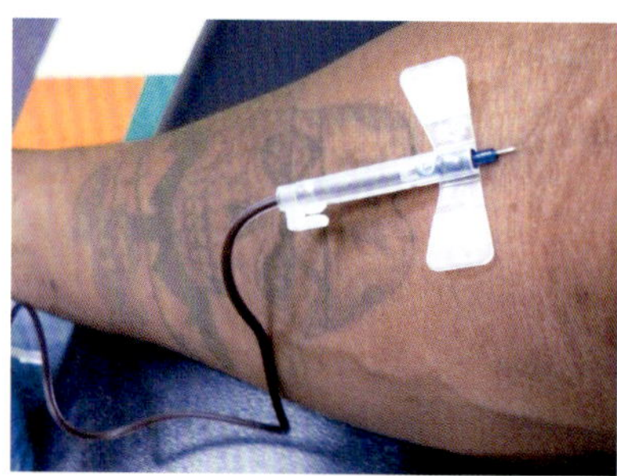

When I was seventeen, my grandmother and I got into a big argument over the dumbest thing, 'cause I wouldn't wash her dishes. She was like, "Fuck you, you faggot. You're going to end up just like your mother."

But I think I would be dead if I hadn't gone back home to my grandma. When I came back to live with her, I was so sick with meningitis. I had dropped all the way down to 109 pounds and I wasn't eating. I couldn't hold myself up. After two weeks of living with my grandmother, I gained weight, I got back on my medicine. It's bittersweet.

Growing up, my grandfather was the only man in my life. He taught me how to take a shower, how to shoot a gun. When he found out I was gay, it broke his heart. But he didn't act like anything was wrong. He said, "Hey, if that's what you believe, I ain't going to knock it. I don't feel comfortable with it. But I do love you." I like my grandfather. He's my buddy.

Everybody always asks me, "Are you scared to die?" No, I'm not. The only fear I have in life is to waste it. To have no meaning. I don't think that I'm a failure. I don't doubt myself. I try to stay positive.

My friends are all I have, since my family isn't really there for me. My friends all look up to me. They ask, "You always smile and stuff. Why? Life ain't that happy." And I'm like, "To me it is."

Jason

I have a tattoo that says "Made In Puerto Rico." I'm proud of being Puerto Rican. For one thing, the island is progressive when it comes to acceptance of the LGBTQI community. My family had no problem accepting the fact that I was gay. Some of the kids that I've hung out with that come from El Salvador, Honduras, Guatemala—

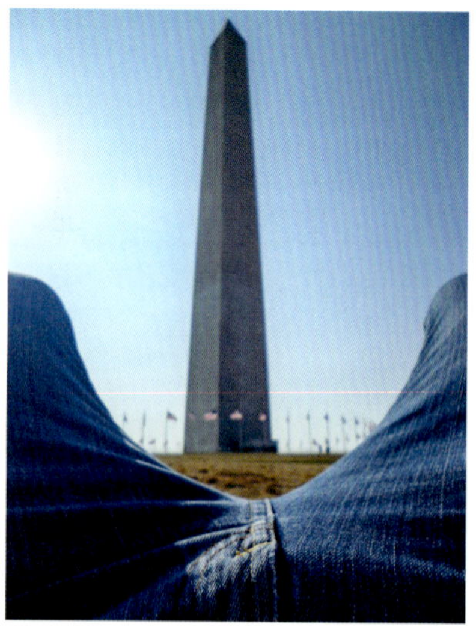

their parents all think being gay is a mental disorder.

I recently came to D.C. to make a fresh start. I'm twenty-five and I'd been in Kissimmee, Florida, pretty much my whole life. I was just sick and tired of it. I wanted to go somewhere and make new memories, meet new people, and just start everything brand new. D.C. has a lot of universities, so I figured it would be a prime place for me to go to school, as compared to central Florida. I want to study biology and then go to medical school.

The first time I moved out on my own I was nineteen, and basically everything that could go wrong did. I mean, my car broke down. I didn't have money. I was living off noodles. I was diagnosed with HIV and was in the hospital for a while. Everything went horribly. And when I came back home, my mom said, "I told you so." But when it came to moving to D.C., I was just like, "Well if I don't do it now, I'll never do it." So I did.

If you look at all the young people who are having sex, I would be willing to bet over ninety percent of them have at some point engaged in unprotected sex. So I haven't done anything different than most of my peers. It's just that there's a higher percentage of HIV in the gay community, which put me at a higher risk. A white girl in South Dakota might sleep with twenty guys and get chlamydia. However, because I live in a more populated area in Florida—which is the state with the third-highest HIV rates—I could sleep with two people and one of those two might end up being HIV-positive.

I always felt like I was swimming against the current of life, that life was full of hardships and I was being pushed back. But since I've been to D.C., even though my life is sometimes a chaotic mess, I feel like I'm in the right place, at the right time.

Kyle

I found out I was HIV-positive in 1987, when I went to my doctor for a regular check-up. Within a couple of years I had full-blown AIDS. I had five T-cells and I named them all: Lucy, Ricky, Fred, Ethel, and Little Ricky.

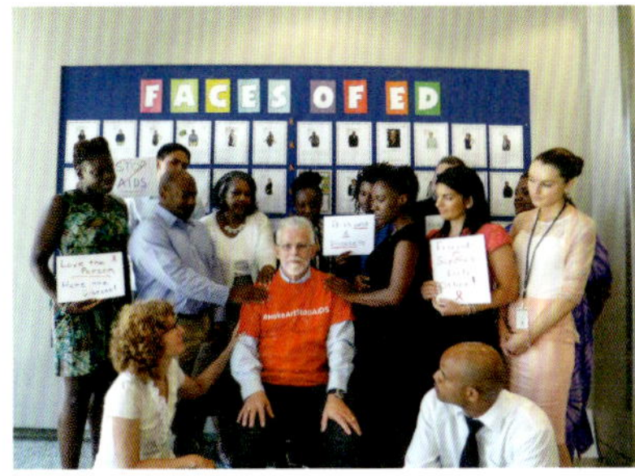

When I got to my sickest, I was in the hospital one night with a mystery fever. My temperature was up to 107 degrees and they were ready to lose me. All of a sudden I saw this brilliant bright horizon, and I saw my two grandmothers and my great-grandmother. It was so peaceful. I was so excited I started walking toward them. One of my grandmothers stopped me and said, "It's not time yet. We want you to know that it's beautiful here and we're waiting for you. You need to go back and tell your family that it will be OK." Then I woke up and my fever broke, just like that.

I'm fifty-seven years old and was born in Paris, Texas, and I now live in Washington, D.C. Before I got sick, I had three very successful careers. I was an officer in the Air Force. I was a college professor for three years. I worked for Texas Instruments. HIV took all that away from me. At first I was devastated. But after the near-death experience, I started a spiritual journey. I saw wonder in everything that I did. It's not like I got on my knees and prayed all the time. I didn't. I just lived my life, and I always knew somebody was looking after me.

Now I have a job in arts education for underprivileged children. I love what I do. I asked my office if they would pose for a picture, and, man, they jumped on it! I'm sitting in a chair and they are laying their hands on me. I can see in their faces it wasn't staged. I can see the compassion in their faces.

Yes, I am HIV-positive, but I'm so many other things. I'm a gay man and I'm a father. I'm a grandfather. I'm a husband—my partner Anthony and I have been together for over eighteen years. I am many things. HIV is just a little part of me.

Sharon

I'm pretty much a loner. I like things that are quiet, that give me a chance to think.

In the environment where I come from, there was a lot of poverty, and a lot of shootings and robberies. Everything I learned, I learned from the streets. Earlier in my life I chose drugs. I chose a destructive lifestyle. But now, I've been clean sixteen years. I'm fifty years old.

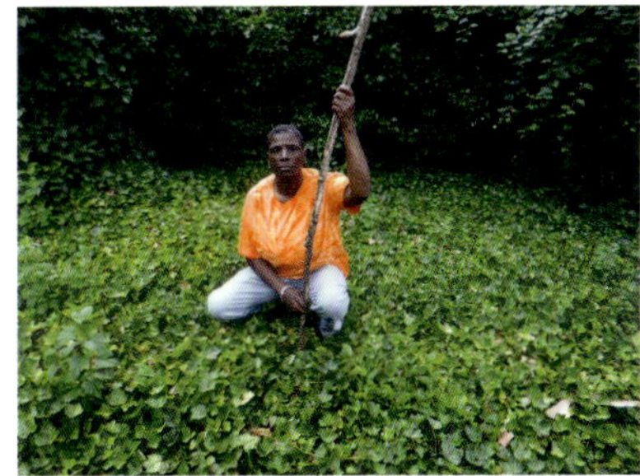

I think I contracted HIV intravenously, through drugs. I found out in 1986, when I was diagnosed with AIDS. At that time, I was in jail. I took sick and was transferred to a quarantine infirmary. I was terribly ill, but they still had to handcuff me to the bed.

I got out of jail real early, on "merciful release," where they let people out who are terminally ill. I went to this house for women living with HIV and AIDS. Then I began to take my medications. People around me were dying, so it just struck me that I needed to get educated about this disease if I got to live with it. So I needed to get involved with my life.

And from then on, my life took off.

Something that interests me now is how the stigma is different against women living with HIV and AIDS. There's lesbians who are living with this disease, but it's not many of us who would actually come out and say so. And then I read today that the HIV infection rate is triple among African-American women as compared to white women. And I'm thinking, what is going on? People are going to have sex—you know that—but they're not telling the truth about who they're having sex with.

And teenagers—who don't have to catch this—they're just not listening. You know, a young woman, she's fifteen, and she meets an older guy at the mall, he winks at her, he looks good, so she relates to it. He's going to get her that iPod she wants. And eventually she's going to have sex with him. But he's not telling her anything about himself—he's just having sex with her.

I just think it's very important for me to speak up for women and try to remove the stigma and ignorance surrounding AIDS.

Tori

My name is Tyranny but everybody calls me Tori. I found out I was HIV-positive on June 8, 2010, in Atlanta. I called my mother in D.C. and told her, and she was like, "Just get back here." She called me again in ten minutes and said, "Your flight leaves Sunday at 7 a.m., and you have a doctor's appointment on Monday." So I moved back to D.C. five days later and went into treatment June 14. When I talk about my mother I always cry, because she is the biggest influence on me. I lived with her and she made sure I stayed on the treatment. Now my virus is undetectable.

Part of having HIV with me is having neuropathy, or nerve pain. Sometimes I can't walk, and it feels like I've just stepped on nails. But having medication honestly helps a lot.

I really have nothing to complain about. I mean, I'm a lot healthier than I was two years ago. And like I always tell people, I got my HIV from being in love with someone and someone saying they loved me. We were together for three years. I didn't use a condom because, you know, we've all been taught to use condoms, but nobody teaches condoms and love. But what I've learned is even though you're in love with someone, you still need to use condoms. Even if you've been together for five years, you should still go and get tested. And that was one thing I didn't do. That's why I found out so late.

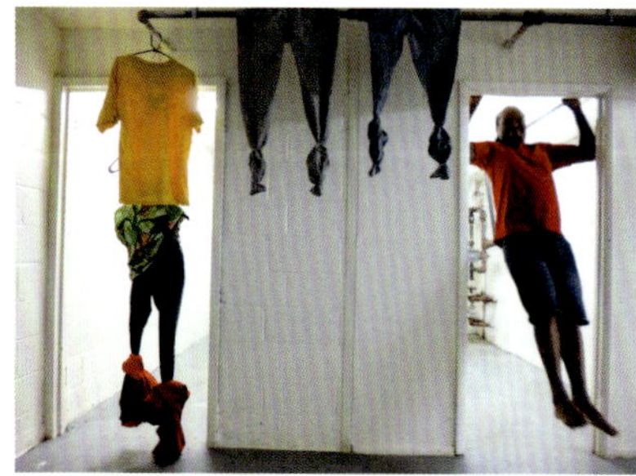

Now I work for Us Helping Us as an HIV advocate for young adults who are recently diagnosed or who need to get back into treatment. My doctor calls me and she'll say, "I have a newly diagnosed person who's scared of treatment." So I go in with them for their first meeting and help them with any kind of support services. When all this was going on, my mother said, "You know what? This is your calling."

I do feel as though my purpose is to show people that you can live with HIV, and to help people out with it. So that's why I always have a smile on my face—because I found my purpose and I love what I do.

Mumbai

Affording and accessing treatment was a key theme of the December 2012 *Through Positive Eyes* workshop held in Mumbai, India. Many participants in the workshop told of scrambling to afford medication, needing to share doses with family members in order to scrimp and save, or facing egregious stigma from medical workers at government hospitals. Another focus of the group's discussions was the blatant injustice of unknowing young women being brought into arranged marriages with HIV-positive husbands. Two faith leaders—one Hindu, one Christian—took the opportunity offered by the workshop to publicly disclose their own HIV-positive status, opening important dialogues within their religious communities about the treatment of people living with HIV and AIDS.

India's AIDS epidemic, as of 2012

Number of people living with HIV:	2.09 million

HIV prevalence

Adults (15–49 years):	0.28%

Epidemic is concentrated in key populations, primarily sex workers and men who have sex with men, but data is not available for 2012.

Treatment

Free antiretroviral treatment is available but access is not universal.

Numbers on treatment:	630,000
% of those needing treatment who are receiving it:	36%

Key events

1986 *The first cases of HIV diagnosed, among female sex workers.*

1987 *The first government National AIDS Control program begins.*

2001 *Cipla, a generic medicines producer in India, offers treatment for less than a U.S. dollar a day.*

Update 2019

In 2017 there were 2.1 million Indians living with HIV. HIV prevalence was higher among female sex workers, men who have sex with men, transgender people, and injecting drug users (1.6 %, 2.7%, 3.1% and 6.3% respectively). 56% of Indians living with HIV were on treatment.

In 2018 homosexuality was decriminalized as a result of a prolonged campaign by LGBTQI and human rights activists. In the same year, legislation criminalized discrimination against people with HIV.

Through Positive Eyes in Mumbai was organized in partnership with MAKE ART/STOP AIDS and Godrej Industries. Major funding was provided by The Herb Ritts Foundation, with additional support from the Heroes Project, Gere Foundation, and UCLA.

Raju

I told my wife, "It's up to you, you can live with me if you wish. If not, I will give you a divorce. It is your life, your choice."

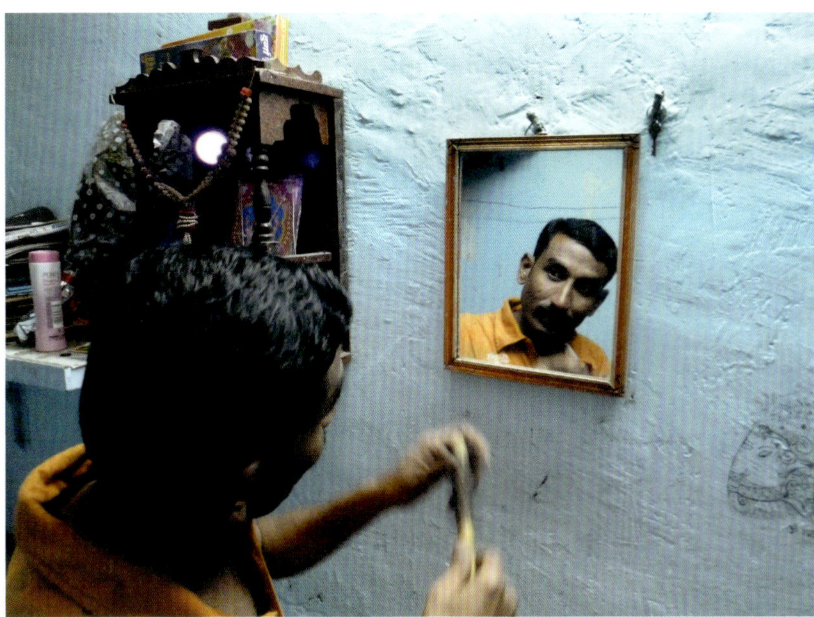

When I found out that I was HIV-positive, my life went dark.

Two years after I got married, my wife and I were unable to have a child. I was diagnosed with low sperm count. At the hospital I had a blood test, which was positive for HIV. I started wondering how this could have happened.

I remembered that I had gone out one evening. I was intoxicated and made a mistake—even though I was aware of HIV at the time. I thought I had safe sex, so I don't know how this happened, but the mistake must have occurred there. I felt like because of one mistake my whole life was ruined.

I went to the top of a building to commit suicide. Then I stopped and said no, there must be thousands of people like me. I thought: let it go. A new life has started for me now.

Afterwards, I was wondering how to tell my wife. I took her out and calmly talked to her. She was worried after I explained it. I took her to the hospital for a test. Her results were negative and I said, "Thank God, at least she is safe!"

I told my wife, "It's up to you, you can live with me if you wish. If not, I will give you a divorce. It is your life, your choice."

My wife has been remarried for a year now. We had been together for ten years, five before HIV and five after. We still talk on the phone and she still loves me. Her parents must have forced her to leave me.

Now I am a community volunteer and I am living a normal, joyful life. I want to be somebody. I am earning and sending money to my mother. I want to take care of my family and also help and inspire others to live better. My life is all mixed up—happiness, sorrow, darkness, light.

To people who are HIV-positive, the message I want to share is this: If you are unhappy about something, look at me and live happily. My life is hard, but still I am living with joy and so should you.

Hari

When I was very young, my father signed me up to a wrestling team. It was through wrestling that my willpower and confidence increased, until I realized I could be stronger than the average man.

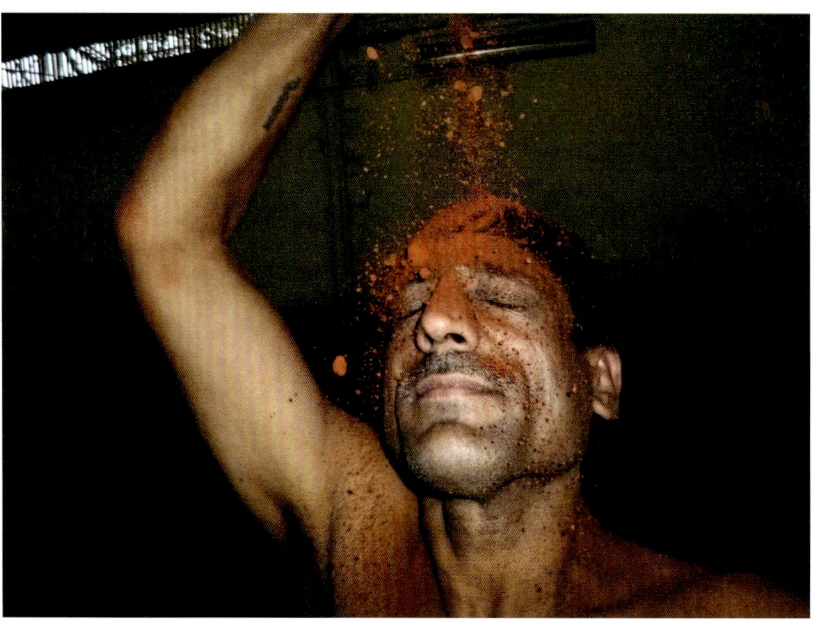

In 1994, I was diagnosed HIV-positive. When I heard this, it was a big blow. The body language of the person who informed me of this news indicated that he didn't even think of me as a human being. I thought I would die in a few days. I told my wife and we stayed at home for several months and didn't tell anyone. We later found out that my wife and two daughters did not have it, which was a relief. But to afford medication, we had to sell our house and take out a loan.

Incidentally, when I was very young, my father signed me up to a wrestling team. It was through wrestling that my willpower and confidence increased, until I realized I could be stronger than the average man. After becoming HIV-positive, I restarted my passion. I began my life for the second time, exercising and playing games. The people who were wary of me since contracting HIV—who didn't talk to me, or invite me to their weddings—these people began to accept me.

With exercise and with good care, my life has been prolonged, my CD4 cell count has grown, and the HIV has become dormant.

In May 2004, United States President Bill Clinton visited India to open a clinic, and a doctor invited me to inaugurate the clinic with him. I was nervous but very happy to meet President Clinton. He was doing such good work for us. After the inauguration, I joined an organization called Delhi Network of Positive People. There I met many people with AIDS, many of whom were living in poverty. I decided that I would work for these people. This is my work now. I became a counselor. I was trained by UNDP, the United Nations Development Program. I learned how to work for the community and how to use a computer, and I fought a case against the Novartis Company for an open market in India to make medicine more affordable. I am able to travel, walk, and run. I am healthy. When I fly, I wear my "HIV-Positive" T-shirt to tell hundreds of people on the plane and in the airport that I am HIV-positive. I want to reduce the stigma and discrimination that comes with HIV and spread awareness that being HIV-positive doesn't mean death.

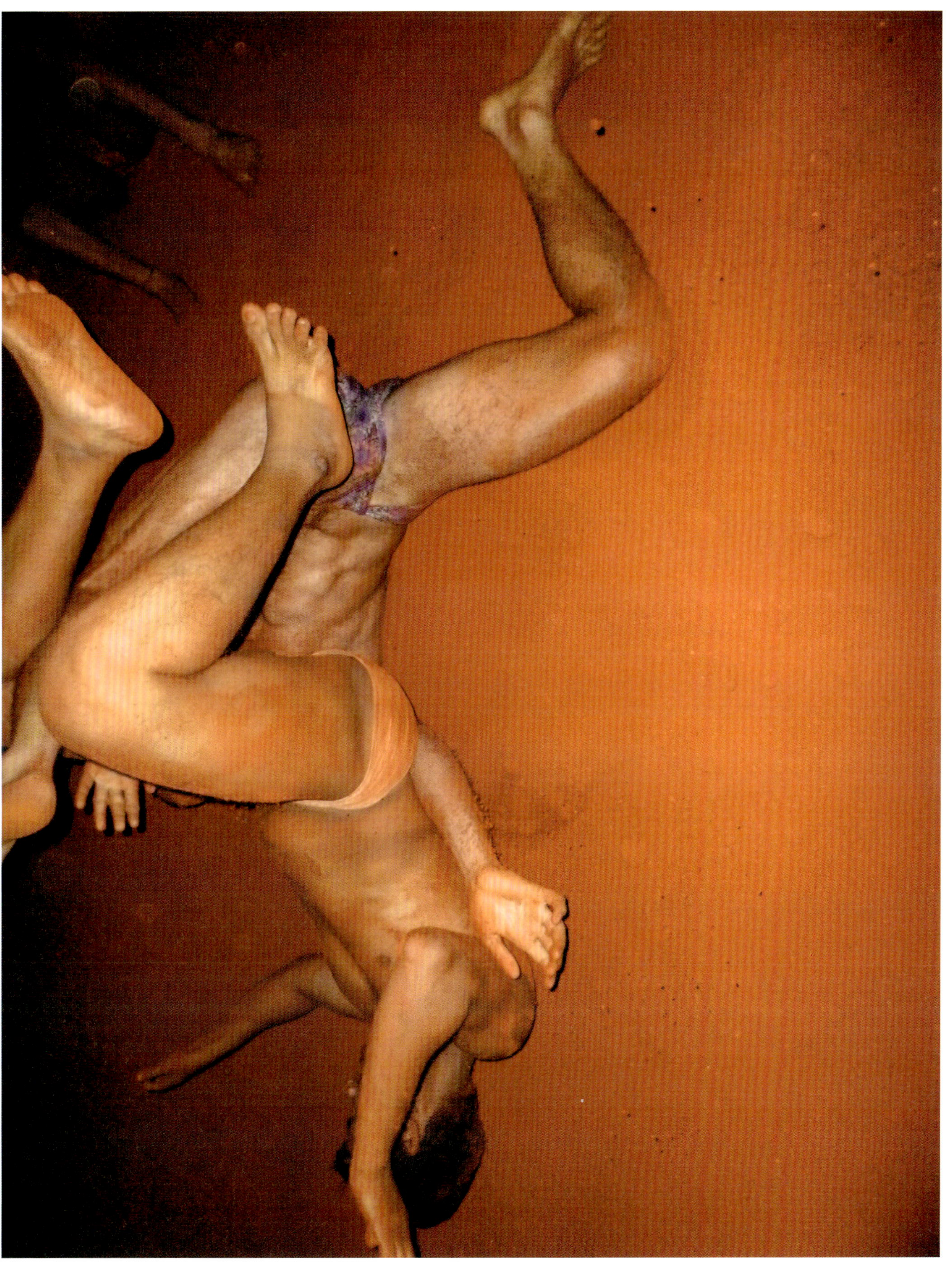

Suman

If you are HIV-positive and you get married, then you need to tell your partner. It is their right to know.

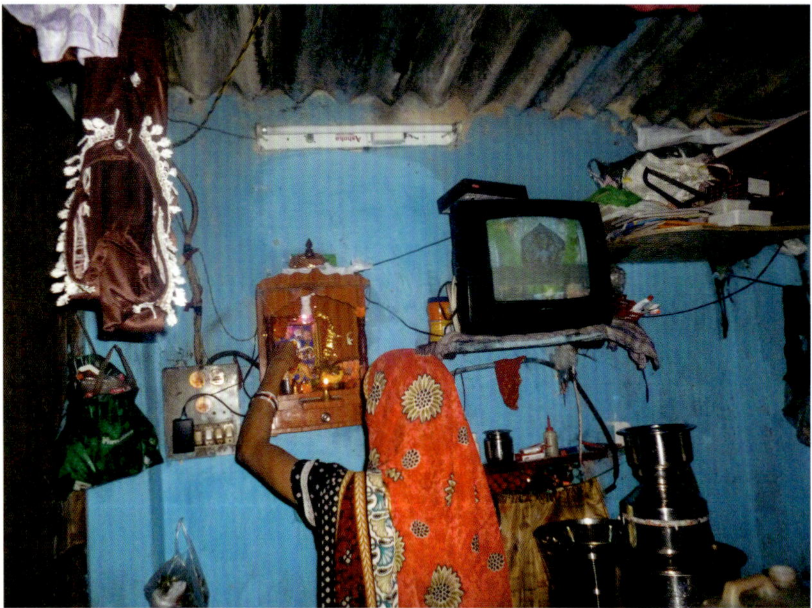

I got married when I was sixteen. When I was pregnant with my first child, I was tested for HIV and found out I was positive. I'm sure my husband already knew his status, because when the hospital asked him to get tested, he refused. If you are HIV-positive and you get married, then you need to tell your partner. It is their right to know.

To my husband, my life was finished. I did not see it that way. I thought it was like when people get diabetes and take pills and continue to live. I tried to make my husband understand this, but he just drank more. In the middle of this, I had my baby boy.

I went on to have two more children. The first two were not infected, but my third son was HIV-positive. I found myself at the hospital all the time because my husband and son were so ill. Because of lack of money, I couldn't buy any pills for myself. Eventually, my husband passed away. I went to live with my parents. Doctors would not treat my son until I gave them money, despite my telling them I did not have any. A man saw my struggle and paid the Rs. 500 [$10 US] necessary for my child's medicine, but my son died by the time we got his treatment.

I still have two children, and I discovered my husband had been married before and had three children from that marriage. Those children's mother had died, so I began to care for them. Now I think of his children as mine.

I began to go to the hospital to get treated again, even though the people there tried to chase me away and made it very difficult for me to get medicine. They said I needed a ration card, which I did not have. I met someone and asked him to give me a ration card because it was urgent. He gave it to me, but when I returned to the hospital with it, the counselor demanded to know how I got one on such short notice. I was very angry and said, "Who are you? Why do you trouble me, saying there's no medicine and that you need my name on a ration card? A person can die and still you don't give them medicine?" From then onwards, they started to behave better.

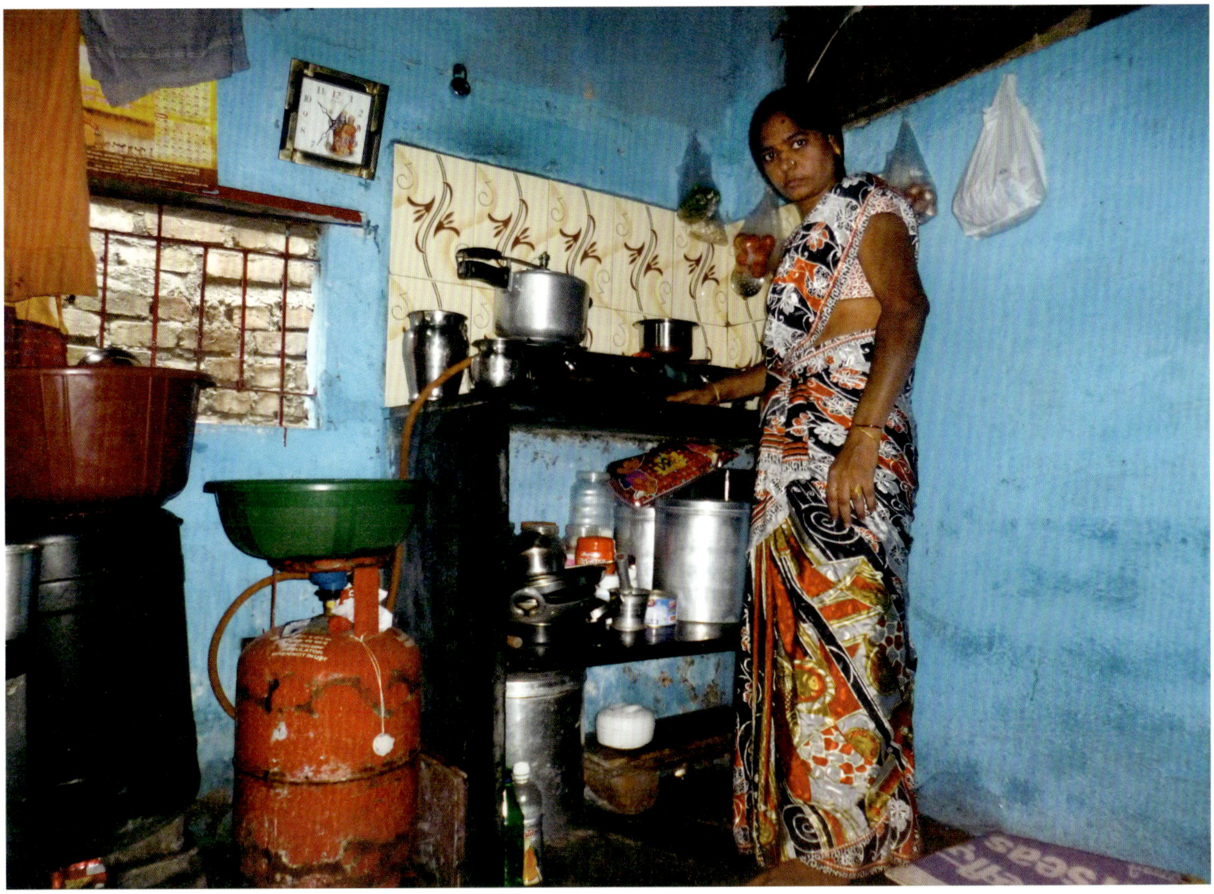

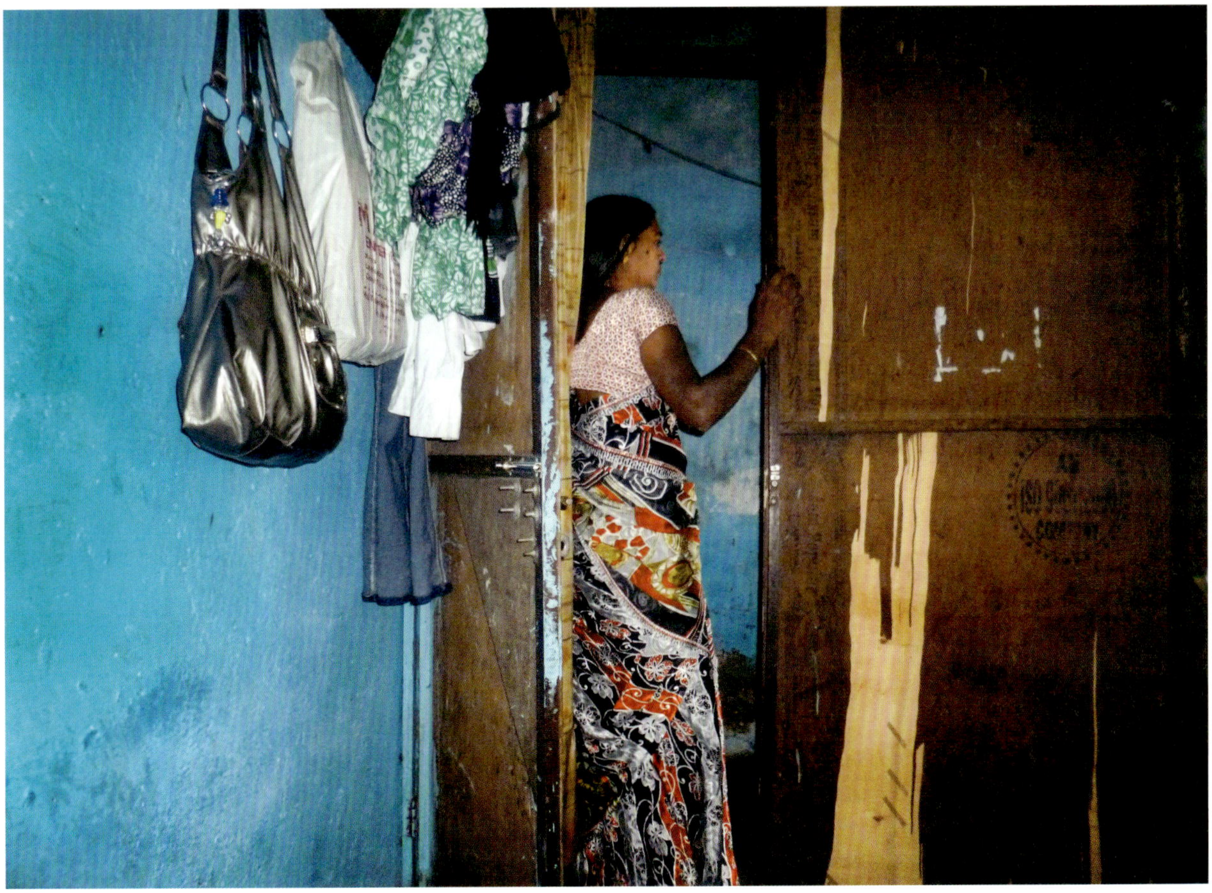

Dolly

I do not dress as a woman while I am on duty as a social worker in the hospital. I make patients feel comfortable to share their problems with me.

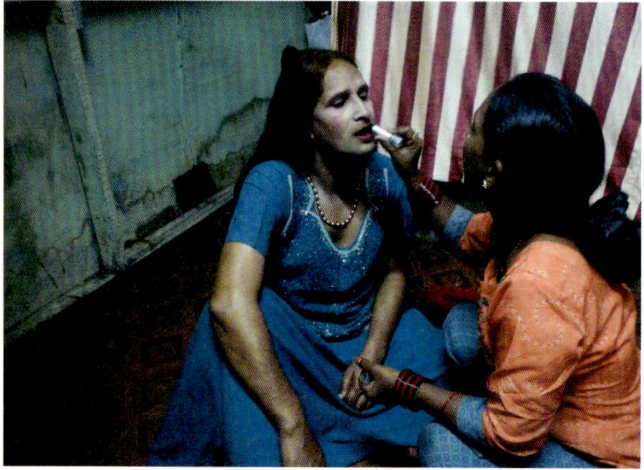

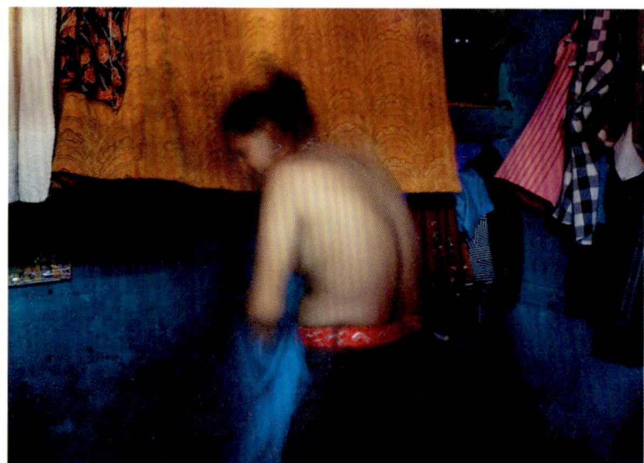

I am a Hindu Punjabi. I was adopted by a Muslim family. And I am transgender.

I have faced many difficulties in my life. I had an accident. My mother could not handle seeing how injured I was. She fell ill and passed away. Following that, my father committed suicide.

My accident had left me unable to pass urine. After an operation, however, I was still unable to pass urine through my genital organs and did so through a hole on the side of my body. I felt upset but continued to live as normal a life as I could. Complications arose and I was put back in the hospital.

There, I met a Muslim man who mistook me for a relative of his named Pappu, who had gone missing. When his family met me, they began to cry, saying my features and my mannerisms were like Pappu's and that I was their son. I thought that being a part of their family might help me, so I lied and said yes, you are my mother and father. They took me to their house. I thought they would be rich, but they had nothing.

In time, I moved to Mumbai. Although my Muslim father knew I was gay, my Muslim mother did not and she forced me to marry a girl. My genital organs were still not functional, but my mother had seen that my wife was well-to-do. On my wedding night, I told my wife my story. We were very worried and didn't know what to do. Family members pressured us to have a child anyway, and we had a test tube baby, a daughter.

Afterwards, I tested positive for HIV. I felt guilty. I was worried and cried a lot and thought I would die soon. I went to the hospital and asked them for work. They said I could look after patients in the ward. I got food in return. I became famous there as Dolly the caretaker. Slowly my health improved, and I began to look better.

With God's grace I remain strong. I am very happy and live by society's rules. I behave and dress according to what society will approve. I am not excessively sexually active. I do not dress as a woman while I am on duty as a social worker in the hospital. I make patients feel comfortable to share their problems with me. Now society is on my side, and how they see me is how I want them to.

Priya

My animals are my human beings. My family, my husband, my children, they have all betrayed me, but these animals have not.

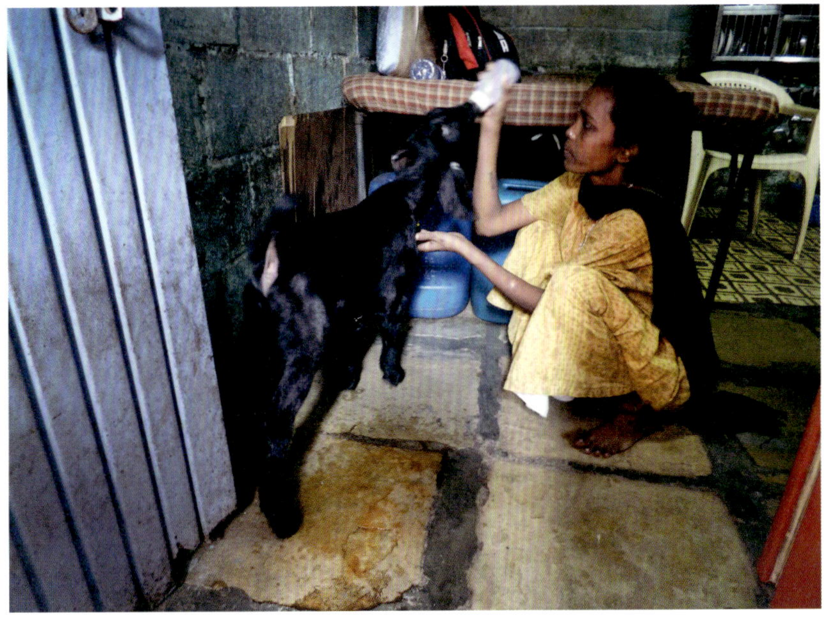

When I told my husband that the hospital informed me I am HIV-positive, he said, "How have you contracted HIV? Who have you been with? My children don't have it and I don't have it." And with these words, he left me. As soon as my parents heard about my illness, they abandoned me too. I have four children, and they have left me as well.

It's been thirteen years. Now I am financially independent. I work as a maid.

At the time when I fell ill, people used to call me names. They used to say, "She is diseased. Don't go near her." It was then that a lady came to me wanting to sell her goat, and I bought it for 2000 rupees ($40 US). I decided that I would look after animals. The lady who sold me the goat didn't realize it was pregnant and, six months later, it had a kid. I was made even happier.

Now I have three animals with me: Julie, Mariye, and Shera. I take care of them and play with them. I enjoy playing with them and taking care of them, even more than I did with my own children. The four of us, we live like a family. My animals are my human beings. They are my god. My family, my husband, my children, they have all betrayed me, but these animals have not.

I was very nervous when I began taking photographs. I have never held a camera in my life. The thought of taking a photograph even with a phone frightened me. I wondered what to do with the camera, but I remembered what my instructors had told me about the timer, so I thought I'd give it a go. I set up the tripod, attached the camera, and set up the ten-second timer. I went to lay my head on the pillow. Julie came to me, nudging me, and fell asleep in my arms. So I held her. She pushed her head up, the timer went off, and this is the photo you have.

No one has supported me before. I pray to God to give his blessings to this family that I have now.

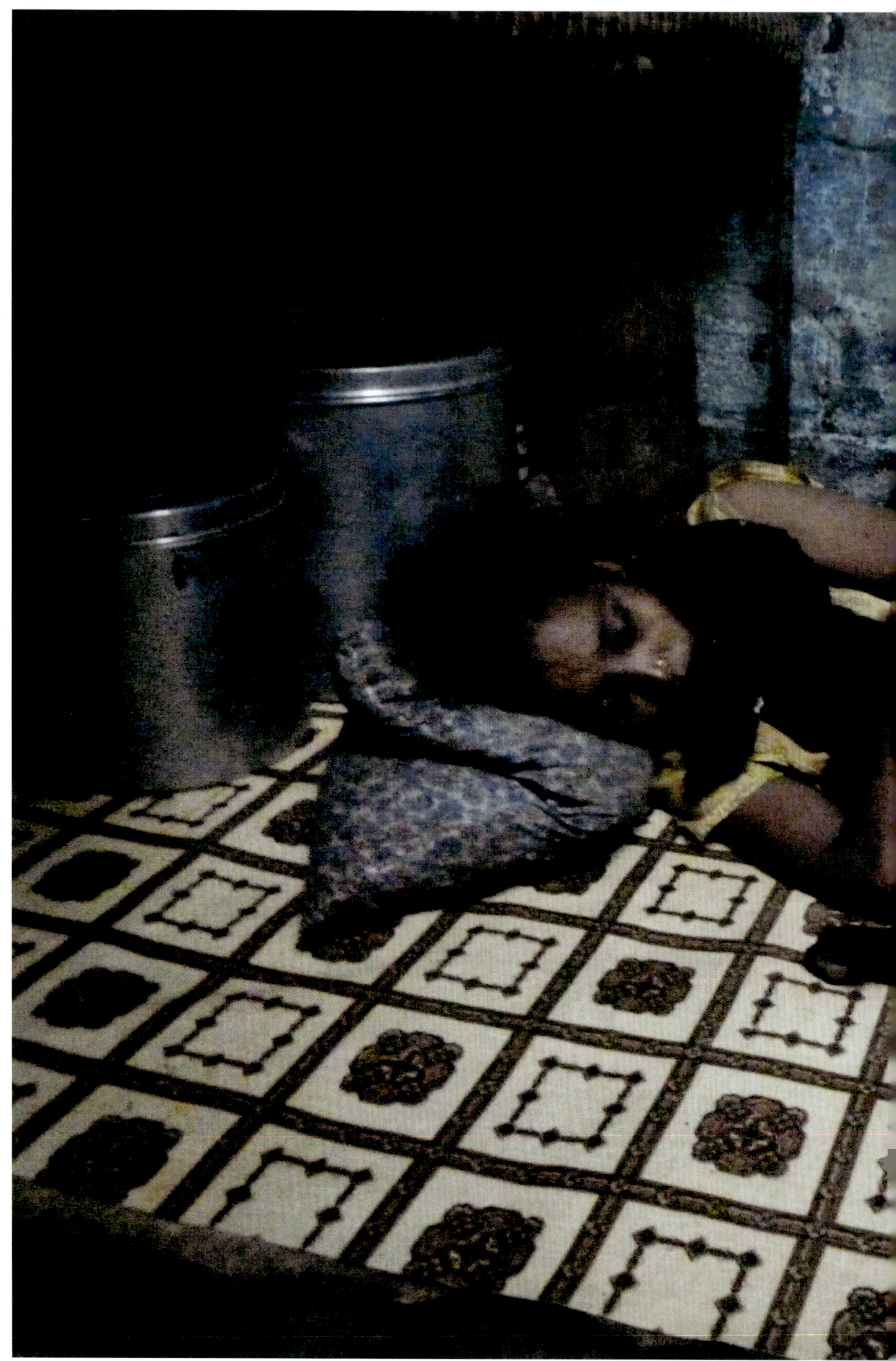

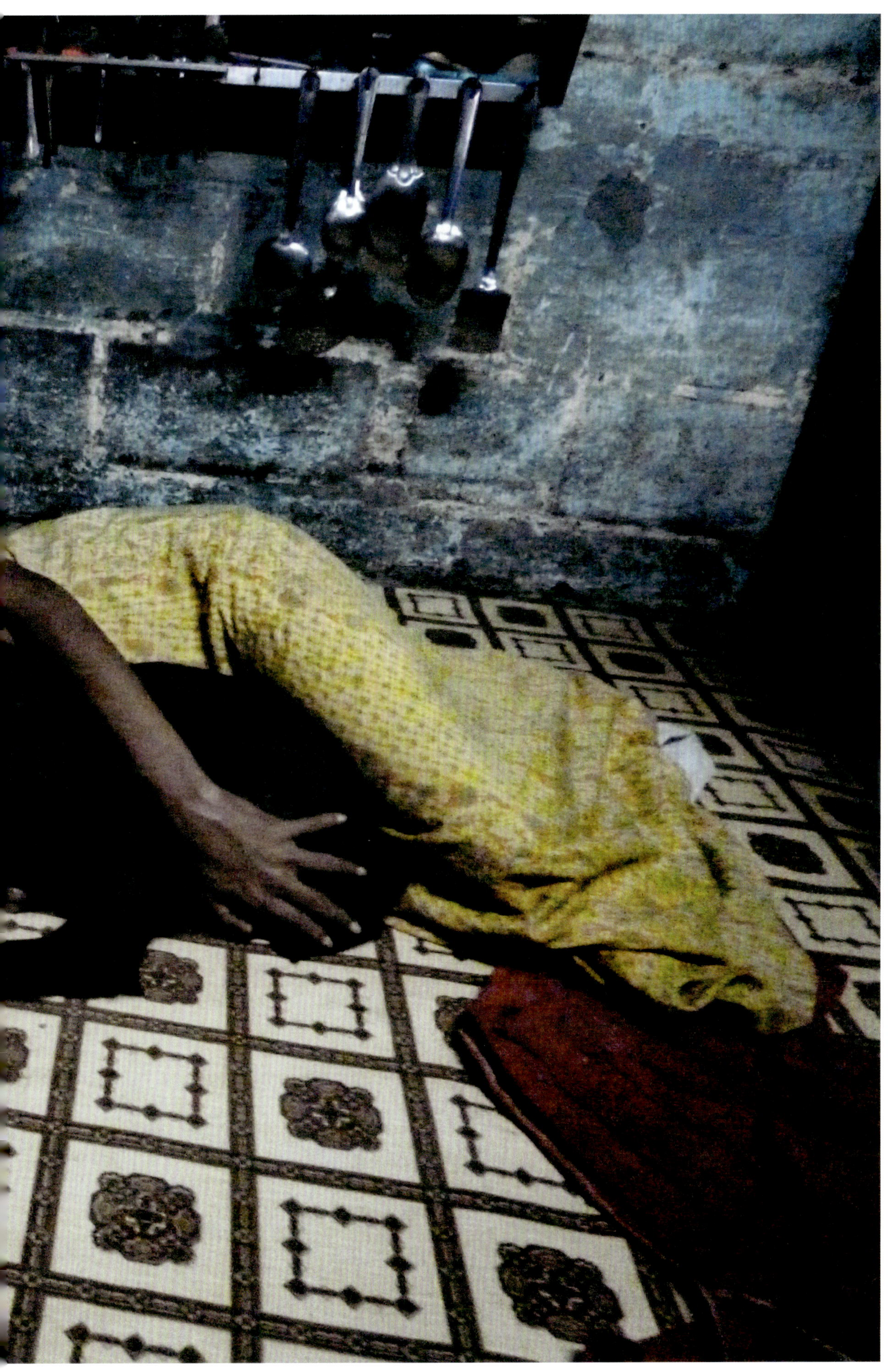

Sudesh

I had to tell the doctor that affording medicine was difficult, and that I had sold my house. He gave me a month's worth of medicine. I could not believe his kindness.

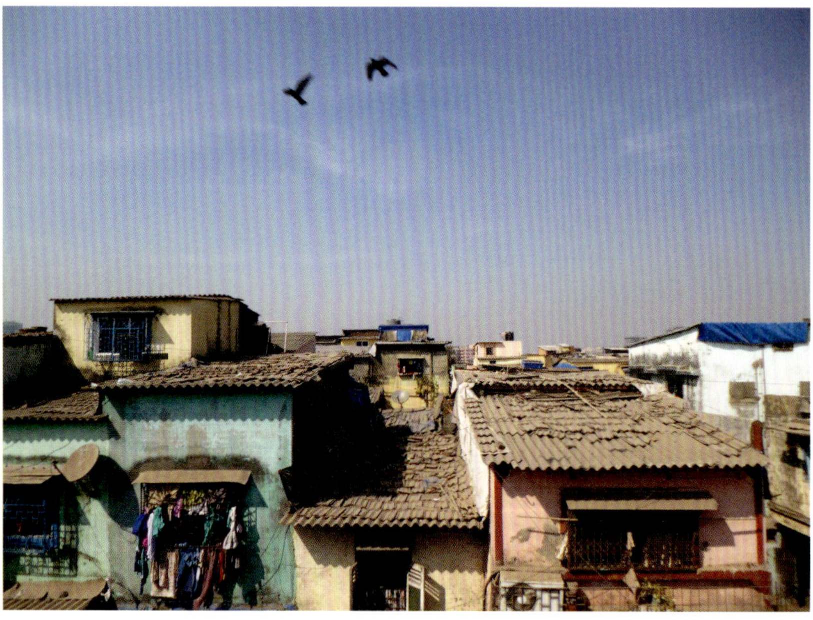

I have faced a lot of problems. In 2005, my wife died—of non-AIDS-related causes—and I thought, "What have I got in life other than misfortune?" I distanced myself from everyone and was very worried that my children did not have a mother. I wondered how I would look after them, but I realized that I had to, so I did not think about anything else.

In 2008, my body was becoming thinner and weighed just thirty-two kilos [seventy pounds]. I suspected that there was something wrong with me, so I got my blood tested. The doctor said I had HIV. I did not know how I had gotten it. I hadn't gone anywhere. I once got an injection, and I suspect I got HIV via the injection needle. I think the doctor had not changed it for a clean one. I told the doctors that I did not have money. My children said not to be stressed. From 2004 to 2007, I spent most of my money on treatment. After selling my house, my money ran out. Again, I had to tell the doctor that affording medicine was difficult, and that I had sold my house. He gave me a month's worth of medicine. I could not believe his kindness.

That is how my life has been—spending all my money on medicine, taking pills, and raising my children. I take care of the home and, after this, if I get time, then I do a little business. I buy and sell kerosene. I have not been ill in the last eight years and my weight is up to fifty-five kilos [121 pounds], but I do not work. People help our family. We have a place to live, which my father built. All my earnings go toward my medicine.

My children know that I have HIV. My daughter told me that everyone takes medicine, and it is OK if I do too. As for the people around me, I have not said anything to them. They think that I have tuberculosis. My children are happy now. I got three of my daughters married, which is one stressful thing finished. My son is in his last year of school, and in two to three years he will be able to stand on his own feet.

Meanwhile, I am alone. I don't have a partner. I fold my hands and accept this. This is my life, and my life will go on.

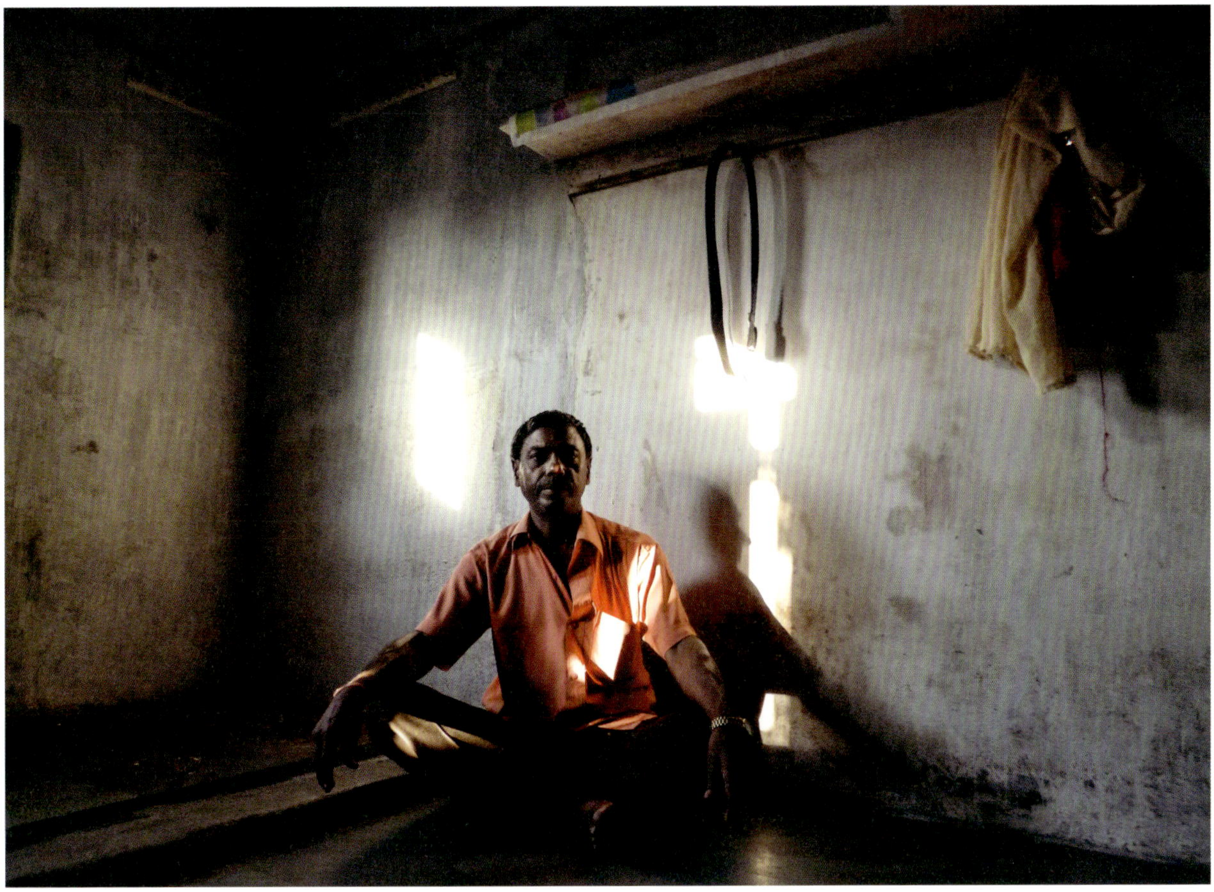

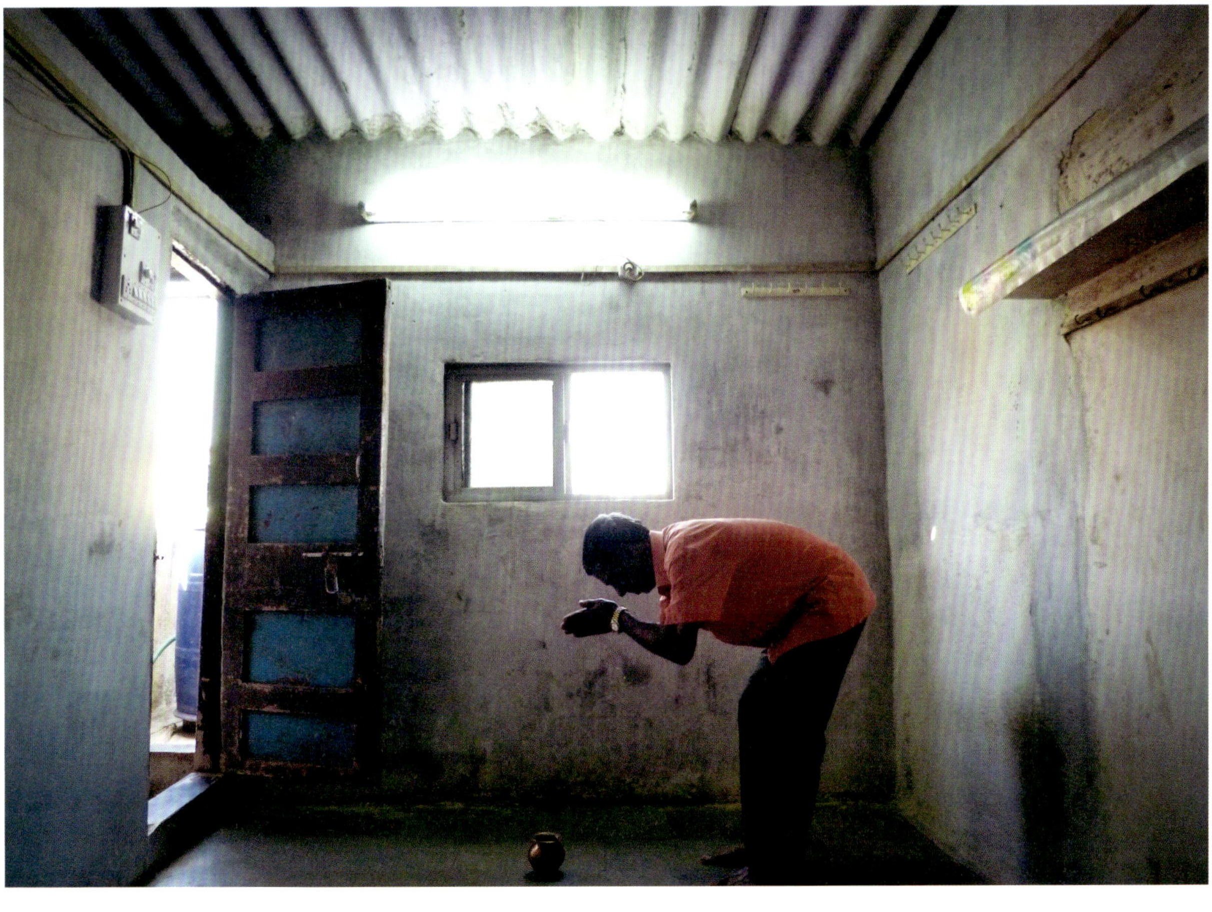

Gautam

If we had learned in school what HIV is, how it is spread, and what a condom is, while our bodies were changing, I may not have become HIV-positive.

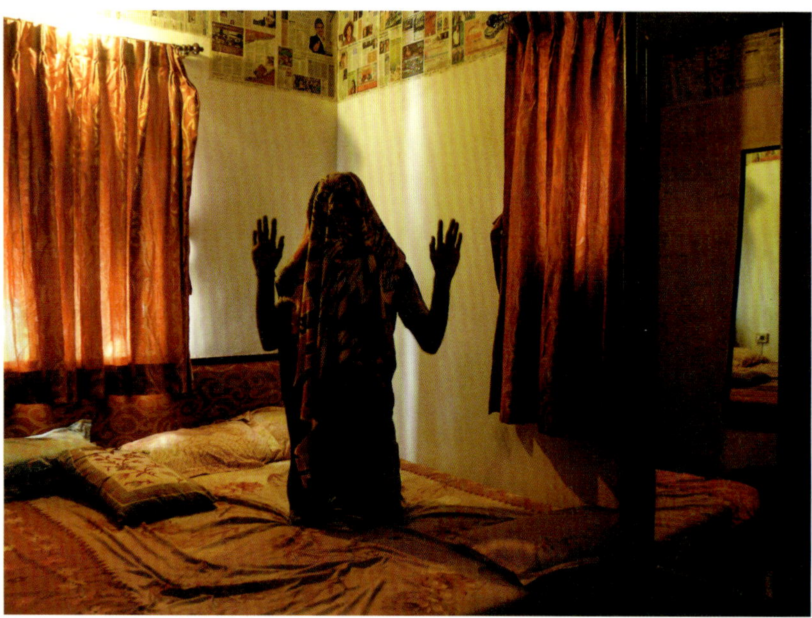

When I was in the fourth grade, I realized I was attracted to men. I was quite confused at the time. I didn't understand whether it was an illness or whether I was the only person facing this issue. Why did nobody else come forward with it? I was bullied, and I stopped going to school.

I was eighteen when I found out I was HIV-positive. I was in shock. I started to cry loudly and didn't know what to do. I thought that being HIV-positive meant my life was going to end. Perhaps I would live for a year or two and then I would die. I was thinking, my life is just starting. Now HIV can't leave me and I can't leave it.

I am a lucky person in that after realizing I was gay and becoming HIV-positive, my parents and family still stood by me and supported me. My sister said, "HIV is nothing. It is not a problem. You be as you are, how you were before you knew you were positive." Coming out was absolutely perfect. I felt just like everyone else.

I have also realized that education is important in life. I eventually completed twelfth grade, and am now doing a bachelor's degree in social work. In the future, I would like to change the education system in India. If it is only during your graduate degree that you learn about HIV and AIDS, gender, sexuality, and sex, then that is not the right age to be informed. If we had learned in school what HIV is, how it is spread, and what a condom is, while our bodies were changing, I may not have become HIV-positive.

If at times I get depressed, I begin to write. I write that if there are no problems in life, life is no fun and has less meaning, because with every problem, you learn some good things and become strong inside.

For me this is a bold step, to come out in front of people and say, "Gautam is HIV-positive." There is no more need for me to lead dual lives. Now I can take my medicine in front of anyone, eat anywhere, sit anywhere. I don't have to worry about who to tell, who not to tell, who to be with, and who to avoid. Anything can happen.

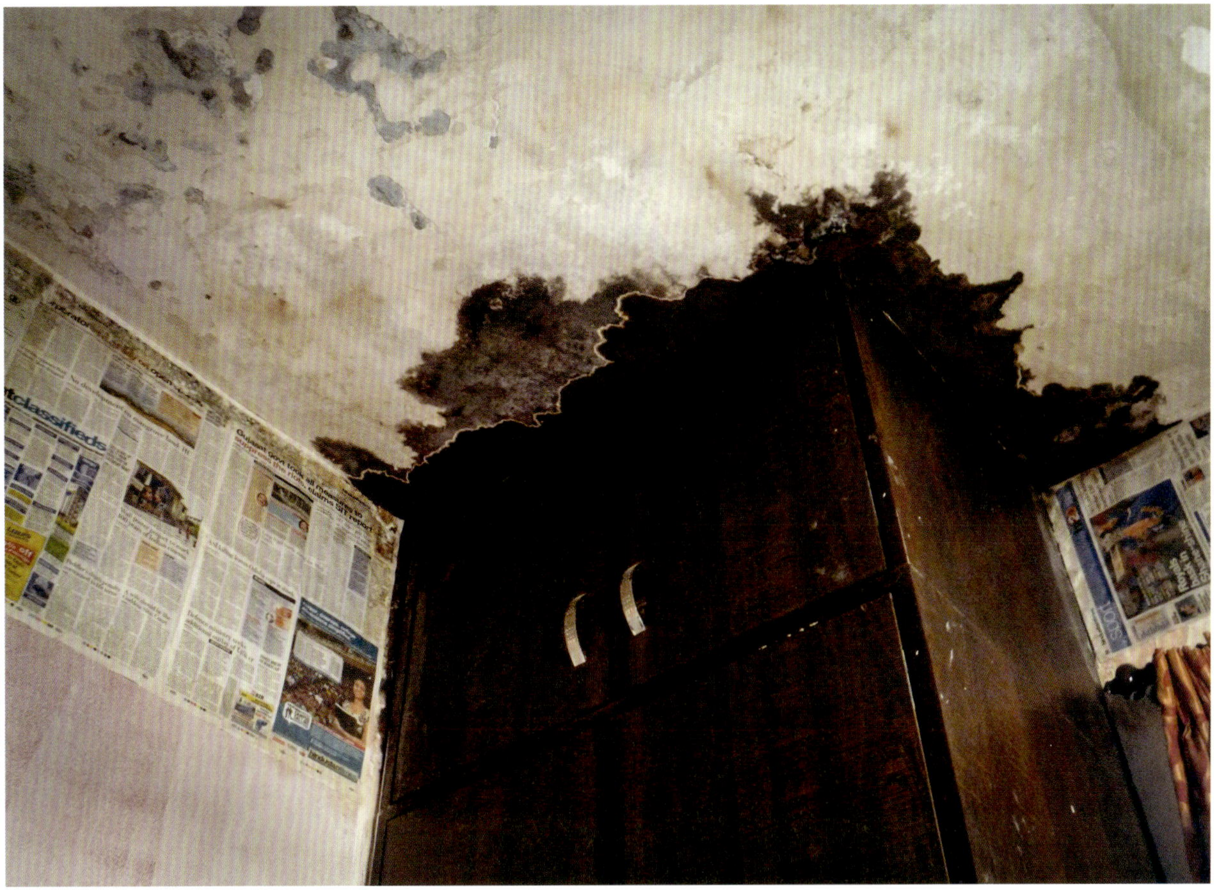

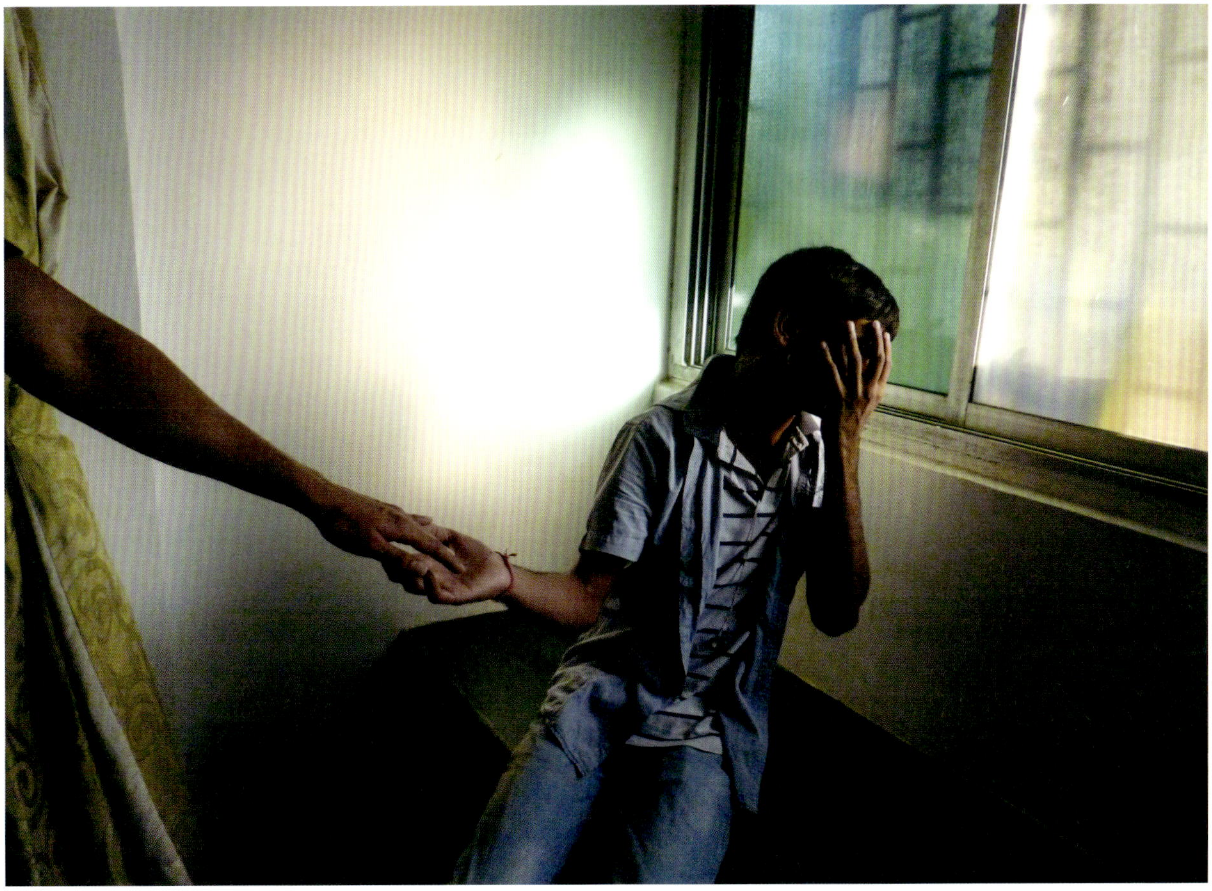

Anthony

There was a girl who came into my life. She had another boyfriend with whom she was in love but, whenever she fought with him, she would come to me and tell me, "I have left him." Finally, one day she came to me and said, "I have cut all ties with my boyfriend. Will you come and ask my parents for my hand in marriage?"

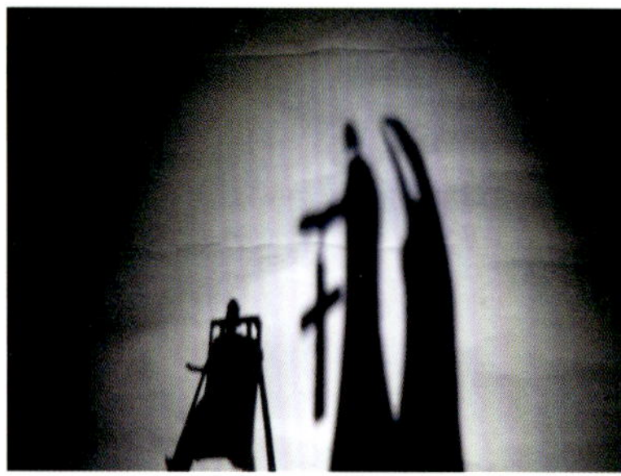

It was her birthday and I took her a cake and a nice dress. After a while her boyfriend and his father came in and began engagement proceedings of their own. Right in front of me, they cut my cake, she wore the dress I gave her, they were offering the engagement cake to her boyfriend, and I was watching.

I was so shocked that I didn't want to live anymore. I began to drink and started to live very carelessly. I lost my common sense and began to visit sex workers. One day I fell very ill and I was admitted to the hospital. That's how I found out I was HIV-positive.

I felt that I was going to die. People from church who came to my home to visit me—the way they looked at me was very wrong.

Over time, my desire to live slowly returned. After visiting the jaws of death twice, and returning from that, I realized the value of life and how it is often wasted. Now I have a wife and children, and my dream of doing social work is a reality. My wife is an HIV-positive person and my good friend. I met her at the organization where we were working together. Since then, my life has become more colorful. I have a guru who says that only when we accept ourselves will other people accept us.

Although I was scared, with the support of my friends and family, and only because of that support, I am standing here today. HIV has not killed me. For those people who are scared or who are keeping their illness a secret, I tell them to come forward, get tested, accept who they are, and keep their family and country safe.

Fatima

My husband found out about his HIV-positive status in 1997. He was already in the advanced stages of AIDS and was in a very critical state. He died of cryptococcal meningitis in 2000.

When my husband found out that he had AIDS, his doctors advised that my son, who was around three years old at the time, and I would need to be tested too. I was breast-feeding my son and was told to stop. I was not worried about myself, but I was worried for my child. If my son tested positive, I would never forgive my husband or myself.

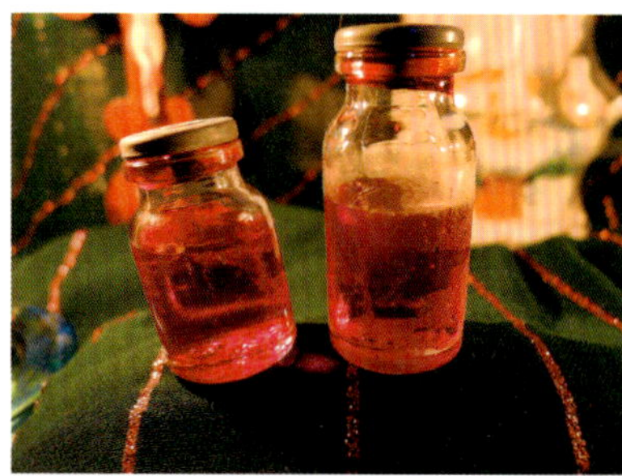

Before going to get tested, I went to the church to pray. I took the bottles that they had given me for the blood test to a prayer center. There is a place there at the church for special prayers, prayers for healing. We got the bottles blessed by the priest.

I tested HIV-positive. Luckily my son was negative. So in that happiness, I did not feel my sadness. I thanked God because my son was safe. Nothing had happened to him. Now my son is eighteen years old and I am grateful to God for not giving him this illness.

In the years that my husband and I had HIV together, I experienced a lot of discrimination. The doctors' attitudes were very bad and shameful, which greatly angered me, because if doctors would only change their attitudes for the better then so would other people, automatically. If doctors were scared, however, everyone would keep away. I saw how the families of other HIV patients would not visit because of this.

I stood strong for my husband and supported him. I was also very lucky, because my entire family gave me their moral and financial support. Sadly, my husband slowly became drug resistant and died. I am very happy, though, that God has given me this opportunity to live after so many years of being positive. I am happy that I will be with my children until they grow up.

Jyoti

After finding out I was HIV-positive, I was very afraid of the stigma, the discrimination, and how I was going to face society. My health started to fail. I was very tired, so I was not able to do housework properly, which my husband did not like. I was emotionally and physically unwell and my husband was not always able to provide me with medication because his mother is diabetic and he was taking care of her as well. In this way, he began to put me in the background, fell in love with someone else, and divorced me.

It took me five years to come out in the open as HIV-positive. I came out because of an HIV activist in America who inspired me through Facebook. I already had to cope with another disability—hearing loss—along with having HIV. It is not easy, but I have no choice. I have learned to live with both.

For me, being HIV-positive is a blessing in disguise. I accept it. Whatever is happening to me now or whatever is going to happen in the future is for the best. I have a virus.

That is me. If you don't like me, that is not my problem.

I meditate and chant to connect closely with God, which helps me. Meditation empowers me to do good and purifies my whole soul. What food is to the body, chanting and meditation are to the soul.

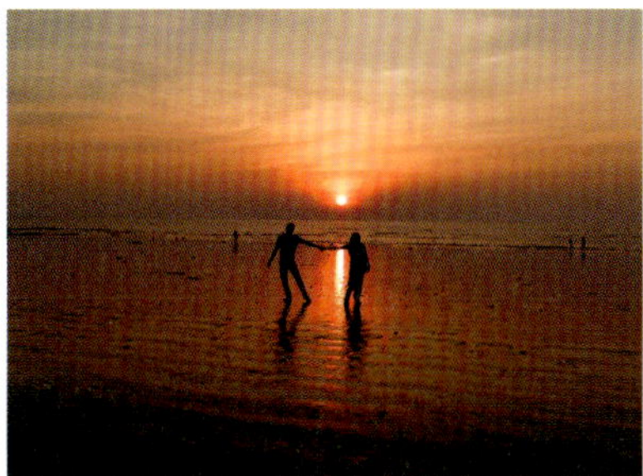

Today, I am an information technology professional, a computer engineer, an Internet blogger, and at the same time I devote my time to serving people with HIV and AIDS. I always say that viruses don't discriminate against anyone, but people do, so my message is this: Don't judge us because of the virus. We don't want pity or sympathy, just love. Being HIV-positive is a new beginning, the new start of life, a fresh hope. Don't let the virus destroy you. Life is short. Live it. Love it.

Manisha

The truth is the truth. I tell everyone that I am HIV-positive, especially those who are close to me. "If you want to be with me, that's fine. If not, you can happily leave. It is not a problem for me."

Around two months after my marriage, I started suffering from a sexually transmitted infection. Then I got pregnant. I had a blood test done when I was in my seventh or eighth month of pregnancy and found out I was HIV-positive. At the same time, my husband became seriously ill, and the doctors said he too was HIV-positive. I believe I contracted HIV from him, but I cannot say how this happened. I tried to ask my husband about it, but I did not pursue it because he was very sick and greatly troubled.

During the time of the Ganapati Festival, my baby son died. My husband was more distressed than I was by the loss of our child, and because of this stress his health worsened. He died barely a month later.

I asked my in-laws for help and they kicked me to the curb, as if I were a beggar. I felt like a drowning person clutching at straws. I was so stigmatized that I could not even kill myself.

Those with HIV are not lesser than anyone else. We can live and work. We must eat and drink. We have the same rights as anyone else. This is important because I believe that there is too much discrimination towards people with HIV among those who do not have the correct information. Those who are aware about this virus do not discriminate.

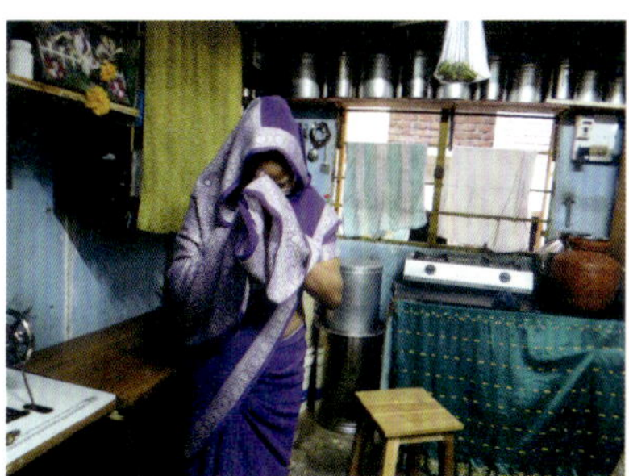

Now I live my life in a carefree manner. I am completely fine. I am able to earn, to feed myself, and to stand on my own two feet. Sometimes when I feel I am losing my courage, I take advice from my elders so that I may regain my strength.

Going forward, people must raise their hands and voices. They should not be held back by fear and oppression. And they should not believe that we have HIV because we have committed a sin. Everyone who finds out they are HIV-positive should immediately start getting medical treatment and take their medicine regularly.

Renukah

After I was engaged, my future husband told me that he was HIV-positive. He did not know whether he contracted HIV in a hospital when he broke his foot and there was blood, or from taking drugs. He said, "Don't marry me." But I just would not listen. I said that I loved him and would marry him and prove my love. I told him that if I were to get married, I would get married to him alone and no one else. Our families agreed to let us marry, but I did not tell my family anything about him being HIV-positive.

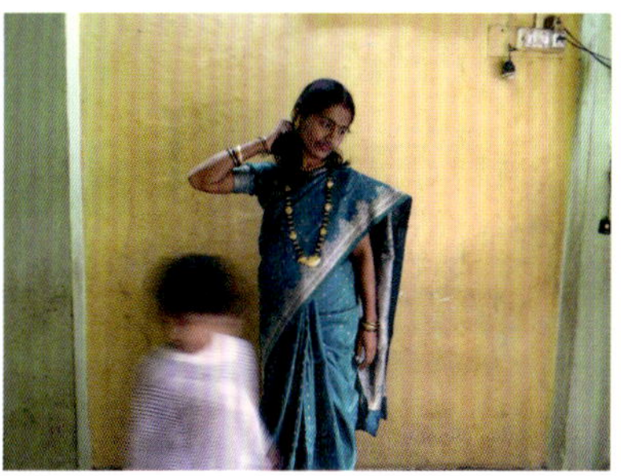

A year after marriage, I tested positive in Bandra Bhabha Hospital. My husband was very sad about this and began to say, "I have ruined your life." But I did not feel that way. I felt I had saved someone else's life. I told my husband we would be together and help each other to live well.

When I was pregnant and had a child, my family was a bit wary of me. (By then, they knew I was HIV-positive.) They kept my towels separate, along with my soap and glass. Everything was kept separate. I wanted to cry when I was bottle-feeding my child and saw other babies in the hospital being breastfed. My doctor, however, would hold my hand and say, "You don't have to be scared of HIV. You look so happy—you should continue to be happy." Eighteen months after I gave birth, we tested the child and she was negative. Then I had another baby. I didn't breastfeed him either. Even he was tested after eighteen months and his report came out negative as well. I was so happy and relieved that all of my own sadness was forgotten, looking at their reports.

As for my extended family, I asked somebody from a nearby care center to come home and explain that HIV is not transmitted through food or friendship. Not by living together, not by sharing soap.

I am not scared of being HIV-positive. I want to live openly and I want others who have HIV to come forward too. When HIV-positive people come to me, I tell them to be like me—or even happier.

Shimray

I am a religious leader, a pastor, in Manipur, India. I was brought up in a Christian boarding school and belong to a Baptist denomination.

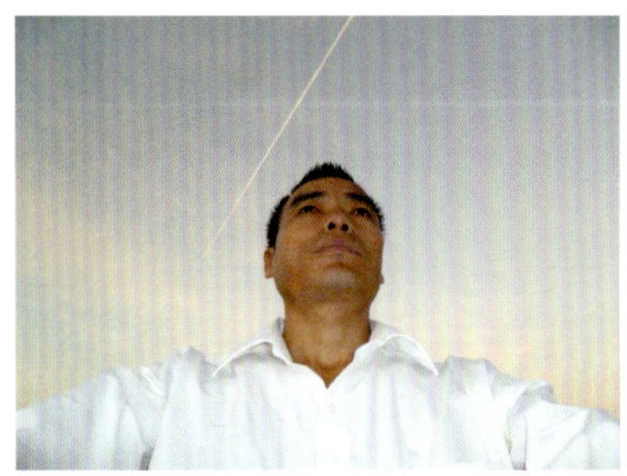

There was a time in my life when my relationship with the Lord was not that good. I was a chain smoker and used to drink a lot. I was into drugs. If ten people came together and there was only one syringe, we would share. I guess the mode of transmission for my HIV was injecting drug use.

In 2001, one of my college friends was sick and I was taking care of him. He went to the hospital and tested positive for HIV. After that, it was made compulsory for all the students to test for HIV. I had my checkup and my blood was screened HIV-positive. I was in denial when I found out. It was very hard to imagine or believe. I felt lost and had many sleepless nights.

Two years later, I came to accept myself as an HIV-positive person. Nobody would ever think or imagine that a pastor would have this virus.

Although I am HIV-positive, my wife and children are all negative. This is what God has made possible in my life. If God wills me to go public and speak about HIV in front of the congregation, I am there.

Before I became HIV-positive, I remember the way Christian leaders treated people living with HIV and AIDS. It was unimaginable. Now, as a person who has experience with the ministry, I feel that I should break my silence and speak out as an advocate for other people who face social stigma and discrimination. This is what I want to request of friends and family and my congregation: Please, treat me as you have treated me before. Do not discriminate against me.

When I break my silence, I will be free like a bird, freed from its cage. That is what I pray and hope. I am sure my being an HIV-positive person has a purpose. I see that most HIV-positive people my age have all died and I am the lone survivor. God is preparing me in some way or another, and I will do what He wants me to do.

Swamiji

Being from Reunion Island, a French territory in the southwest part of the Indian Ocean, I was raised in a Christian family. As an adult, I converted to Hinduism. Life took me that way. Similarly, life brought me HIV. HIV is socially dangerous because it is linked to sex, but most of the time people don't know that you can get HIV without having sex—by injection or by blood transfusion.

And so now I have HIV. Should I commit suicide because I am positive? I considered it, thinking about what people would say. I kept my status quiet for eighteen years. Over time, however, I have come to love my HIV. Although the infection is there in my body, I appear healthy. I take a yogic approach to it.

One of my meditation techniques is to go inside myself and reflect on how many billions of cells we have, just like the Milky Way's billions of stars. Are you a universe of cells or a cell of the universe? I teach my yoga students to feel all the cells of their bodies when they move, and to start moving like stars. The mind is a powerful tool to feel this energy potential and, if you can discover and use this potential, it can help you manage your HIV. It is my scientific and spiritual challenge.

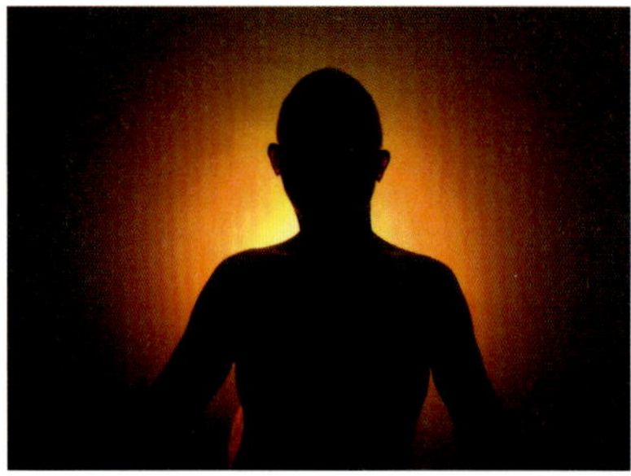

I love my HIV because, if I fight it, I lose energy, whereas if I love it, I gain energy. Plus, I have found the courage to speak about HIV to people and I enjoy helping. Once I became open about being HIV-positive, so many opportunities came to me. HIV has brought me around the world.

I have known stigma since childhood. My father passed away when I was a baby, and my grandmother spoke badly about my mother. I moved to France as a teenager and people at school would say, "You are Zulu. You are from Africa. You are cannibals." As an adult, I came back to Reunion Island. Being a white man, I was judged for going to the Hindu temple. And now, I am talked about for being HIV-positive.

Therefore, I am used to stigma, and my experience helps me go beyond it. Stigma exists because of ignorance. Through knowledge, we can remove it.

Bangkok

The *Through Positive Eyes* workshop in Bangkok was held in December 2013, amid massive political unrest in Thailand's largest city. Months later, a coup d'état would establish a military takeover of the country. Against this tense backdrop, the participants in the Bangkok workshop shared their experiences facing the stigma associated with drug addiction, prison life, and sex work, as well as their determination to find the beauty in their own bodies and in their lives.

Thailand's AIDS epidemic, as of 2013

Number of adults living with HIV:	451,258

HIV prevalence

Adult HIV prevalence (15–49 years):	1%
Female sex workers:	2.2%
Men who have sex with men:	7.1%
People who inject drugs:	25.2%

Treatment

Treatment is provided free as part of Thailand's universal health insurance and has been provided according to WHO guidelines.

Numbers of adults on treatment:	232,816
% of those needing treatment who are receiving it:	80%
% of HIV-positive Thais on treatment who have no detectable virus:	95.35%

Key events

1989	*Ministry of Health conducts first national HIV surveillance.*
1991	*"100% condom campaign" promotes safe sex nationally.*
2000	*People living with HIV demonstrate in front of Parliament, and Minister of Health agrees to double the budget for antiretroviral treatment.*
2002	*Introduction of universal health coverage.*
2013	*Treatment eligibility extended to all Thais living with HIV, regardless of CD4 count.*

Update 2019

A 2014 study showed that early Thai prevention programs had averted around 10 million HIV infections between 1990 and 2010.

By 2017, 440,000 (1.1%) of Thais were living with HIV. Of these, 320,000 were on treatment and 270,000 (62%) had supressed viral loads.

HIV prevalence among female sex workers had declined to 1%, but prevalence among men who have sex with men and injecting drug users had increased to 9.15% and 19% respectively.

Through Positive Eyes in Bangkok was organized in partnership with Space Bangkok, with assistance from Rainbow Sky Association, Red Cross—Bangkok, Tantawan Group, and the Bangkok office of UNAIDS. Major funding was provided by The Herb Ritts Foundation, with additional support from The Ford Foundation, Gere Foundation, National Endowment for the Arts, UNAIDS, and UCLA.

Aoi

Sometimes I feel that the dogs love us more than humans do. They never complain—unlike human beings, who are apt to scold or judge us.

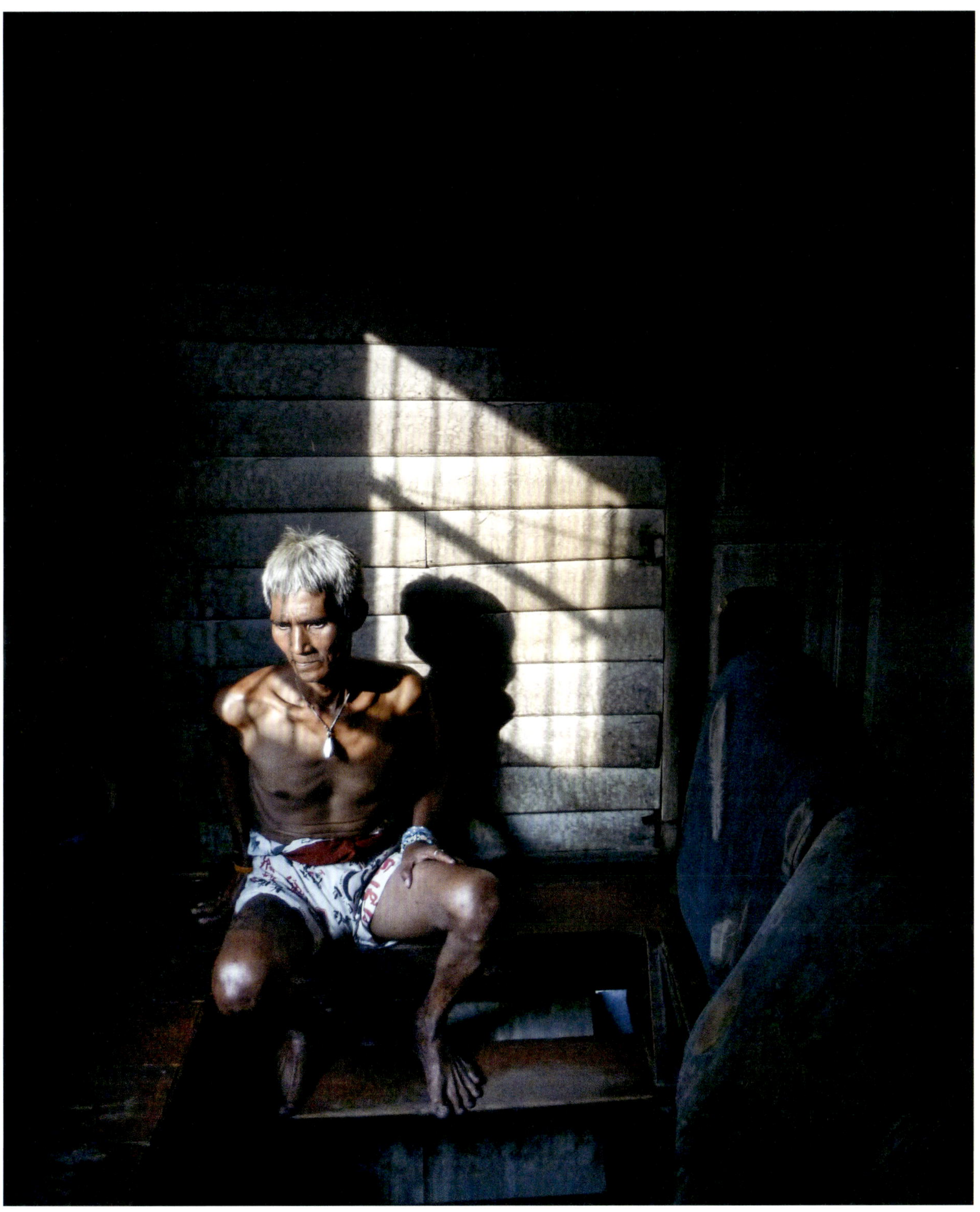

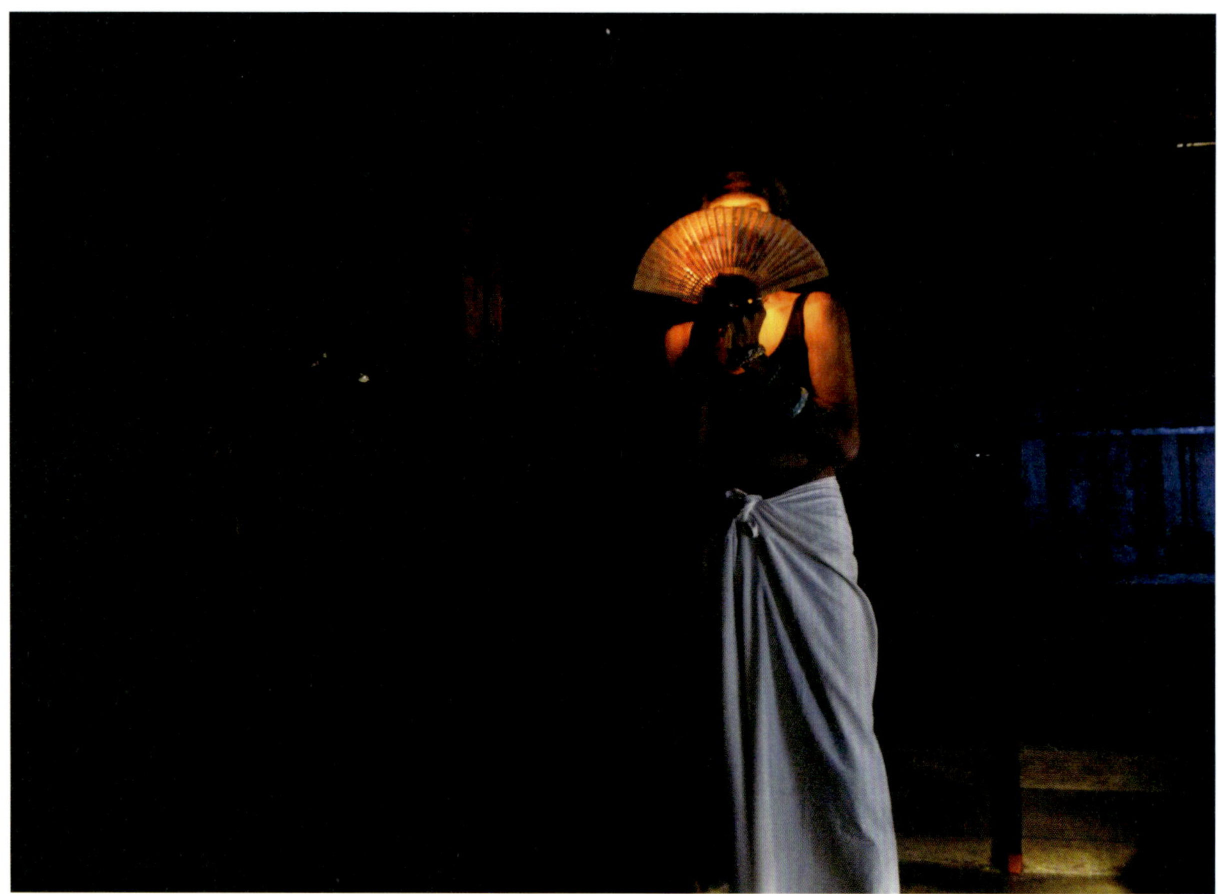

Growing up, I misbehaved a lot. I shared needles and drugs with others. I got arrested for selling. After five years in a provincial prison, I was sent to the main prison. I got a tattoo while I was in jail. My prisoner friend gave it to me by using a sewing needle and ink we collected from a prison guard. The tattoo is an image of the watchtower I saw everyday while going back and forth in jail. My last time in prison was the longest: seven and a half years. There, I began to get sick from tuberculosis. The doctors checked deeper to discover the cause. That was when they found I had HIV.

On my last day at the prison, staff from Alden House, a home for people living with HIV, picked me up. Our country's policy is to send infected people like us back to where we came from. They don't understand the dilemma that puts us in. Even if our families accept us, our neighbors may not.

Now I live with No, another *Through Positive Eyes* participant, whom I met at Alden House. We take care of one another. We have been together more than ten years. We are both estranged from our families and have no children, so we have added dogs to our family. No loves animals. Dogs make her happy. Sometimes I feel that the dogs love us more than humans do. They never complain—unlike human beings, who are apt to scold or judge us.

Every morning, around 8 or 9 a.m., I go to the clinic to receive methadone for my addiction. I also have hepatitis C, which destroys my liver and makes me breathe unevenly. It causes my health to deteriorate. No is afraid that I will pass out when I come home after the treatment.

My greatest fear is departing from No. If I died, who would take care of her?

Before I began taking my HIV medication, I looked very sick. My weight was forty-two kilograms [ninety-two pounds]. I now look so much better. I can go out and work, selling jewelry, without having to worry. And I like dressing up. I dress to impress passersby when I sell in the market. If someone stops to talk with me, that makes me happy, even if they don't buy. Some days I earn money, some none at all, but I feel happier this way than doing illegal work again. I hope people see my goodness.

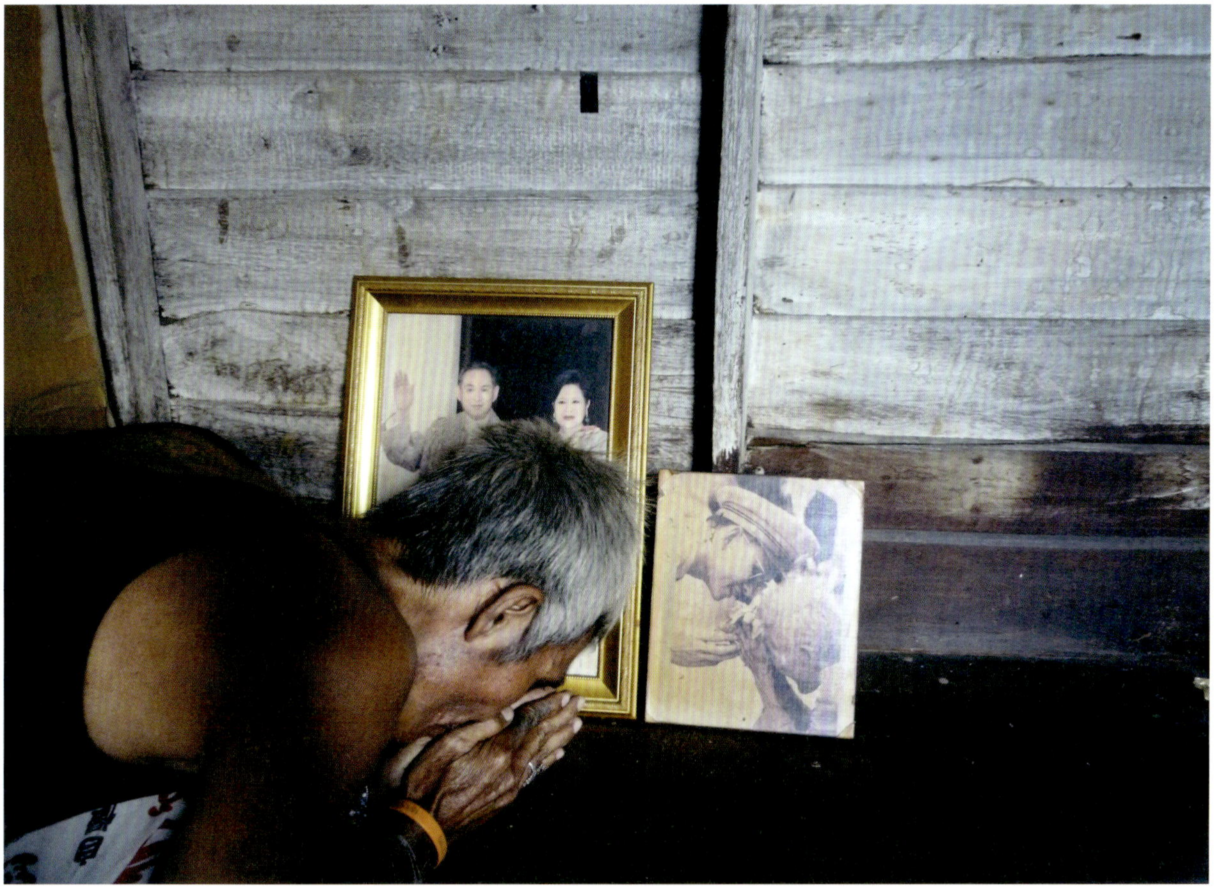

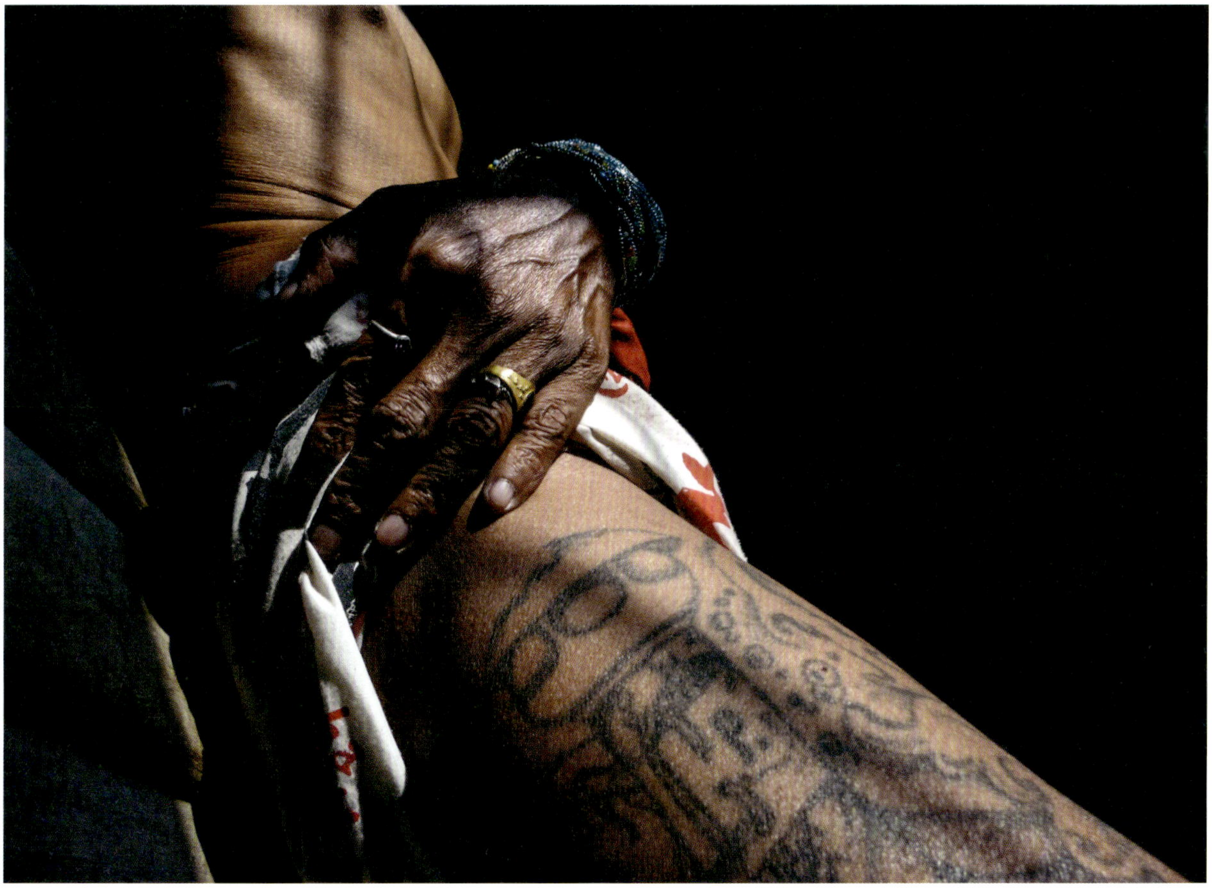

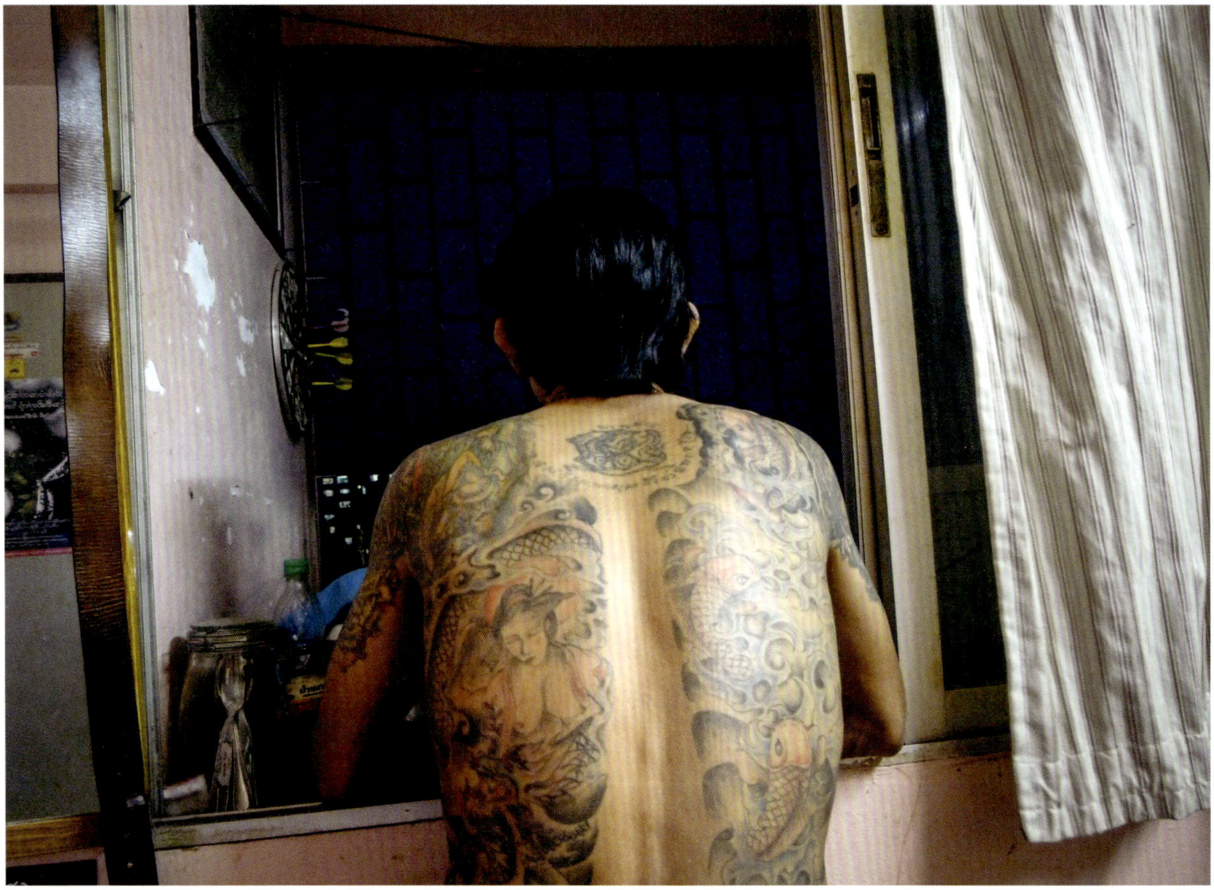

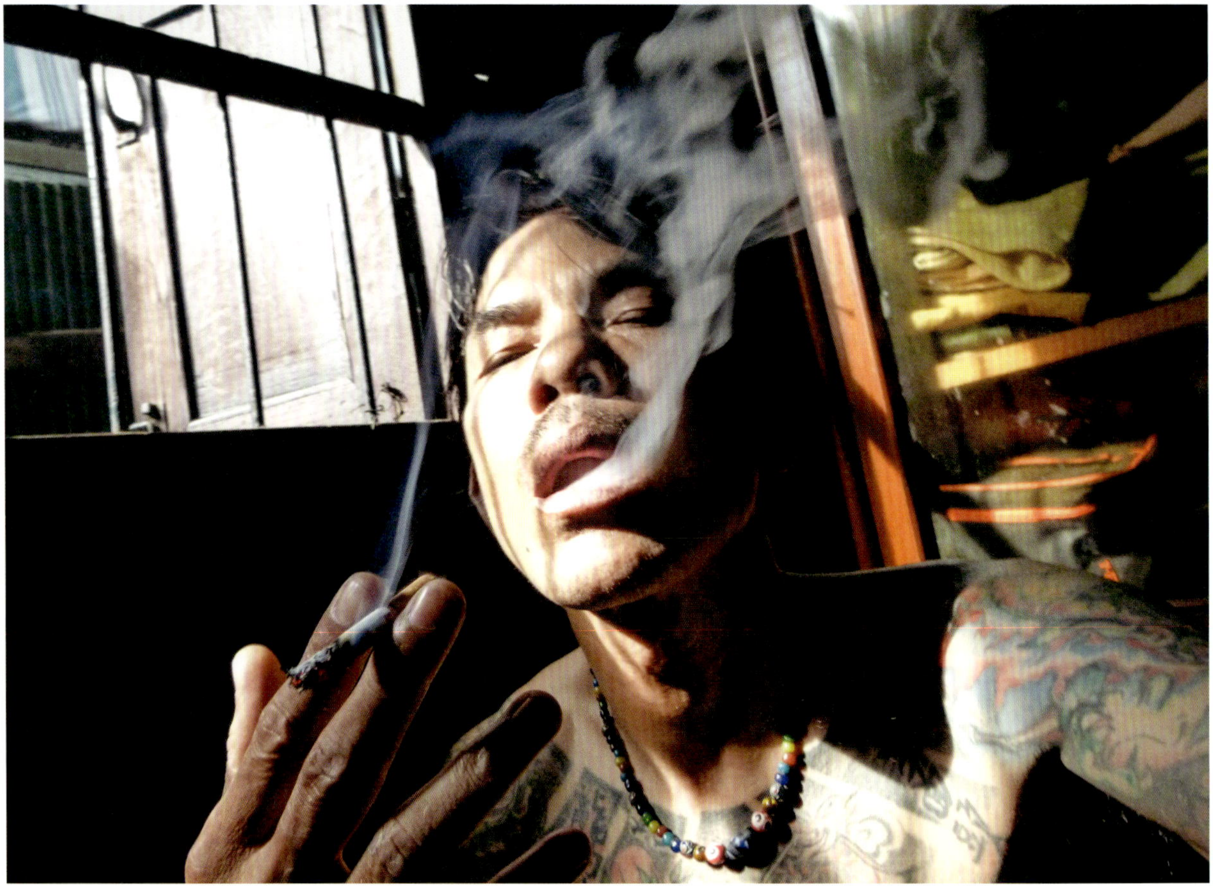

Jo

Heroin was easier to find than needles. Possession of needles was against the law. This situation practically forced drug users to share needles. One needle would be used by seven to eight people.

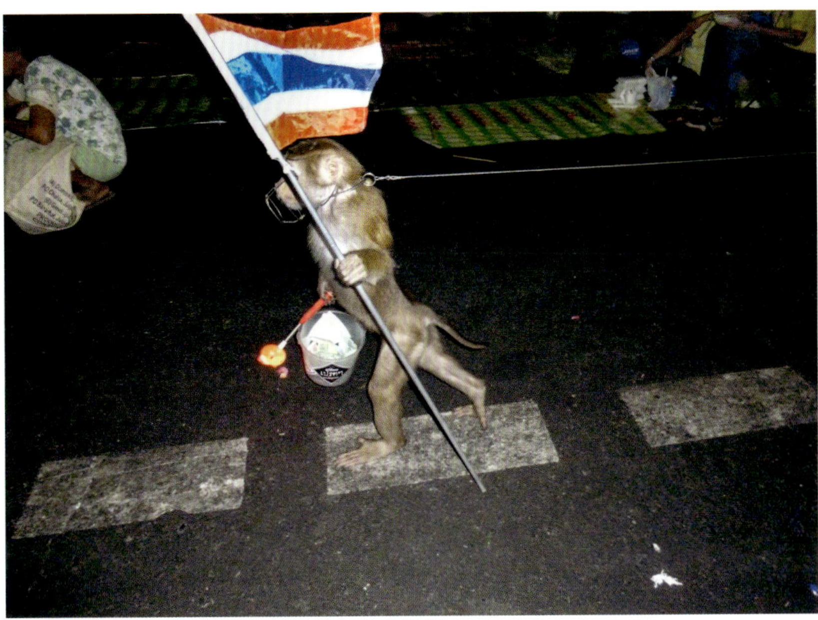

I grew up in a broken family. My uncle raised me along with my cousin, but it seemed like all the love went to his own child. So I acted out by doing drugs to get attention. I was a bad boy. I tried all kinds of drugs. I always said to myself that it was only once, that I could always quit. But it didn't turn out to be as easy as that.

The year I turned twenty, I entered the military. My new friends at the base had access to all sorts of drugs. By the time I finished service, I was fully addicted, had no job, and no money. I was enslaved to drugs. I didn't care how I got money for drugs. I did anything, from robbing to stealing to picking pockets. I was in and out of prison nine times.

Eventually, I switched from smoking heroin to injecting it. I shared needles with others without knowing what a bad idea that was. Heroin was easier to find than needles. Possession of needles was against the law. This situation practically forced drug users to share needles. One needle would be used by seven to eight people.

I kept my HIV diagnosis a secret from my family. Well, no one would have paid attention anyway. None of my family members ever came to visit me when I was in prison. Five years later I felt so ill that I knew I was in a critical stage. Opportunistic ailments attacked my body. So I decided to tell my family. They couldn't accept my bad news. I contacted a support group for people living with HIV and AIDS and told them I needed a place to stay. There I received the right medicine and got better after two years.

I am a loner, no one from my family wants me. They are disgusted with me because I am still a drug addict receiving methadone treatment. I speak the truth about my life now so that others in society know about the behaviors that can transmit HIV. I try to raise awareness among youth by using my life as an example. Anyone who takes risks like I have has a chance of getting HIV too. But as long as I am breathing I won't give up.

Aoy

Even though I'm HIV-infected, it doesn't mean I don't care about my personal beauty. I can make myself look good. I don't want society to see HIV as something pathetic. I don't want them to feel sorry for me.

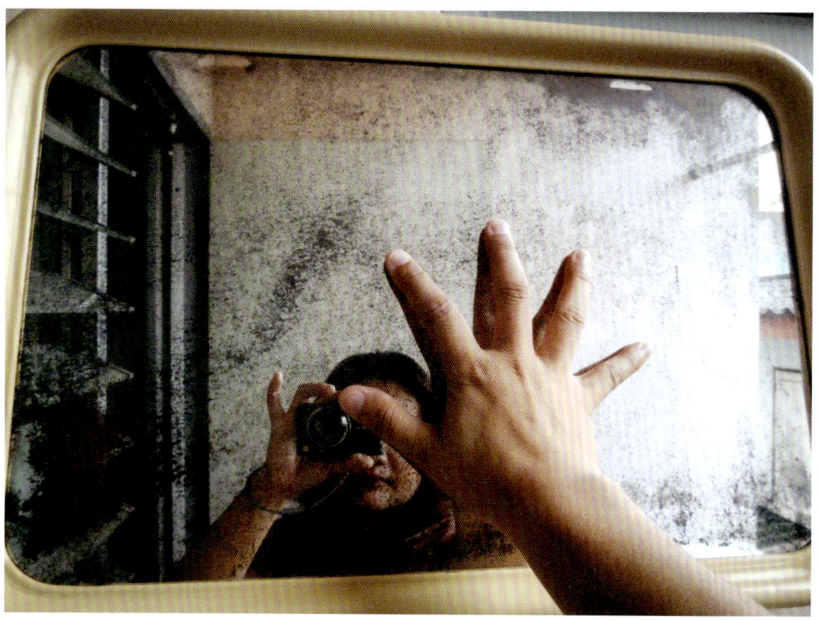

I became infected with HIV ten years ago, when I was thirty, from sexual intercourse with my boyfriend. At first, my reaction was just as you would expect. I was shocked. And also, I was worried that people would judge me. But then I met a group of new friends living with HIV. I realized that people with HIV can live for so many years. And I thought to myself, "Why can't I stay alive too?"

I take my medicine and care for myself, both body and soul. That's why I'm still here now. I have to be very careful about the timing of my medication. I wish there were a cure, so that I didn't have to take it anymore. Each medicine has a different side effect. As a result, my body has changed. I do exercises every morning to help get a better shape, to help reduce my lipodystrophy—body bulge is a common side effect from taking HIV medications. It's not like I'm fat, but it's not natural. When I look at myself naked in the mirror I feel that I look like a monster. Before, I had the normal curves. Now, I have a hump on the back, and I have a distended tummy. My right fingertips feel numb. I can't even make a fist. Nobody knows the pain that I get from my HIV medication. Nobody else feels it. But I know it, and I feel it.

If we don't want people to stamp HIV on our foreheads, then we have to take better care of our appearance. Even though I'm HIV-positive, it doesn't mean I don't care about my personal beauty. I can make myself look good. I don't want society to see HIV as something pathetic. I don't want them to feel sorry for me.

My personal space is my home. Home is the happiest place on earth for me. I feel relaxed and refreshed when I enter my door after a long day at work. I enjoy my time watching TV, relaxing, listening to the music, cleaning the house, and doing my hobbies. I am a neat person. Every morning, even if I'm running late, even if I'm in a rush, I sweep and clean my room. If my room isn't clean when I come back from work and I'm tired, I can get very annoyed—so annoyed it can cause me a migraine.

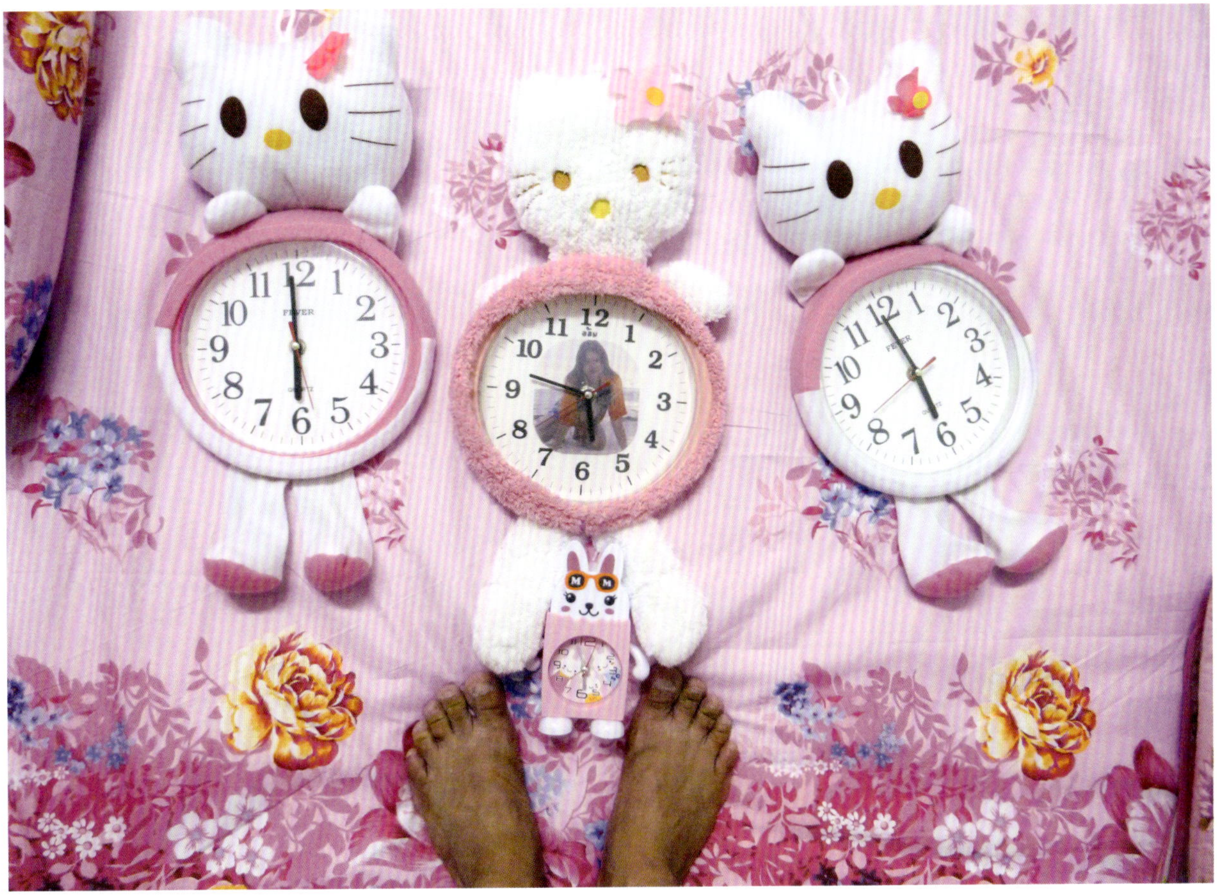

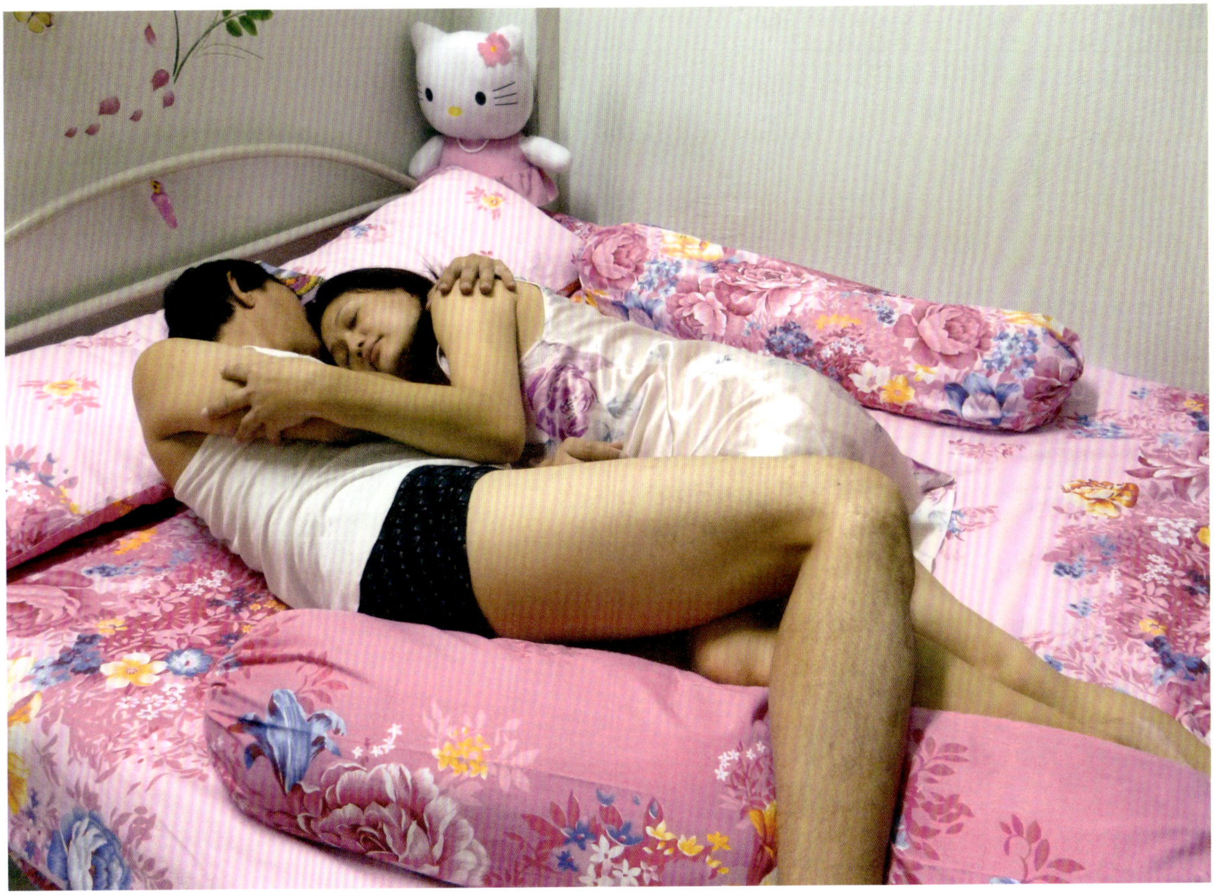

Keng

The big question for me now is, how can I live happily while having HIV in my body? If you can't win over your own mind, you can't win over HIV.

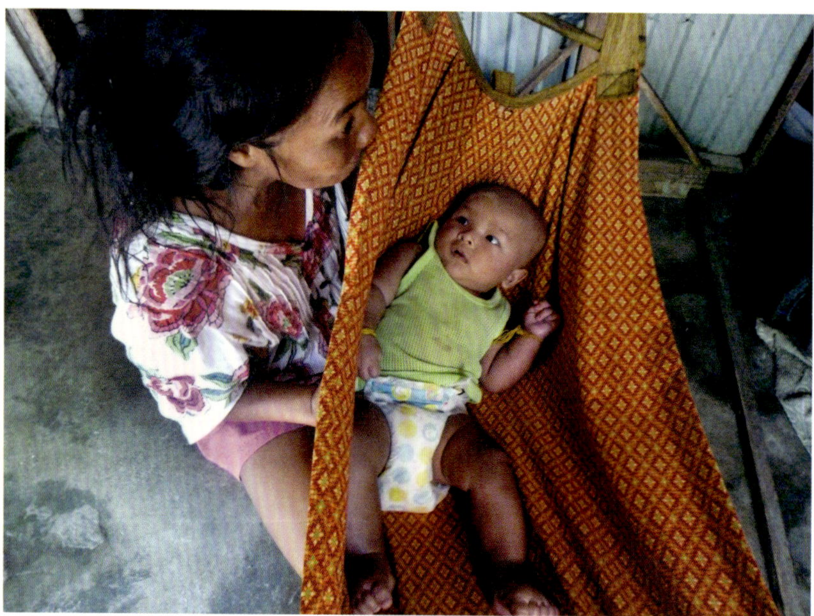

In my teens I was addicted to drugs. I think I got HIV from sharing needles. I found out I was HIV-infected during my pregnancy with Nong Kao, my third child. I didn't pay much attention. I only knew from the media that this ailment was sure to end in death. I was, however, scared by the thought that my kid would get the infection from me. Nonetheless, it seems that the baby wanted to be born, and to live.

The doctor said I couldn't breastfeed and that I had to be very strict about administering drops to the baby every four hours for two months. I paid strict attention to the doctor's instructions. I didn't want my baby to get infected on account of me.

During the time I was very sick, I received love and support from my mother and my daughter. My mother took care of me. Three of her children have died from HIV. I am the only one who survived. One of the staff at the hospital asked me, "Keng, don't you want to live and spend your life with your lovely son?" Encouragement was important. If I hadn't heard those words, I wouldn't have thought about who would take care of my kids and family. I couldn't die now. I recovered so fast. It took me only two months.

My son and I are very close. Little by little, I have explained to him about my illness. The big question for me now is, how can I live happily while having HIV in my body? If you can't win over your own mind, you can't win over HIV.

These days, I love watching movies and listening to music, when I come back home after work, sitting in front of the TV or computer, enjoying programs or games together. Our family routine is to watch movies—at least three—before going to bed. I cook meals for everyone. When I cook, I prepare massive quantities. I love to eat and want everyone to be well fed. When the kids have days off or holidays, we always go out for some fun. They take me to fish and to play in the nearby canal with them. I always go and sit in the sun waiting for them to catch fish. Once they catch one, we release it back. We don't want to kill it. I love to be with all the kids. They make me so happy.

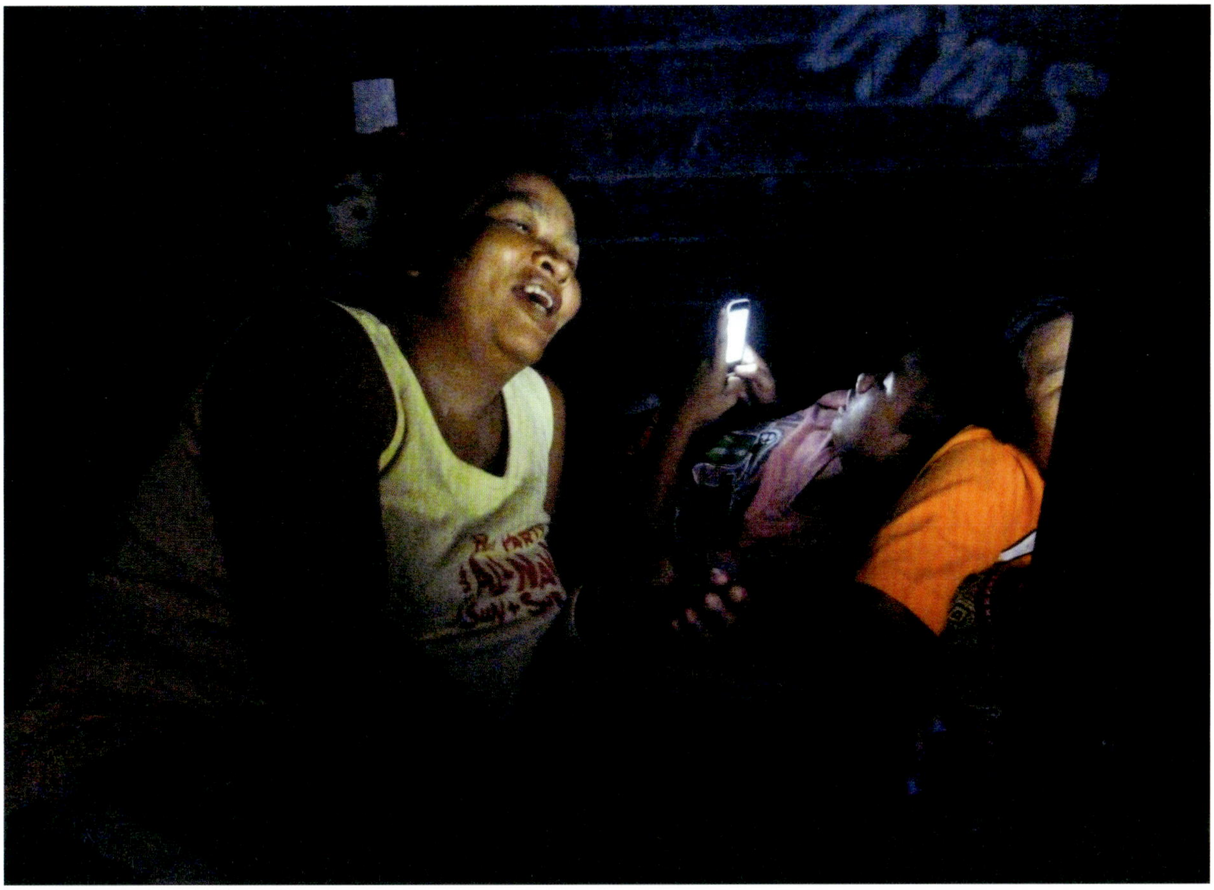

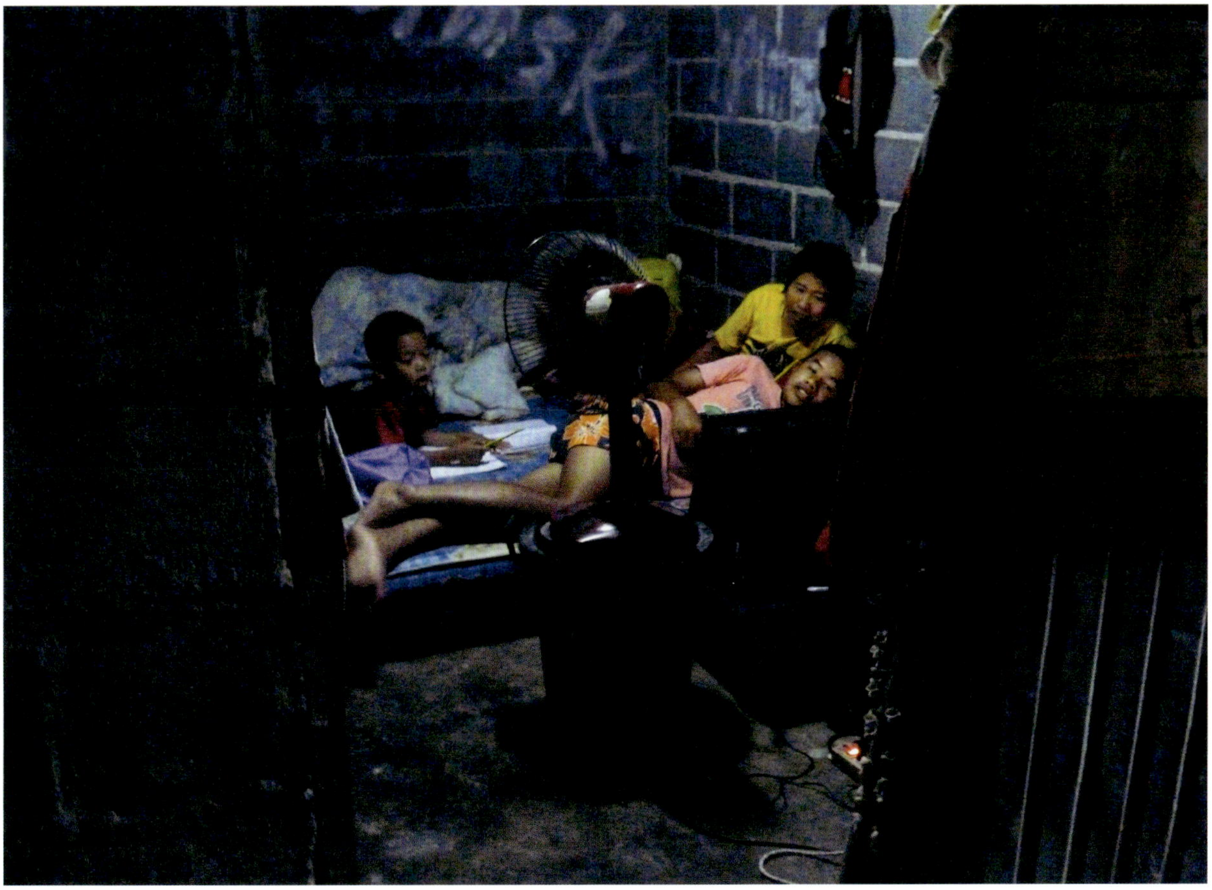

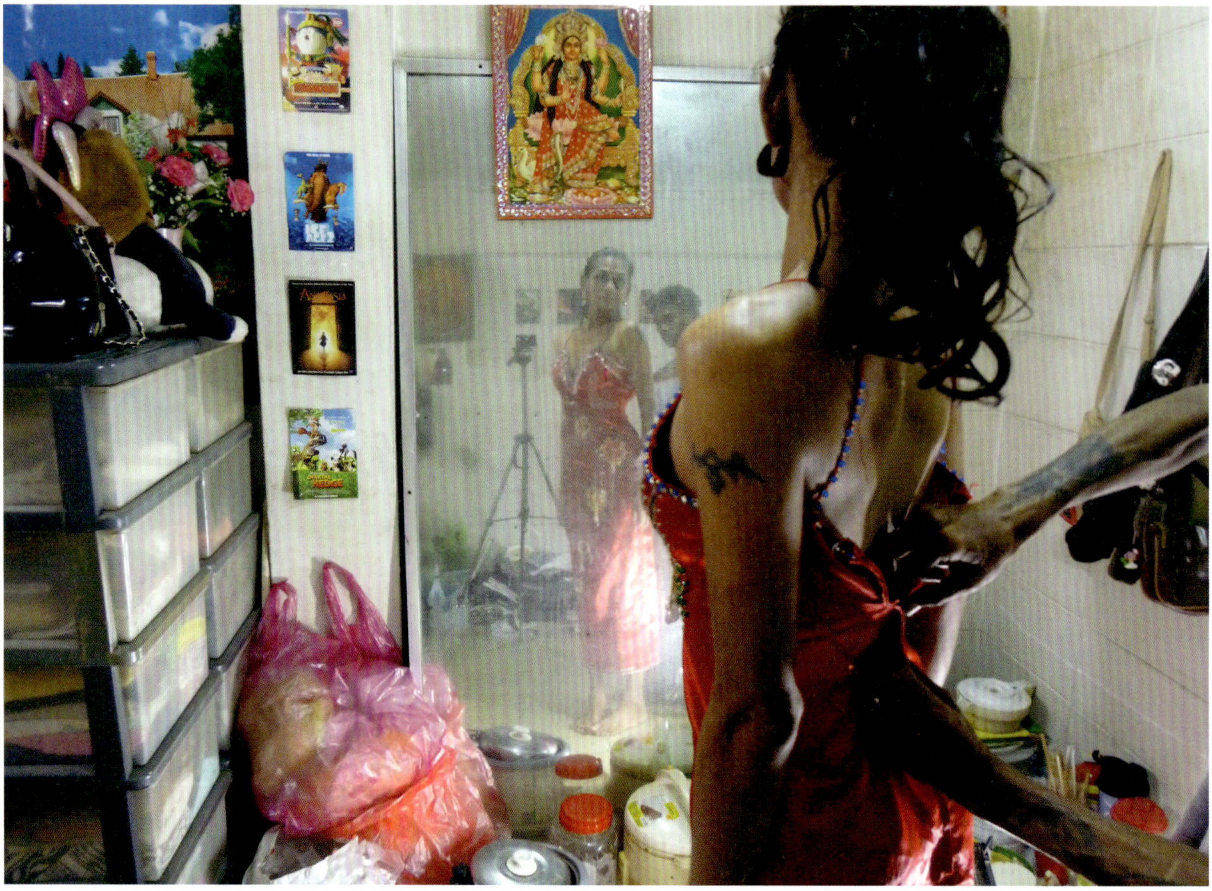

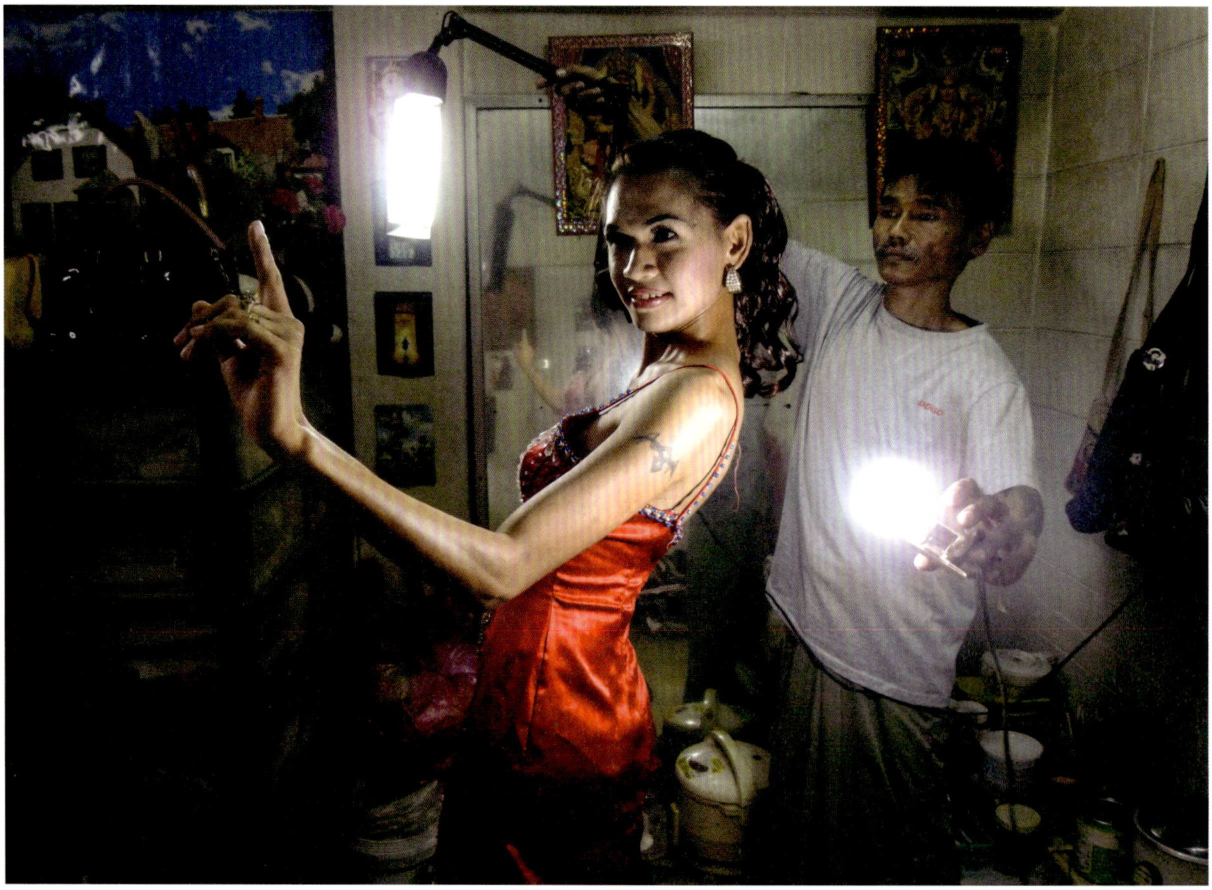

Bee

It's hard to be different from others. But am I afraid? At first I was so scared of HIV, but once I got to know and learn about it, it wasn't that scary anymore.

Some people accept my being a lady boy. I have felt like this since I was a child.

Every lady boy's dream is to be just like a real woman, with breasts and female sexual organs. I dreamed of saving money for the operation when I grew up. But when I finally saved up enough money for the operation, my dream was shattered. The transgender operation was impossible, because I have HIV. My boyfriend at the time was an injecting drug user. And I was a sex worker. So I never knew for sure how I got HIV. In the end, I only got the boob job.

For a time, I felt very down. I used to have nobody with me. My dad and mom didn't want anything to do with me because I'm transgender and HIV-positive. My parents have now passed away.

When I first entered show business, I started as a dancer. Then I got to be one of the lead lip-synch performers. The first song I lip-synched on the stage was "Miss Saigon."

Most people think that a dancer's life is exciting, wearing all those wonderful costumes. I worked as a show dancer and sex worker at the same time. Sex work is the easier way to earn money. I've never seen a job ad for a lady boy, though the lady boy situation has become much more open now than it used to be. For example, flight attendants can be lady boys now. As for military service, in the past they always identified lady boys as mental misfits. Now the policy has changed to identify lady boys as people who inhabit their gender differently from when they were born. I want to use my life as an example to newcomer lady boys, that they should be extra careful.

It made me so happy and proud to be a lady boy when a real man asked me to marry him. I keep this wedding photo to be displayed at my own funeral, in case one day something happens to me. This photo will show that I was beautiful once.

Sometimes I feel despair. I feel lonely. I feel like my life is at a crossroads. It's hard to be different from others. But am I afraid? At first I was so scared of HIV, but once I got to know and learn about it, it wasn't that scary anymore.

Auwn

One day, after overhearing me talk with someone on the phone, my landlord asked me, "Is it true that you have HIV?" I had to move out at three o'clock that very night.

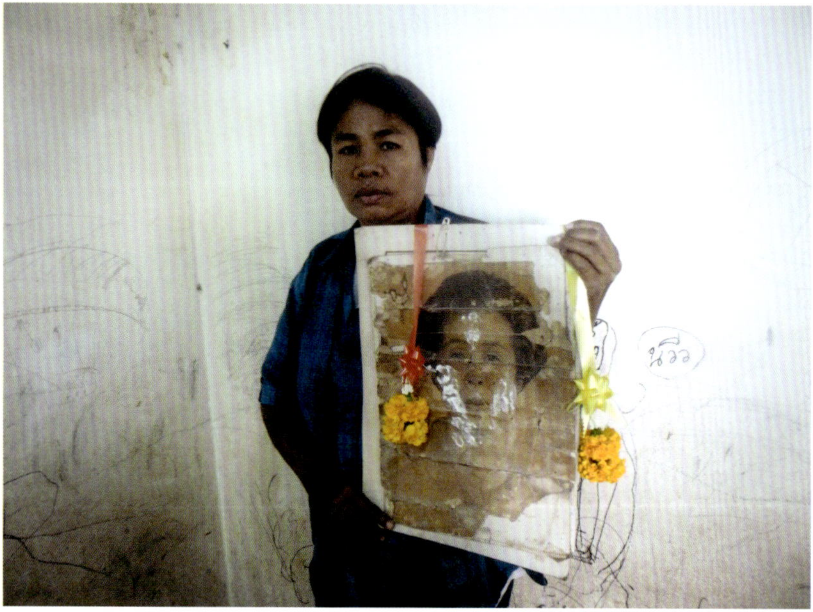

In my family I play the role of mother and father to everybody. I'm always reaching out to embrace and support others.

My partner, who had HIV, was a hard-working man, gentle to me, and he accepted my two children from a previous relationship. I was a good housewife, taking care of the housework and cooking for him. I got pregnant, and that's when the doctor told me I was HIV-infected. When we found out, both of us fell into silence.

My partner would not let me have an abortion. The doctor thought I should, but I kept my baby. My partner told me that whatever happened with the baby, we just had to do our best, until one night he was murdered at his job as a security guard. Suddenly I had no one. It felt like I had been shipwrecked.

I went back to see my relatives in our provincial home. They saw me with my two children and pregnant with a third, and they said, "Don't drop your burden on us." So I took my children, walked away, and got on the bus heading to Bangkok to find work. I drove a motorcycle taxi, taking passengers everywhere, until I had my baby. When my baby was only two months old, I was already working again, as a construction worker. One day, after overhearing me talk with someone on the phone, my landlord asked me, "Is it true that you have HIV?" I had to move out at three o'clock that very night. I moved continually from house to house. My children had to attend many schools to complete their studies.

Nothing is better than spending time with my family. Maybe it's not a lot, but it makes me happy. In my household, my children and grandchildren do not have any problem with my HIV condition. I am satisfied with what I have now. I never have any thought about wanting a bigger house or wanting more rooms. Never.

Now I am forty-four years old. I have been HIV-infected for eighteen years. I am a family lady who has raised three children by myself, and seven grandchildren. From my outside appearance some might think I'm a tomboy or lesbian, but I'm not anything. I just want to have a healthy life. As long as I have my motorcycle I can do anything for everybody. If I were to give up my motorcycle, I would feel lost. It is my body, my life.

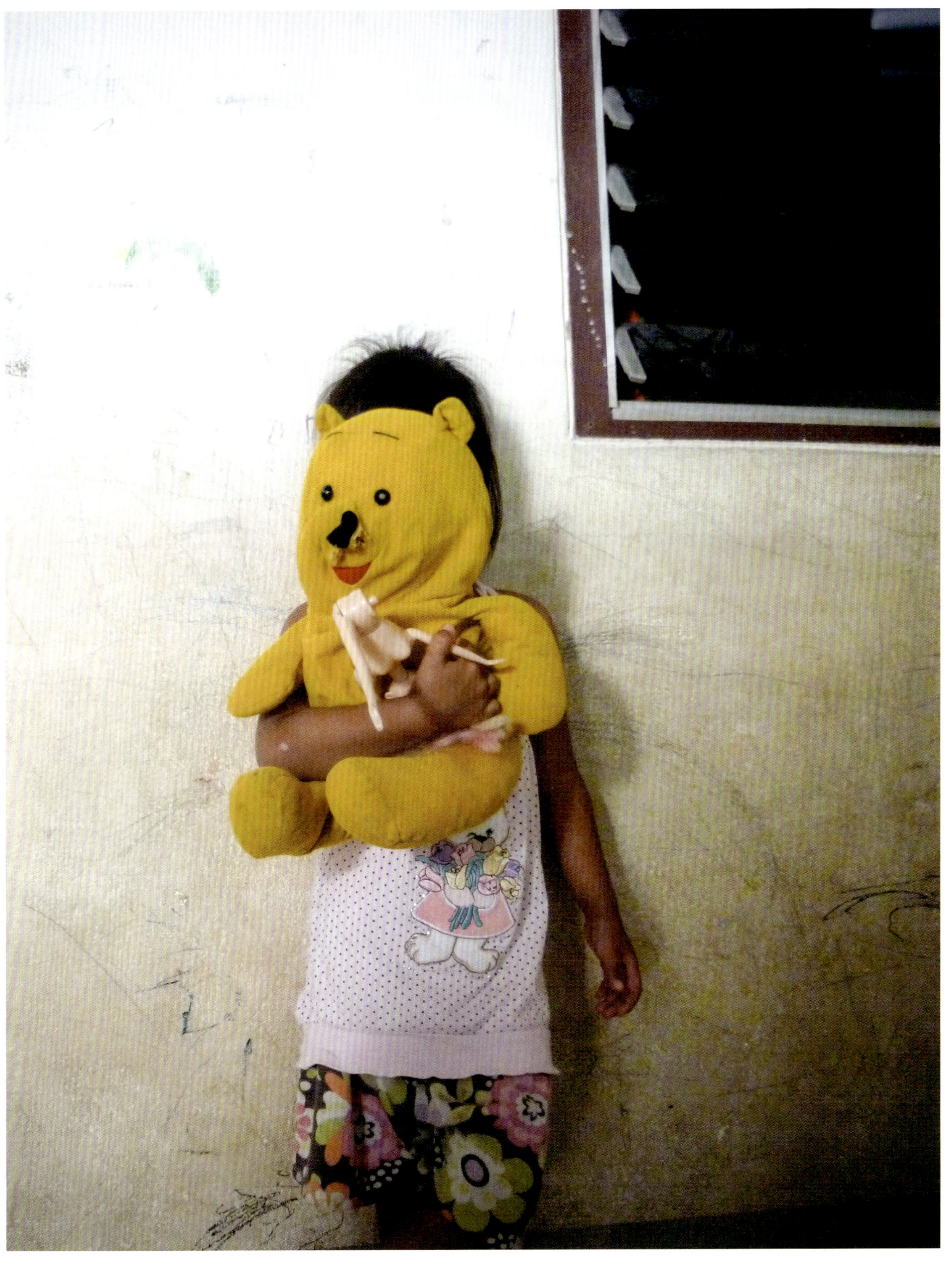

Jai

I got HIV from my partner, who liked buying sex. I told him if he couldn't stop messing around like that, he should at least use condoms. "If you were to get AIDS, what would we do?" Not long after that conversation, when I visited the doctor for antenatal care, they found that I had HIV. Luckily I had not given HIV to my baby.

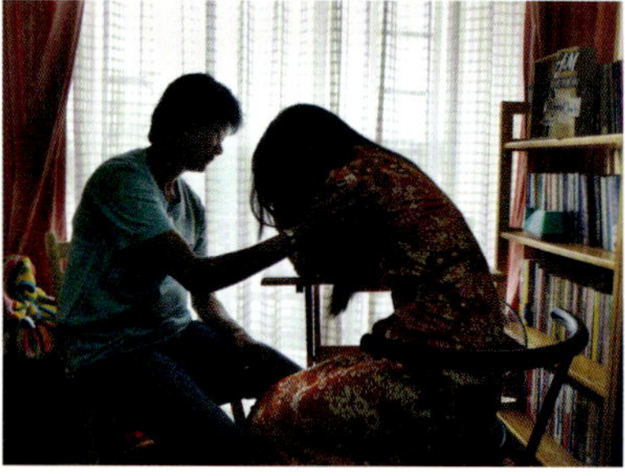

That day shattered my dreams. At that time there was no medication and the information I got was that I couldn't live beyond three years. When I came home I told my partner that I was infected and he said, "If I'm infected too, I'm committing suicide." I was so scared. I thought three years would be the end of my life. Soon after, my partner was diagnosed with fungus on his brain. He lived for another two years and died.

The day before three years was up, I was imagining how I would die, even though I was so healthy. I couldn't sleep at all—it would be my last night and last day! Then the morning came—I was still alive. I thought, well, I can continue to dream then. So I started to focus on raising my children. I would aim for them to go to school. I wanted them to graduate from primary school, junior high, high school, even earn a bachelor's degree, which my eldest child accomplished. I have faith. I want to live until fifty—I'm forty-three now so that will be another seven years.

Now I'm a counselor. I am often the first person a woman speaks to after finding out her HIV-positive status. I have to have a lot of self-control. I must be stable and not succumb to any personal emotions, because if I break down, it might trigger more sadness for the client. I have to encourage her, give her support.

When a woman comes to see me for counseling, she carries an emotional burden and needs to talk to someone. She doesn't know where to turn. But here, with me, she can talk about anything, and I will keep it secret. I wanted to do this counseling work because I remembered how I felt, how I needed to have someone to trust and talk to.

I am a giver of support, but I also want to be the receiver because I am also living with HIV. When I worry about myself I need somebody to listen to me. I need somebody to nurture me too.

Joe

In Bangkok, gay life and society means extravagance. I spent money on expensive stuff and, to be frank, I slept around. But every time I had sex with anyone, I always used condoms. That's why I'm not sure how I got infected. I guess it happened when I got drunk one night. On account of my drunkenness, I don't remember what happened.

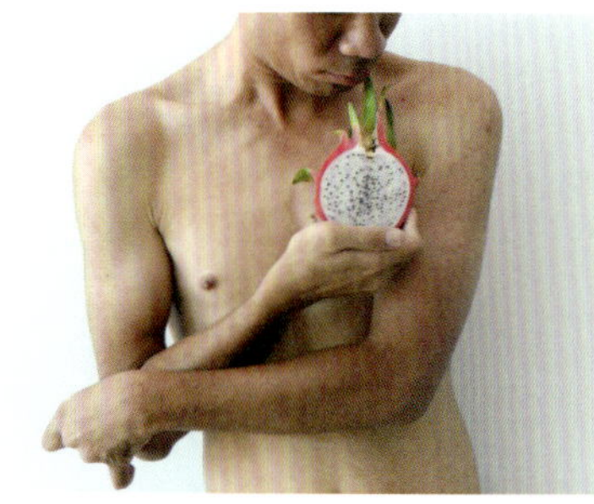

Everything drastically changed when I got HIV. After my diagnosis, I decided to be ordained. My father is a Buddhist monk. We went to Chiang Rai and stopped at Wat Rong Khun, a Buddhist temple. We had a photo taken there, the only photo taken during my monkhood.

Thereafter, I was admitted to the hospital in my hometown, in Chonburi province. I told my mother and doctor that I had HIV. I was close to death. Eventually, when I started to get the right treatment and medicine, I got better.

I joined a Christian group where no one was unwelcoming to me. Everyone comfortably used the same glassware and plates as I did, knowing that nobody would get infected. I have learned that HIV can't spread this way to others. At the church, everyone knows who I am and what condition I have. The church is the most comfortable place for me. I am still a Buddhist. But I don't go to the Buddhist temple. I go to the Christian church instead.

The left side of my body is partially paralyzed due to an HIV-related fungal infection in the brain. If I could walk like normal, everything would be perfect. Although my body is not the same on both sides, I can still do things. I can take care of myself. I don't need to be a burden to anybody. The good half of my body allows me to continue with my life. I can do everything, as if nothing has happened. The whole fruit is completely beautiful but it doesn't mean that the cut fruit won't be beautiful too. It has a different, perhaps greater, beauty. This is my good half. My disability doesn't affect the beauty of my soul.

Maam

When I was pregnant with my third child, the doctor told me they found a problem with my blood.

I cried for seven days. I didn't eat anything. All I could do was cry. Then I discovered more information and realized that there was a way to live. If I took medicine as the doctor said, HIV would not transmit to my baby. I felt so great that she was born in good health. I hadn't done anything to hurt her. My kids know I have HIV, and they give me the strength to live. My eldest daughter says, "Mom, you have to be with us, we will live together. When I grow up, I will take care of you."

My current husband is my third and he is a good guy. We have been together more than ten years and he still treats me nicely. I am so happy. I am happy everyday now.

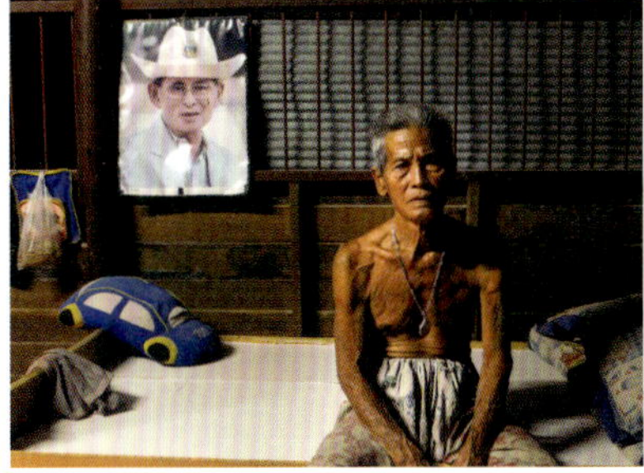

On normal days I volunteer at the hospital. Otherwise I sell fruit in the market. Until photography refreshed my eyes, the produce in the market didn't look interesting or appetizing to me. I lived there everyday. I got jaded. I was so worried at first when I started shooting photos in the market, but I had fun once I got going. When I saw the photos afterward, I felt so alive.

Normally, my father-in-law and I are not close. So I was surprised that he let me take his photo. He likes to sit there, watching TV. I think it reminds him of watching with his wife. Behind him, on the wall, is a portrait of the King, who is a father figure too.

Looking in the mirror I think to myself, I am just an ordinary thirty-six-year-old woman, a mother and wife, but I am still capable of taking care of everyone in the family. The mirror reflects who I am and my life. I have to look after myself. If I don't take care of myself, how can I take care of others?

Sometimes there are four kids sitting on the bed while I am doing other things. You can see the affection among us.

Family is my medicine, healing my wounds. Sometimes I completely forget I have HIV.

No

I was an unruly young person. I ran away from home. I wanted to work and earn money and dress beautifully. When I was about seventeen, I became a go-go dancer—a sex worker—in a bar. My first drug was cocaine. My main addiction was heroin. Later when I was in prison, I began to bleed badly. My friend took me to the hospital infirmary for blood testing. The result showed that I had HIV. I remembered that I had shared needles twice when I was in prison. I'm sure that I got HIV by using the same needle as others. After that, sometimes I sat and cried and almost injected heroin to kill myself by overdosing.

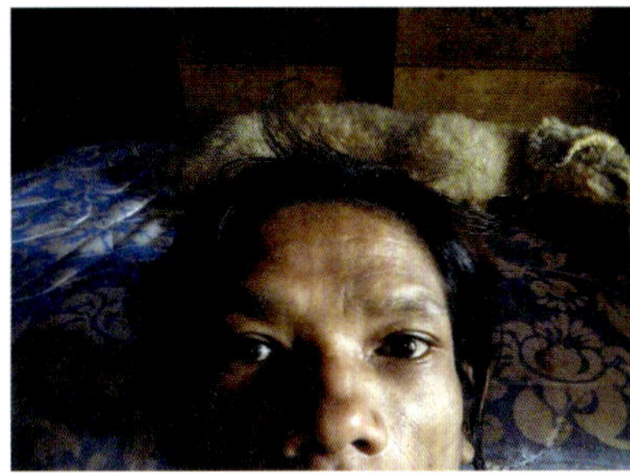

Then I met Aoi, another *Through Positive Eyes* participant. Aoi takes methadone and he doesn't suffer and still can work. So I take it too. I can take care of the house and hold down other jobs as well. When I wake up in the morning, I rouse Aoi to go to the methadone clinic. When we come back home, I let him rest.

At this point, at the age of forty, I have been on treatment for three years. When I don't take methadone, I behave badly. I'm easily upset and moody. When that happens, I feel bad for my dogs. I love them so much and I love my little family here. I don't want to see my dogs get sad.

I sometimes miss my past, when I was being myself, the real Anocha, who could go anywhere, dress any way, and do anything I wanted to. I am thinking of writing my life story, from the beginning, starting when I became a go-go dancer and continuing until I ended up with HIV. If I could turn back time, I wouldn't have run away from home. As it is, I have a broken relationship with my family. I only talk with them on the phone. I never visit them and they never visit me. I just got so lost in the colorful nightlife and money.

The three things that encourage me to live my life are the dogs, Aoi, and my community. I always tell myself to fight for my life and stay in this society without the fear of others looking down on me. Now, wherever I go, I feel so proud that I haven't caused any trouble to anybody, and that I am a good person.

Sam

Hailing from the economically depressed northern part of the country, I always dreamed of having more money and seeking better security in life.

Once I moved to Bangkok, I did things I would never have done before. Attractive people, bright colors and lights, nice clothes, sound and music —these things could seduce anyone. The city was a new experience for me. I could do anything I wanted for the first time in my life, such as traveling, smoking cigarettes, drinking alcohol, and going out at night. Greed made me focus on doing anything that could earn me lots of money—the easy job with a big payoff.

Because of all that money, I told myself, "Just give it a try. It won't hurt you." I am not sure how I got HIV. It could have been from working for a sex service, from the clients, or it could have been from the girlfriend I had at that time. Unfortunately, life is not a game that we can replay when things go wrong.

Today I live life as an HIV patient. As I take my HIV medication, I lean on Lord Buddha. He gives me peace and calm. But I am proud that I have learned a lot about life. I got sick, that's all. What has been done already, I can't change. If I could turn back the clock, I wouldn't want to be infected. I wish I could be healthy, as if nothing happened.

As it is, now that I am twenty-eight years of age, at least my life story could serve as a lesson to others. Some days my life feels empty. At the very end, all humans leave nothing behind. Being born, making money, getting sick, dying—it's all the same. A stable thing can also be unstable. I need love, warmth, and intimacy. Loneliness makes me feel like I am in the dark shadows. So, everyday I make my life as happy as I can. I always think that today is my last day because I don't know how long I will live.

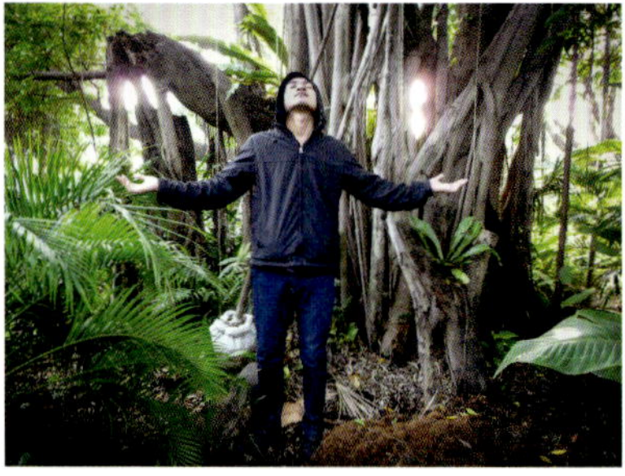

Wat

I fell very ill and had to be admitted to the hospital. I told no one but my mother. My doctor told me I wouldn't live long. But my mother refused to believe it. She said, "I have eight children and I won't let any of them die before I do." I trusted her more than the doctor. What she said made me realize that I wanted to live.

At that time, I asked my mother whether I could pay my respects to her by washing her feet. I thought it would be my last chance to do so. My mom patted me on the head and said, "Stay. I want you to stay." From that moment, I knew I would live. This became an annual ritual. On my birthday, I wash her feet to mark the fact that both of us are still here.

My mother's words made me want to fight. The doctor gave me medicine but my mother gave me strength. After taking medicine for about a year, my CD4 infection-fighting cells increased and my health improved. This proved that the medicine was effective. But at the same time, many other patients couldn't access medicine because of its price. So I joined a treatment access group in Bangkok and was chosen to be a regional leader. Our agenda was to demand that the government finance an HIV medication program by initiating a national tax. We succeeded.

Now, societal stigma is our biggest problem. In Thai culture, HIV is associated with bad karma. People consider it to be the illness of sexual deviants and drug users, who have accrued bad karma in the past. This is why I help distribute meds to people who live far away or can't afford to see a doctor. When people are short on medication, they call me and I help them. I encourage them to take their medications properly, and to disclose their HIV status to their loved ones. It's better that way. One client I work with was sick for sixteen years, but he only just got on medication three months ago because he didn't know about his right to get free medication.

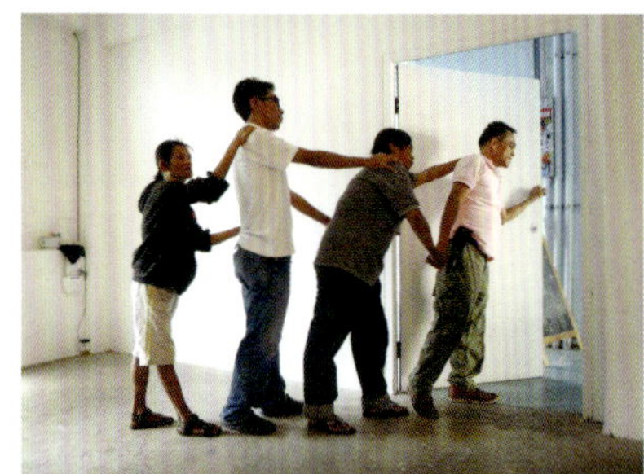

When I'm home I always exercise to be strong. I meditate to calm the mind, allowing it to be empty. We can't control life. We have to set it free. If I don't love myself, who is going to love me? If I get sick, who will take care of others?

Port-au-Prince

From the very beginning of the global AIDS epidemic, Haitians have been stigmatized as one of the originally identified risk groups for HIV infection, alongside homosexuals and hemophiliacs. In Haiti, high levels of HIV stigma—including internalized self-stigma—have continued, as reported by the participants in the *Through Positive Eyes* workshop held in Port-au-Prince, Haiti's capital city, in December 2014. A house being set on fire, a Christian priest rejecting a beloved parishioner, gossiping neighbors, a father who refuses to speak to his son—all these real-life examples attest to the negative impacts of stigma on people living with HIV and AIDS in Haiti. And yet, over the past decade, Haiti has witnessed a 25% reduction in new infections and AIDS deaths, a remarkable achievement that gives hope for an end to unwarranted stigma.

Haiti's AIDS epidemic, as of 2014

Number of people living with HIV: 130,000

HIV prevalence

Adults (15–49 years): 1.7%

There is no data on prevalence in key populations for 2014.

Treatment

Limited treatment provided free since 2003 by Gheskio, with expanded national access since 2005.

Numbers on treatment (2012): 50,000

Key events

1982 *Haitians living with HIV diagnosed in U.S., leading to stigmatization of the country and economic downturn. President Duvalier reacts by making it illegal to mention HIV or AIDS.*

2001 *President Aristide initiates government policies to prevent and treat HIV.*

2012 *A survey reports 58% of Haitians would not buy vegetables from a person living with HIV.*

Update 2019

Between 2010 and 2017, new HIV infections decreased by 25% and AIDS-related deaths by 24%. By 2017 there were 150,000 Haitians living with HIV. Key populations most affected by HIV are sex workers, men who have sex with men, and prisoners, with an HIV prevalence of 8.4%, 18.2%, and 2.7%, respectively.

In 2016 it became national policy to treat all people living with HIV. In 2017 94,000 Haitians living with HIV (64%) were accessing antiretroviral therapy.

Through Positive Eyes in Port-au-Prince was organized in partnership with FotoKonbit, with assistance from Foundation Esther Boucicault Stanislas (FEBS), Gheskio, and Zanmi Lasante/Partners in Health. Major funding was provided by The Herb Ritts Foundation, with additional support from The Ford Foundation, Teiger Foundation, Gere Foundation, and UCLA.

Emmanuel

One day in 2008, I stood up and openly admitted that I was gay and was living with HIV. This was the first time a Haitian had made such a public declaration. A few days later, they burned my house.

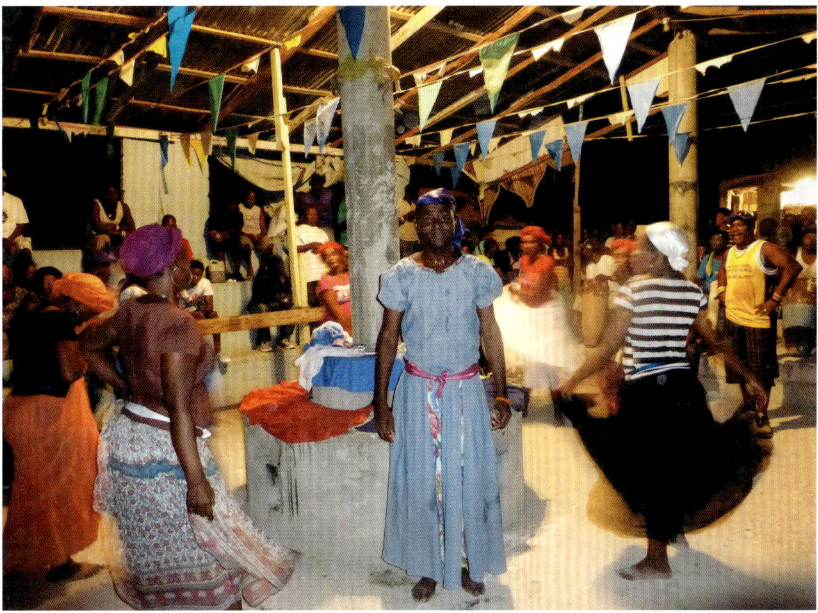

When someone first receives their test results and realizes they have HIV, they believe their life is over. One thing I always say to someone newly infected is this: It's not the end of life. It's more like a new phase of life. After I got my positive test result, I was motivated to get my gay friends to go take a test as well. For every twenty who went to get a test, eighteen of them were positive. A question I had asked myself was, "Why do gay men always die young in Haiti"? And I finally understood that it was because they were infected, did not get the right treatment, and died.

One day in 2008, I stood up and openly admitted that I was gay and was living with HIV. This was the first time a Haitian had made such a public declaration. A few days later, they burned my house, they threatened me. At that moment I gave myself a mission. I dedicated myself to serving my community by telling the truth: Gay life has a danger within it, and this is what we have to do to protect ourselves.

A lot of people think that vodou is the devil and other bad things. But it's a reality, it's a culture that all Haitians have in them. It's in our blood. Vodou is something I love very much. I love the sound of the drum. It makes me move my body, it makes me want to dance. I remember my first experience when I was just starting to dance vodou. The person who was teaching me said, "Vodou came from Africa. That is its history. To dance vodou well, whether you're a guy or a girl, you must wear a dress. There are movements that you will do while dancing and the dress will help you. The dress will move for you."

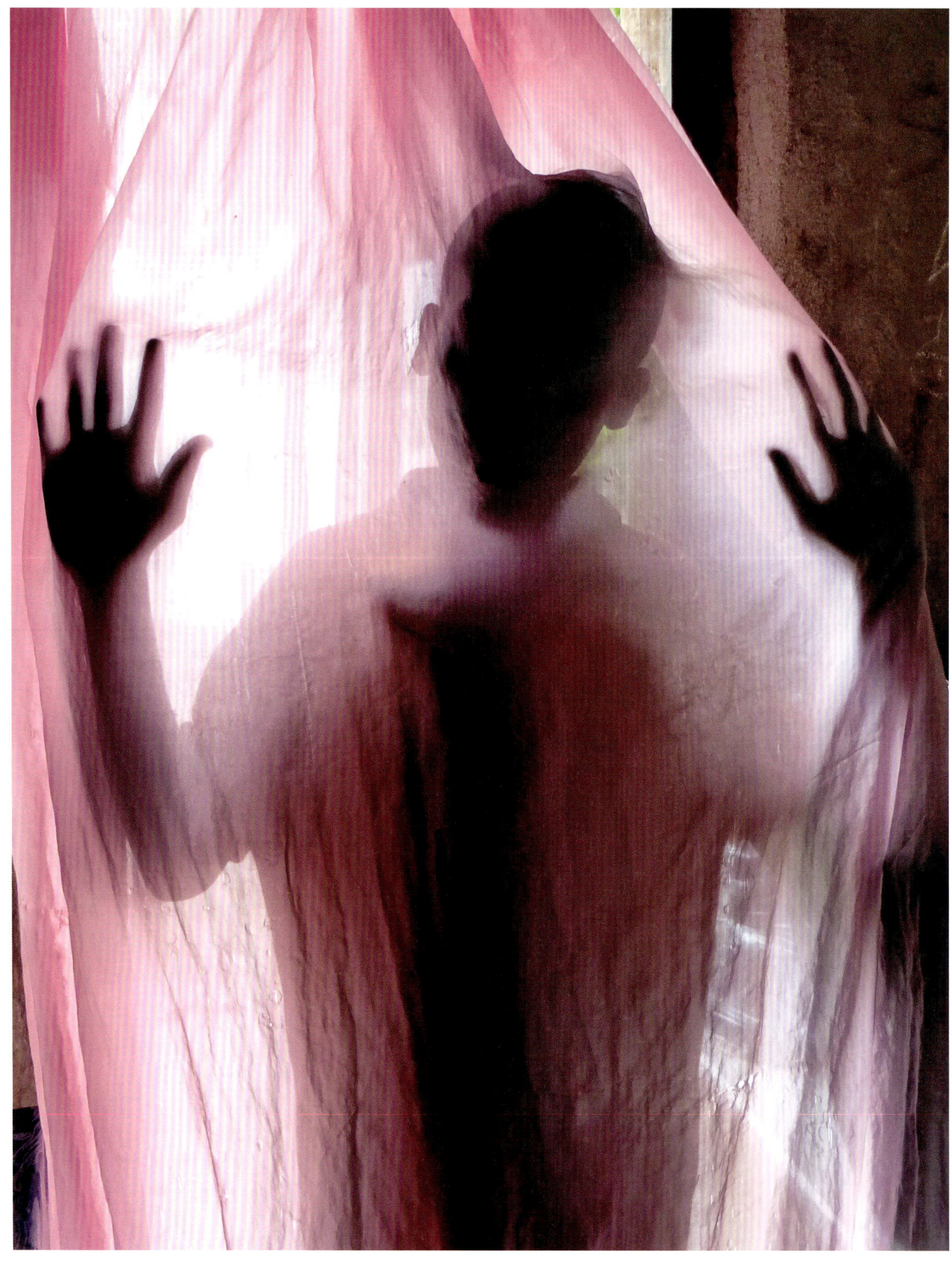

Medina

Sometimes I think, maybe I should have died, like my children's father. But then I say no, life is still beautiful. I will continue to drink my medication.

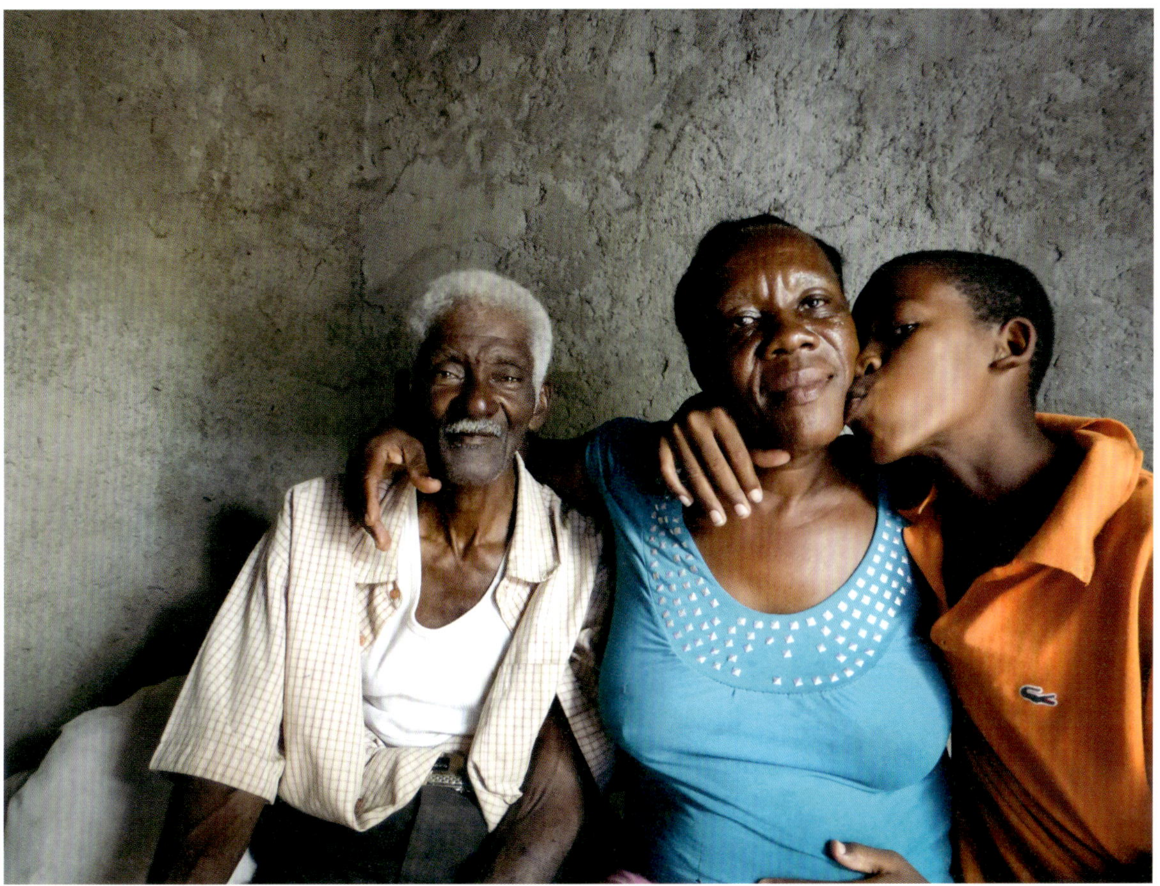

The father of my children died in 2004 from HIV, and that gave me a lot of problems. I cried. There are still people who stay away. They say I have HIV and that I can't live next to them. They are afraid and they talk amongst themselves, always pointing their fingers at me. But that does not trouble me anymore, because I have to take care of the education of my children. I am the only one left. Sometimes I think, maybe I should have died, like my children's father. But then I say no, life is still beautiful. I will continue to drink my medication.

We have an organization that just formed, and the patients say they want me, "Dina," to be the president, to represent them. I tell them all that they must take their medication. Because sometimes when you give them medicine, they put it under their tongue and spit it out later. Why do you think they put it under their tongue? Because they don't have food! When you give patients medicine, they should get something to eat. Give them food so they can really take the medication and not throw it away.

In the photos I have taken, I see how much my younger son supports me. I see he is there with me, everywhere. That makes me want to live.

Gaston

My father called me on the phone and said, "Don't call me again. All I owe you now is a coffin." And from that day on, I never spoke with my dad again.

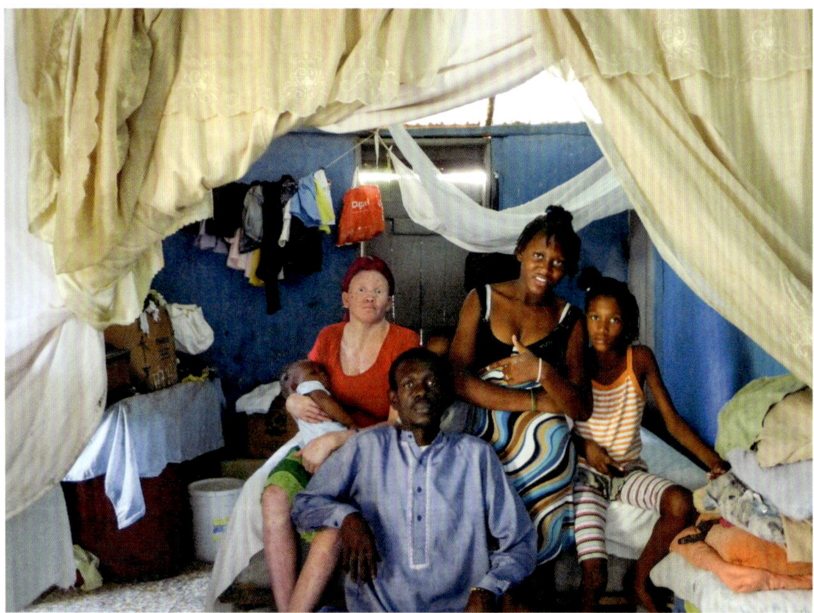

I have never tried to find out how I became HIV-positive. You know why I never wanted to find out? Because that would have made me an angry and mean person for sure.

I am the father of five children. I have known my status for ten years. HIV is in my blood, I deal with it. In 2014, AIDS should not be such a destroyer, it should not give us this much trouble. The stigma that we are subject to within our families is the hardest. My father humiliated me in my own house. Worst of all, he did not even do it face-to-face. He called me on the phone and said, "Don't call me again. All I owe you now is a coffin." And from that day on, I have never spoken with my dad again.

I remember my friend Robenson telling me that he was afraid of me. He was afraid to shake my hand, he was even afraid to walk next to me. Today, he is in my house, eating with me. We are eating off of the same plate, drinking from the same glass. I know that I am HIV-positive. I know how to protect myself and protect others. Today I can remove that veil, and tell other people like me, who continue to hide behind a veil, "It's time to break the chains."

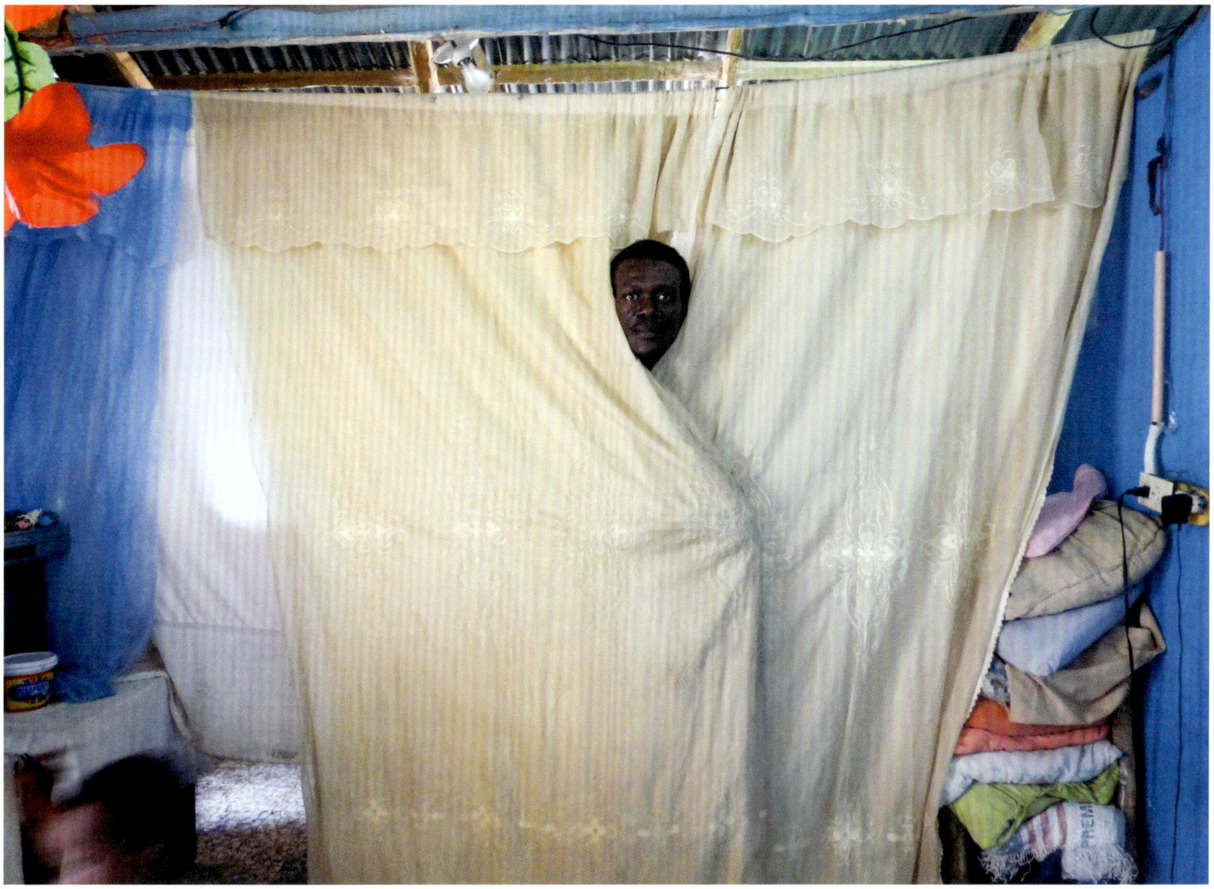

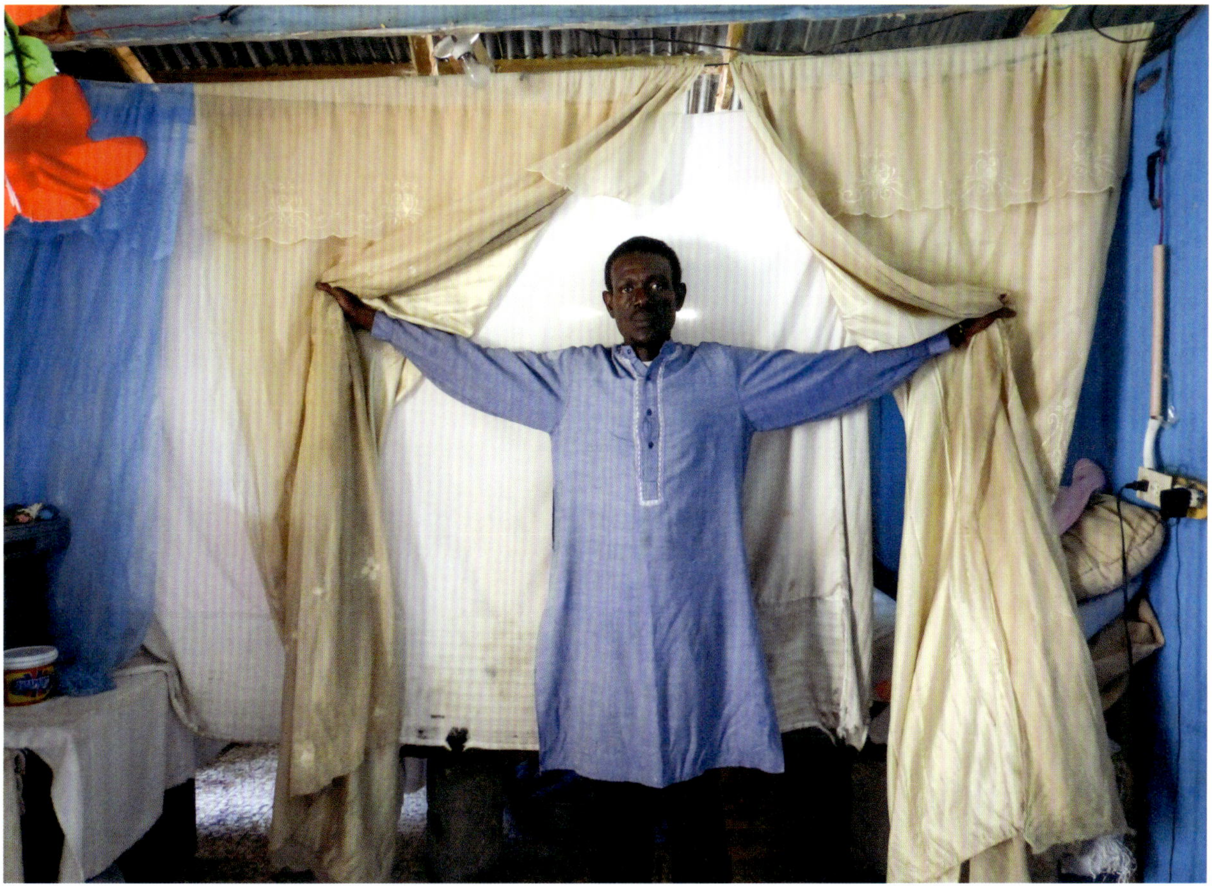

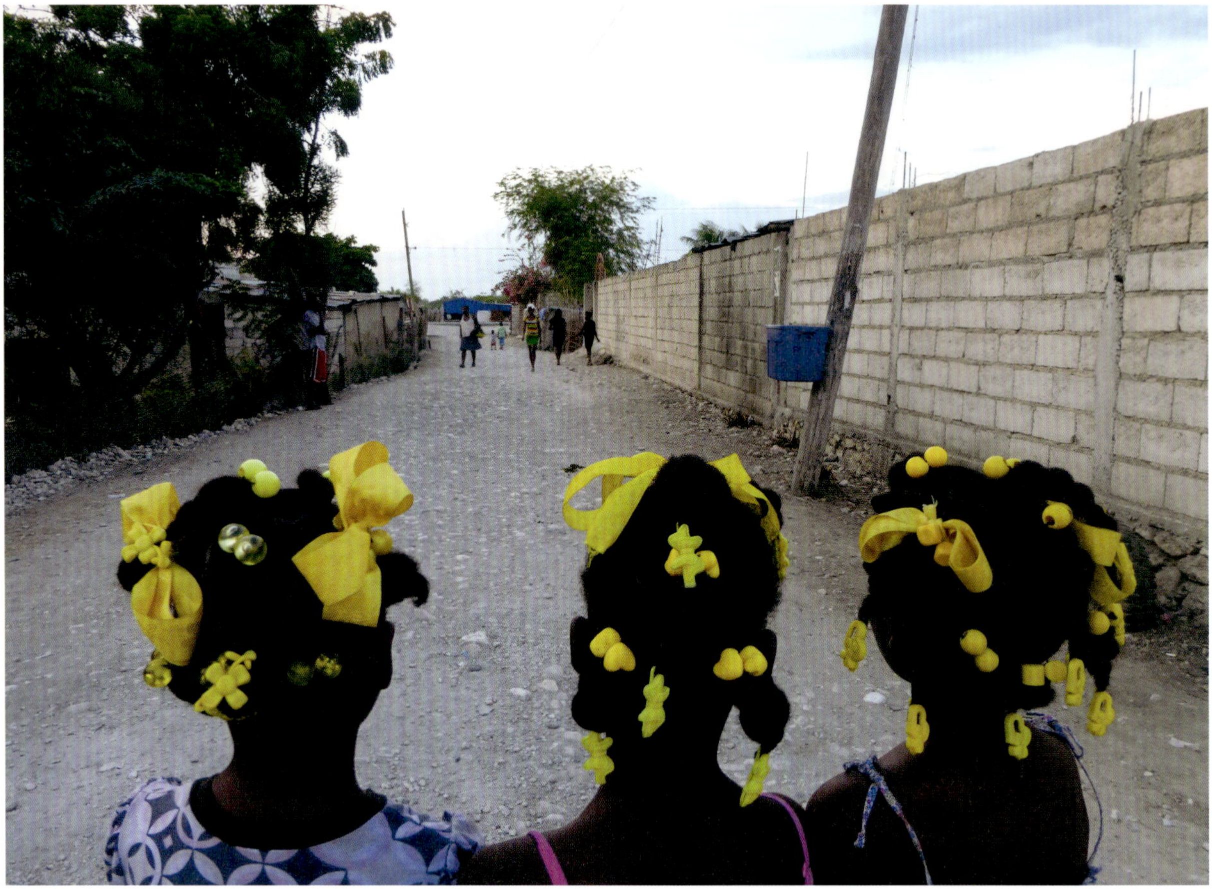

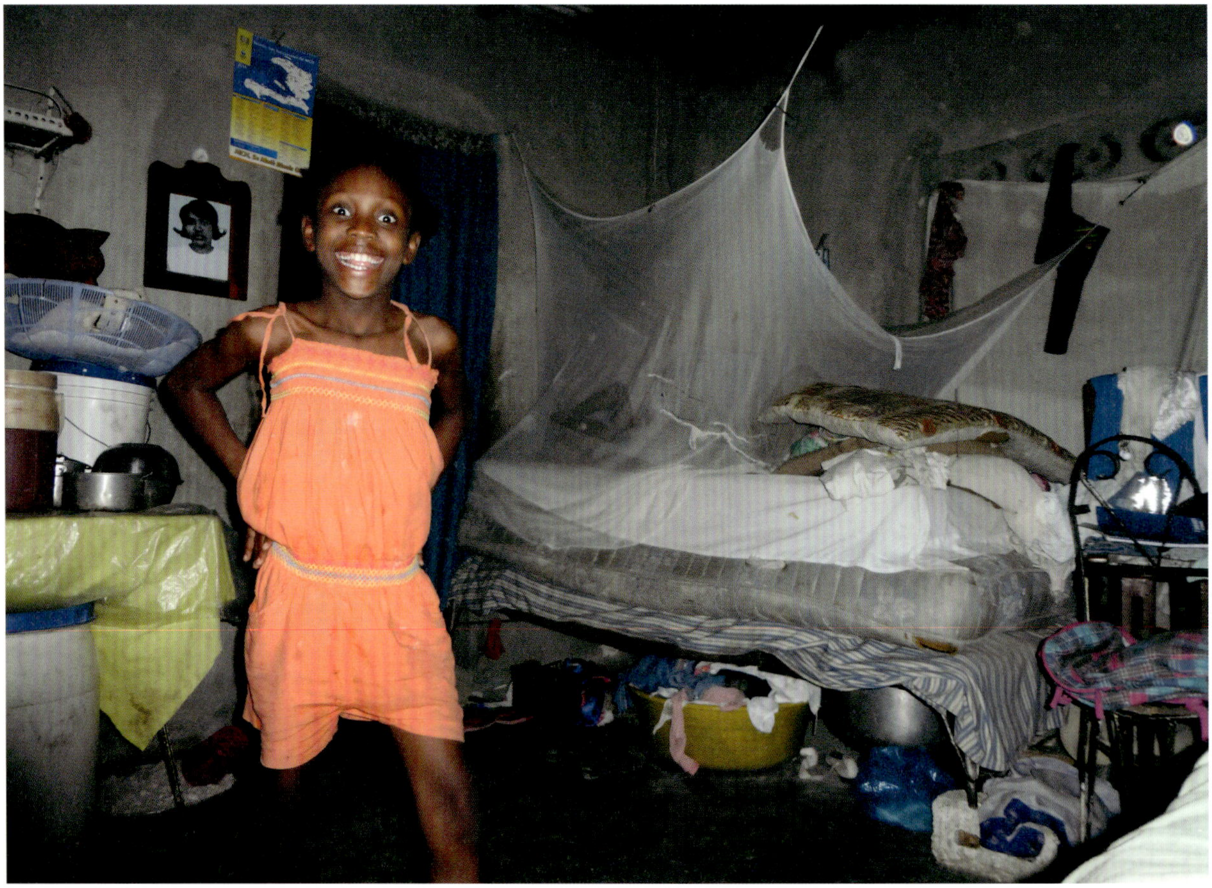

Mideline

People look at us like we are fire. They don't want to touch us because we will burn them. But here I say, we are not fire, we will not burn anyone, they can touch us.

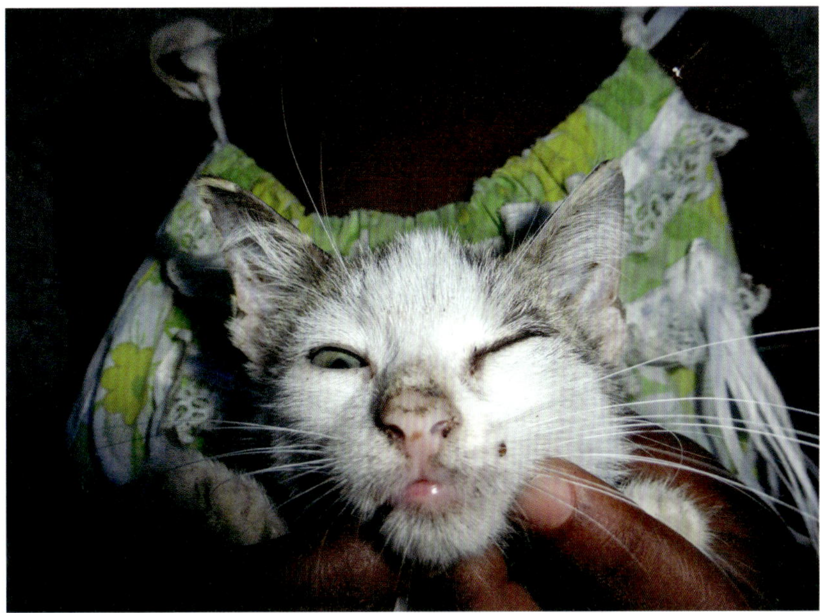

When I found out that I had the virus, I was pregnant with twins. They gave me medicine the whole time I was pregnant and giving birth. They gave my twins medicine and they followed up with treatment. And they turned out to be HIV-negative. It was hard to take them to the hospital. To support them and feed them was difficult, too. To really care for them was really hard. So that is why I put them in an orphanage. But it would be best if the kids were living by my side.

I had no idea about the disease. I kept getting sick, again and again. I went back to the doctor and he said that if I did not take the medicine I would die. After that, I asked questions of my grandparents. I asked them how my mother died, because I did not know. And they explained that it was through my mom that I got infected.

People look at us like we are fire. They don't want to touch us because we will burn them. But here I say, we are not fire, we will not burn anyone, they can touch us.

I used to look at the world like I was not part of it. It's like I was living in another world, with no hope, but after I took control I realized that it is nothing. I realized that I was just like anyone who is alive. Stop stigmatization against people with HIV. We all belong to one society.

Wilda

This daughter of mine, she represents so much for me. I used to worry so much, that she would be infected like me. But she is not.

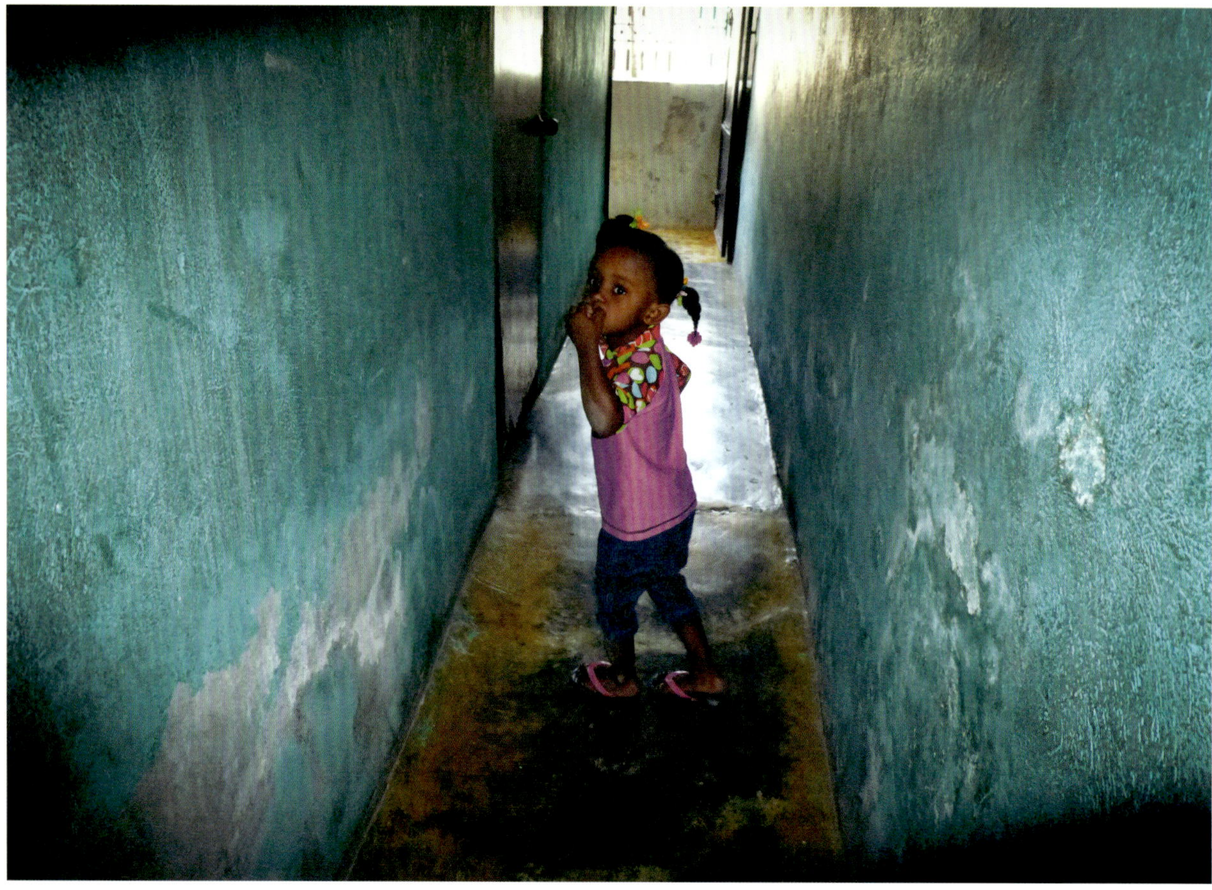

I found out my boyfriend was sick. I loved him. I did not protect myself. We were enjoying life, without protection. In 2008, I started getting sick too. When I found out I had HIV, I thought I was done, already dead, my life was over. I had thoughts of drinking bleach. I wanted to kill myself. I even wanted to kill my baby and then kill myself. I had a cousin who was a big support for me, and she always appeared at the worst moments and talked me out of it.

While I was breastfeeding, the doctor called me and said, "How come you did not come to take the syrup for the baby? If you don't come get it, the baby may be infected just like you. Wouldn't you like the baby to be healthy?" I ran. I took a motor taxi and went to get the syrup for the baby. Then I went to the clinic to have her tested. The test revealed she was negative. That's how I learned that the medication could save our lives. I started taking medication myself and life became what I wanted it to be.

This daughter of mine, she represents so much for me. I used to worry so much, that she would be infected like me. But she is not. I take a lot of care to make sure that she'll never be positive, the way I am.

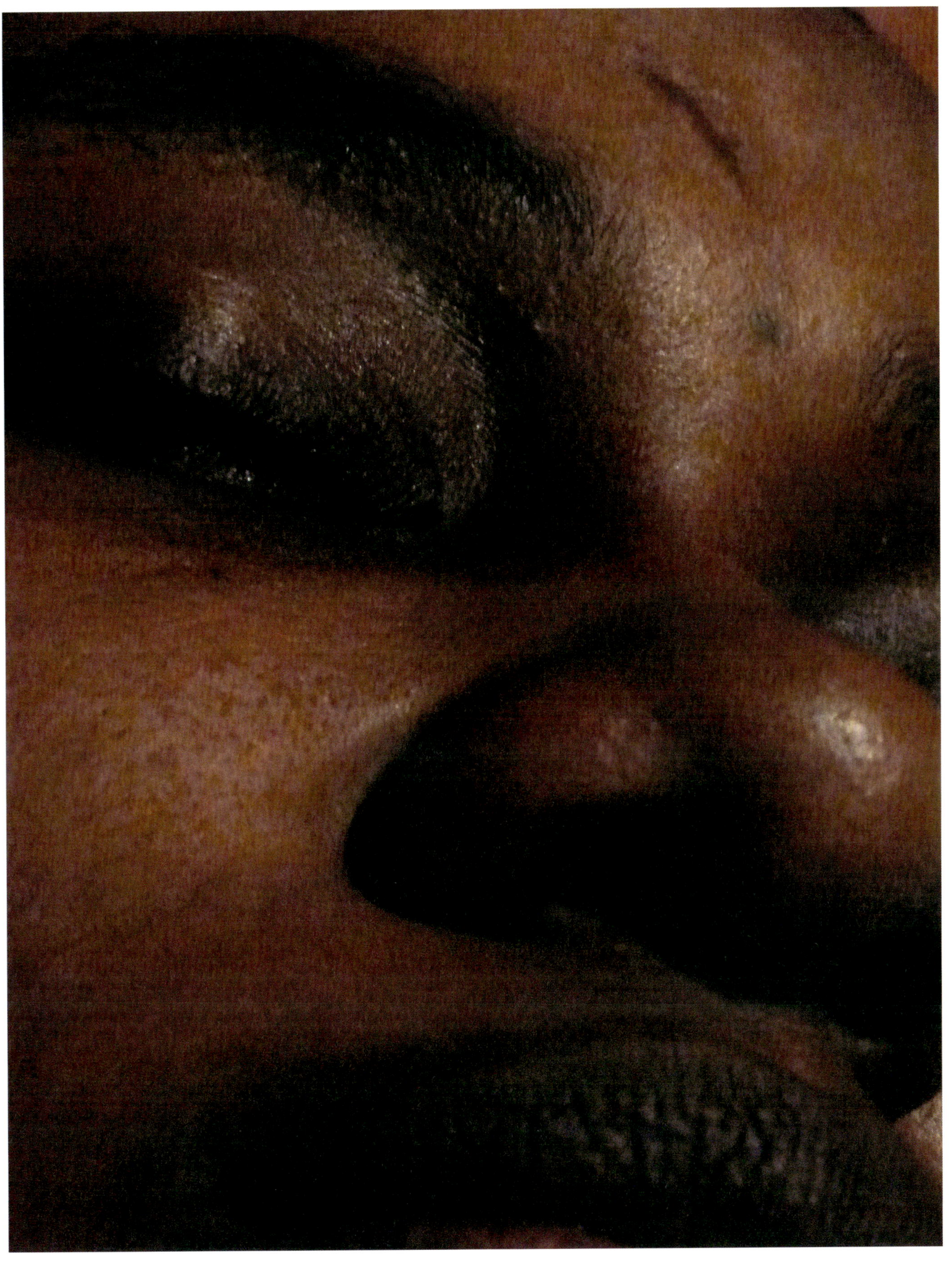

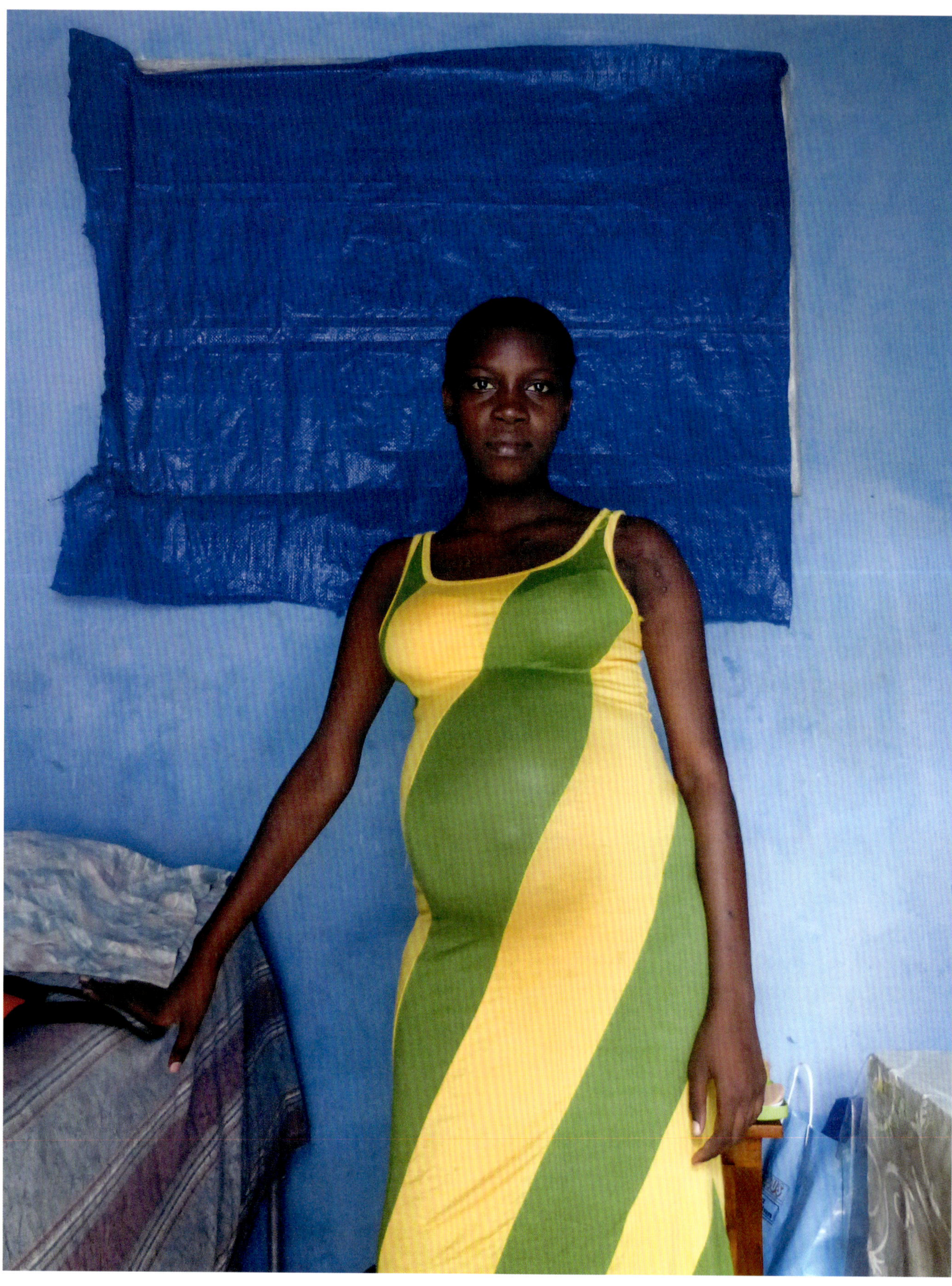

Wideline

What I want, from taking all the medicine, is for the baby to be born healthy. They say that if I take all the medicine, the baby has a big chance of not having HIV in her blood.

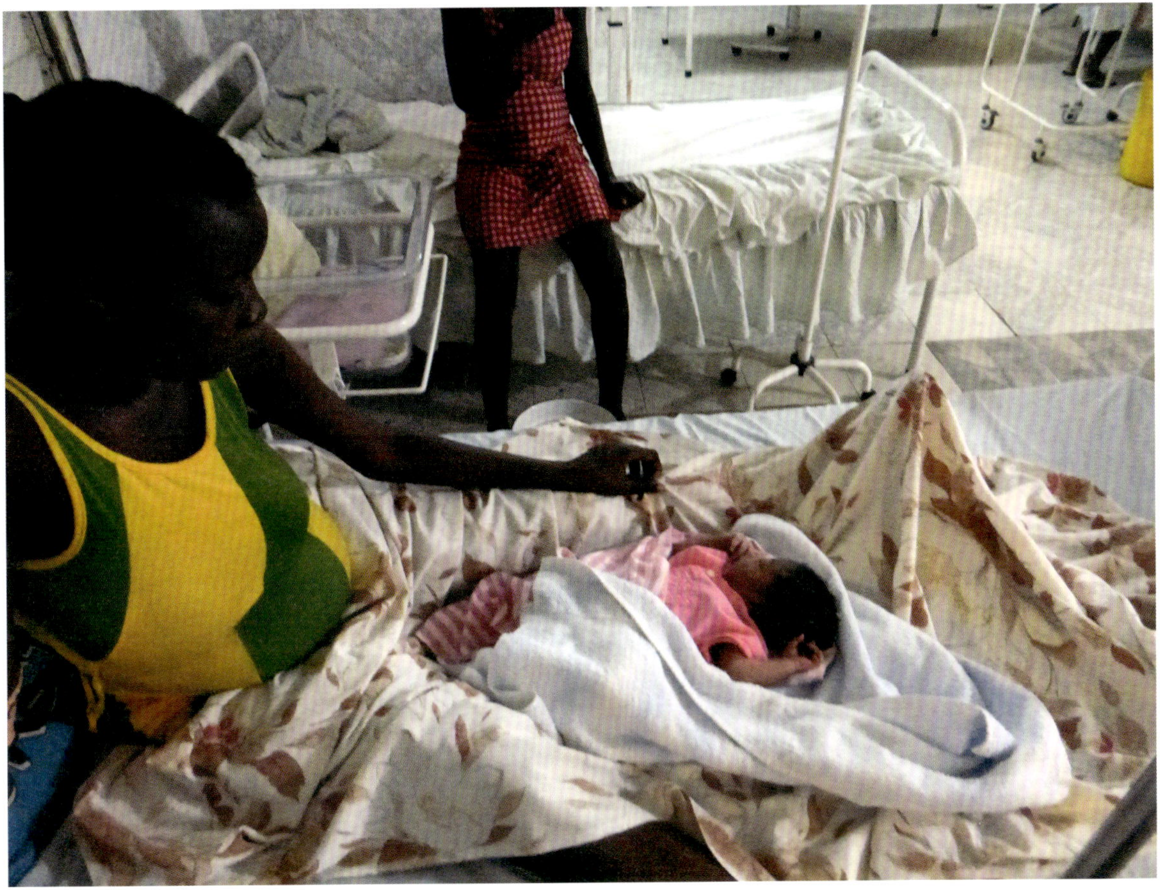

I started sex work when I was sixteen years old. Sometimes clients didn't understand and they got mad. They even curse at you. But the boss would never let anyone hit you. If they are with you for a minute they pay $10, and it could be less or more. I felt trapped, it was hard, but I got used to the job. From the moment I found out I was pregnant I stopped doing it. I found out I had HIV in January 2014. At first, I felt confused and bad, because I had done a test that came out negative, then went back again and the test came out positive.

Some people living with HIV feel they are not part of this world, but for me it feels the same. My friends help me, and my boyfriend is there, too. For me, I see the world the same way I saw it before. I go to the hospital every month, they give me medication, and they also give me other medication because I am pregnant. What I want, from taking all the medicine, is for the baby to be born healthy. They say that if I take all the medicine they tell me to take, the baby has a big chance of not having HIV in her blood. When she grows up, I wish that she will not do the same work I did and that she will be a good citizen.

Raphael

I want to tell people in Haiti to stop talking about things they don't know. Learn what AIDS is before you criticize us.

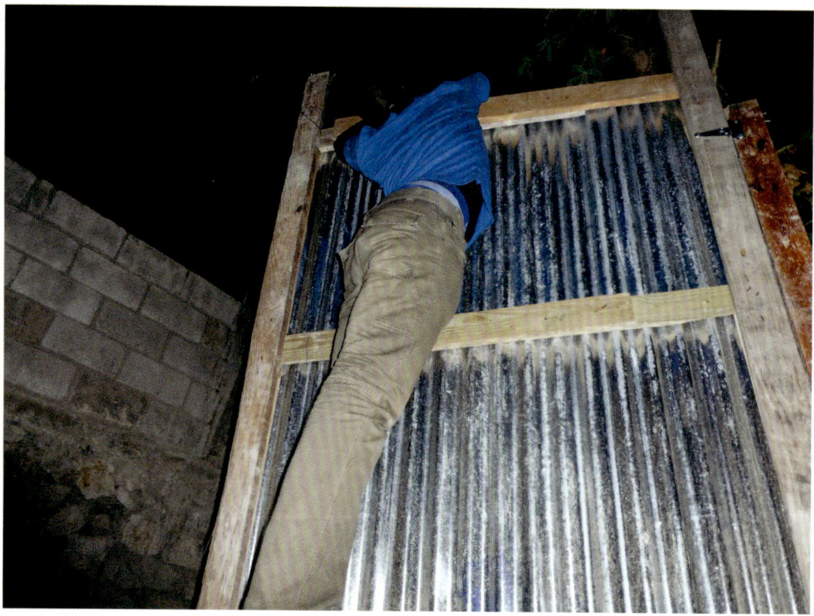

In 2004, I went to take the test and I found out I was positive. When I first found out, since I did not really understand what HIV was, it did not make an impact on me. I took it like a fever, like a cold, like any sickness that keeps you in bed.

I don't really know when or how I got infected. I was in a relationship with a woman. We enjoyed each other, we made love, I penetrated her without a condom, and she said, "Hmm, you did not wear a condom?" When I went to get tested, I remembered that moment and thought, maybe that was the time I got it.

Now when I take photos, I know how to analyze the situation, and this means a lot to me. I use that knowledge. When I take photos by my house, for example, I can't use the tripod at night because I just moved in the area, and security is uncertain. But I found a way to use the camera to my advantage. I hold it steady for a long exposure, which pushes me to take photos in an original way.

I want to tell people in Haiti to stop talking about things they don't know. When you hear that there is a disease that is a force of destruction, learn what AIDS is before you criticize us, before judging us on account of the disease.

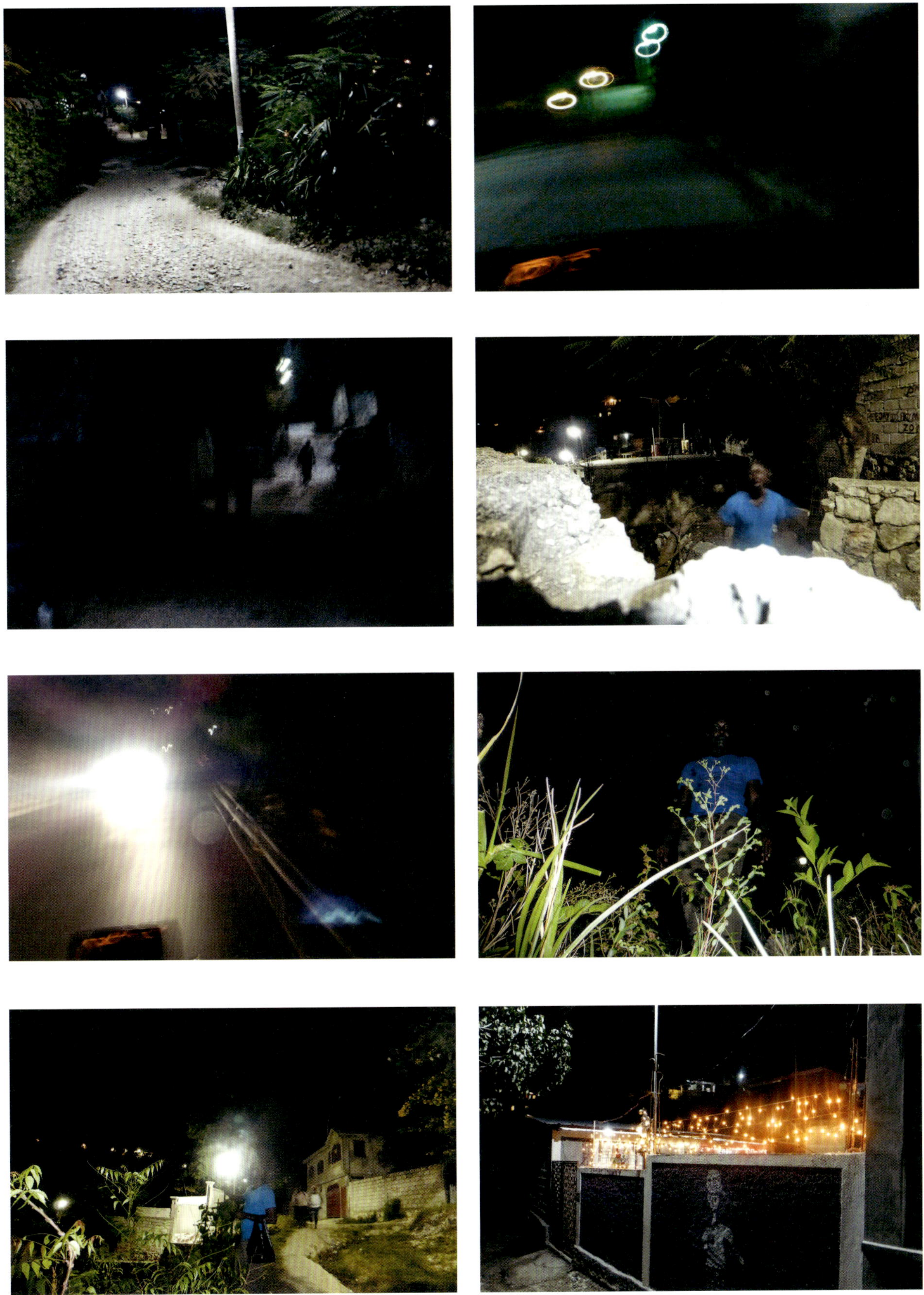

Steeve

I gathered a bunch of my friends and sat them down. I talked to them about my HIV status. I could not hide any longer. I thought that maybe some would stop talking to me.

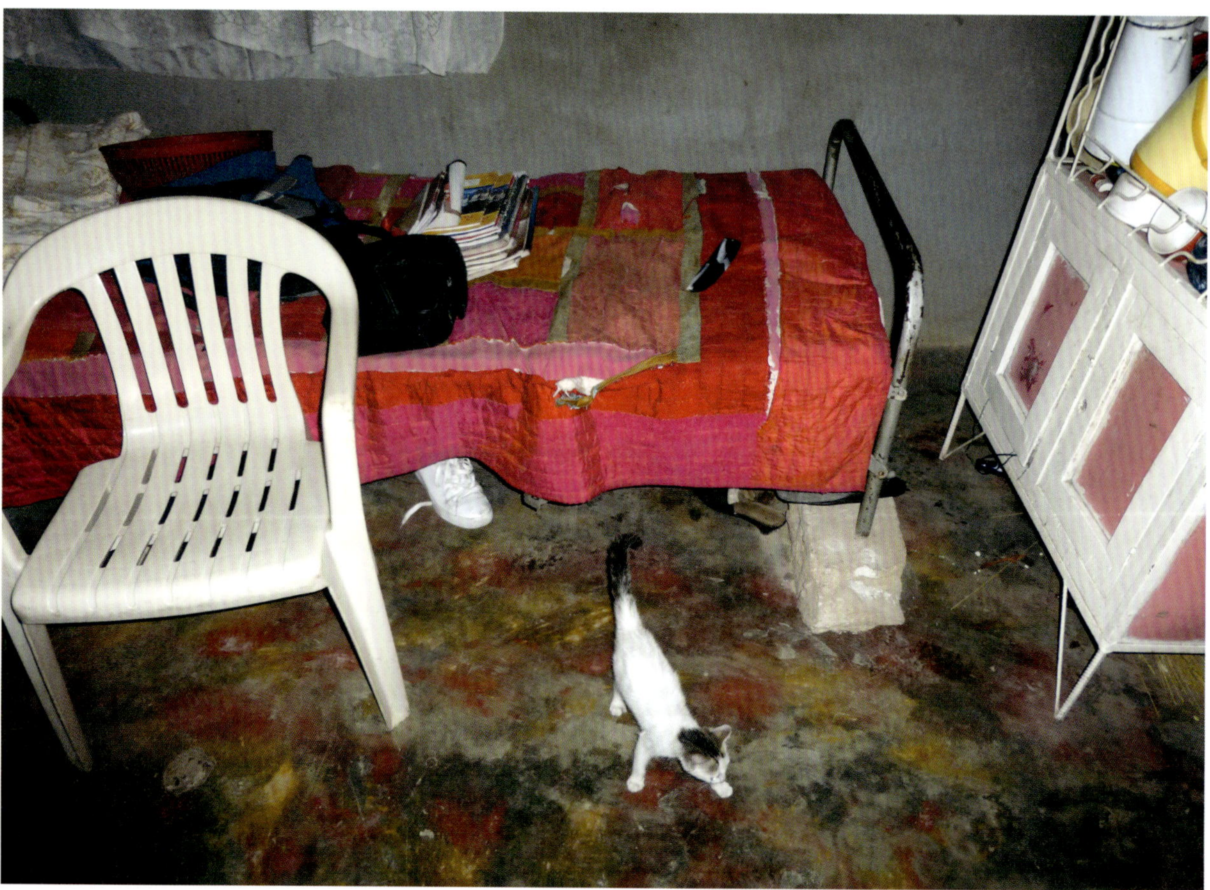

I used to go to a lot of brothels. I had never gotten advice that I should use condoms. One day I woke up and felt an intuition that I had to go and get tested.

When I first heard I was infected, I was very worried. I felt out of place, not normal, agitated inside. I felt stigmatized and discriminated against by my neighbors. I would say hello and, when they found out I had HIV, they would not answer me. Or, if I came to stand next to them to have a conversation, they would move away. That made me feel isolated, like I was not part of this world. I was living in a desert. At one point I even wanted to kill myself, but eventually I found strength and never felt like that again.

I gathered a bunch of my friends and sat them down. I talked to them about my HIV status. I could not hide any longer. If they found out somewhere else, it would give me more problems. I thought that maybe some would stop talking to me. But I realized then that I had good friends and that I had to stay strong.

At the end of the day, my friends and family have never let me down. They are always there for me. I wish for all the people like me to be strong and believe that they are like everyone else, and to not live in isolation. And to always be open to receiving advice, and always going to the hospital and taking the medicine.

Wilder

The priest of my church said to me, "What are you doing inside the church, Wilder? You have this thing and you come and sit among us? Why?" That was a big shock to me.

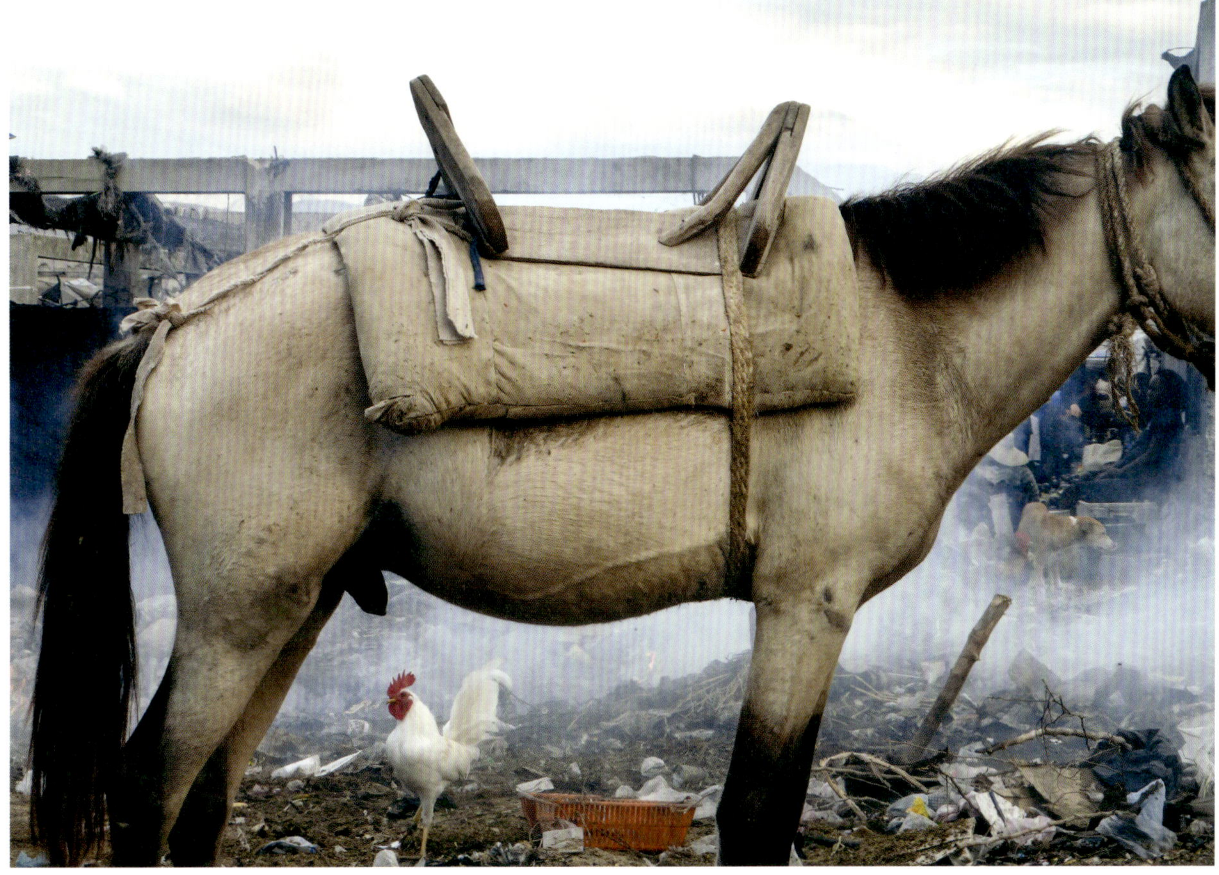

I found out about my HIV status in 1998. I went to see a doctor for my skin. The doctor asked me to get tested, and I found out I was infected with HIV. I wanted to throw myself under a car. I don't know what held me back. The doctor had thrown me out of his office. It was hurtful to me, because he had a lot of people waiting for him, and I sat in front of him crying.

The priest of my church was my good friend. One time after mass, I called him and told him, "I have a big problem. I have HIV in my blood." And he said to me, "What are you doing inside the church, Wilder? You have this thing and you come and sit among us? Why?" That was a big shock to me.

Now I practice vodou, because I have a home there. I pray to God all the time.

This is a message for all people living with HIV and AIDS: Stigma and discrimination can be found everywhere. Therefore, you need to find strength. Do not let stigmatization crush you.

Esther

Poverty is the number one reason why we can't control the HIV virus in this country. I realized that a lot of other people do not have the support my family gave me. That is why I created the Foundation Esther Bousicault Stanislas (FEBS), in order to provide support to as many individuals living with HIV/AIDS as possible.

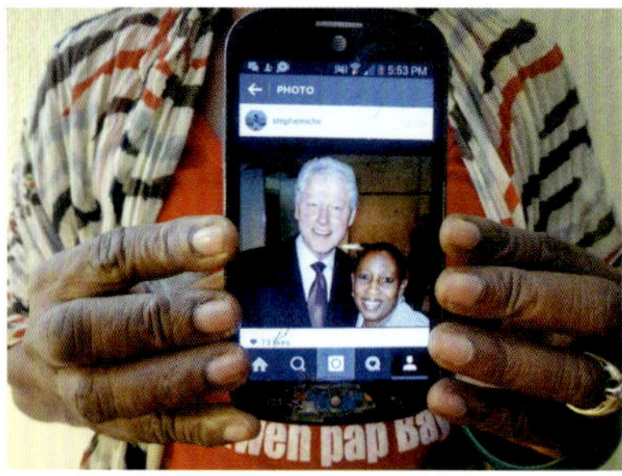

My daughters are always present in my mind, they are the youth, and I recognize the power of engaging the next generation. I have suffered so much. I told myself it was not possible to suffer this much and not be able to say out loud that I have HIV.

First, I decided to go on the radio. It was World AIDS Day and a lot of young people were present. They threw things at me, they cursed at me. That hurt me a lot. But after that I decided to go on TV. I made a documentary on my life, a positive account of my story and how I live my life. I removed the veil. I told myself it was unbelievable that no one before me had done that. If someone had, maybe I would not be sick today.

I wanted to give a face to AIDS, because it was not right to suffer so much alone. This is what gives me strength and the reason why today, after twenty years, I am still alive. I adore my two daughters and the support and love that they give me sustains me.

Riccardo

In 2009, I went to spend a summer vacation in Jeremie, a town west of Port-au-Prince. While there, I contracted malaria and typhoid, which took a toll on me. The doctor made me take a bunch of blood tests, which revealed I was infected with HIV. They called my parents and told them. Everyone wondered how it was possible. My parents did not have it. My sisters did not have it. So how was it possible?

In my imagination, I see a mirror that represents the world. I am in the middle, and the spots are the criticisms I face. I am hiding, I don't want to reveal what I have, I don't want people to know. The suffering I have to deal with— it's better to tell the truth about yourself, than for people to find out on their own.

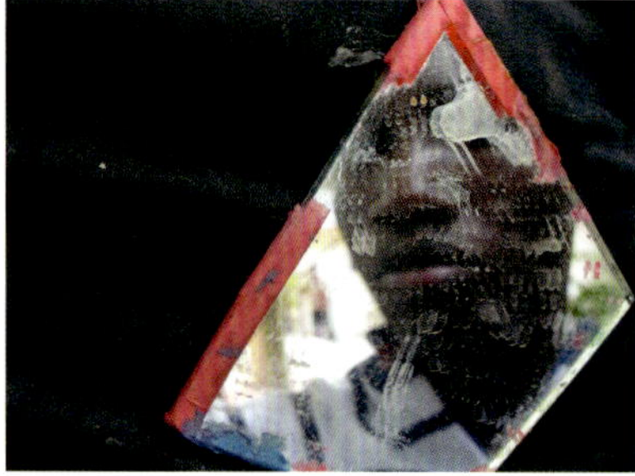

I would like to speak to others like me. For those in hiding, when you stay hidden you put yourself in more danger than when you reveal. Once you reveal, you will feel better, you will feel happier. Here I am free, free of my self-consciousness, free of all criticism, free from all things.

I am free.

Yveson

I met Emmanuel when he first came out as positive. When he went to the barbershop to cut his hair, the hairdresser refused and told him, "I will lose at least fifteen clients because of you." I ran into him shortly after that. We lived in the same neighborhood. And I knew how to cut hair. From then on, I became the one to cut his hair. We have become best friends.

Emmanuel was the one to tell me that it was important to get tested. He insisted. Getting tested was a clear decision. Whether I had HIV or not, I was ready. So when I finally found the courage, the test came out positive. I told Emmanuel right away. After that, he took me to a bunch of seminars. These trainings gave me a lot of strength.

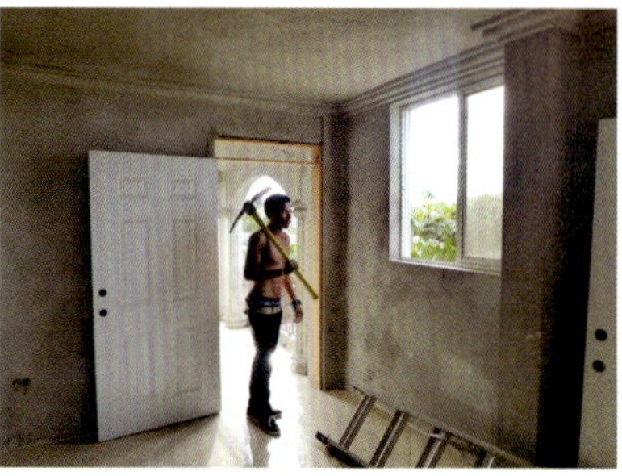

When I take photos as part of this project, I see them as stops on a journey. When people are looking at them, they should see a continuation. I feel very proud. I love the colors of my photos, and I will always continue taking photos. When you have HIV, it is not the end of life, but rather a new relationship with society and with yourself as well.

London

Thanks in large part to the United Kingdom's robust National Healthcare System and strong network of HIV and AIDS resource centers, the London participants in *Through Positive Eyes* were living healthy and productive lives when the workshop took place in March 2015. This is not to say that the London group members do not struggle with stigma and other HIV-related complexities—however, they tell an important story about the impact that consistent healthcare (including mental healthcare) and supportive housing and resource centers can make on the quality of life, treatment adherence, and personal empowerment of people living with HIV and AIDS. It is worth stating, even if self-evident, that greater resources translate to greater health.

United Kingdom's AIDS epidemic, as of 2015

Number of people living with HIV:	101,200

HIV prevalence

Adults (15–74 years):	0.21%
Men who have sex with men:	5.87%
People who inject drugs:	1%

Treatment

Free universal treatment is available from the National Health Service.

Numbers on treatment:	88,769
% of those needing treatment who are receiving it:	83%
% of those in treatment with no detectable virus:	78%

Key events

1987 *"Don't die of ignorance" mass national campaign; Princess Diana holds the hand of a patient in an AIDS ward at London Middlesex Hospital.*

1988 *Section 28 of the Local Government Act prevents teachings that "promote homosexuality" in schools, a statute only repealed in 2003.*

2010 *The Equality Act qualifies anyone living with HIV as disabled, which gives protection against discrimination.*

2016 *Campaigners fight for, and win, provision of pre-exposure prophylaxis by the National Health Service.*

Update 2019

By 2018, adult HIV prevalence in the U.K. had fallen to 0.16% of the population and 98% of people living with HIV were on treatment. Of these, 97% were virally suppressed. In 2018, London was the first global city to exceed UNAIDS 90-90-90 targets. The reduction in new infections has been driven mostly by fewer diagnoses among men who have sex with men, which have decreased by 31% since 2015.

Through Positive Eyes in London was organized in partnership with Positively UK, with assistance from Dean Street Clinic, Baseline, Forum Link, and St. Anne's Anglican Church. Major funding was provided by The Herb Ritts Foundation, with additional support from The Ford Foundation, Gere Foundation, and UCLA.

James

The photos I have taken are indicative of my desire to represent my HIV within a broader context of human intimacy, as healthy, erotic, and sensual, as playful and loving, as sacred and nurturing, because I am all of those things.

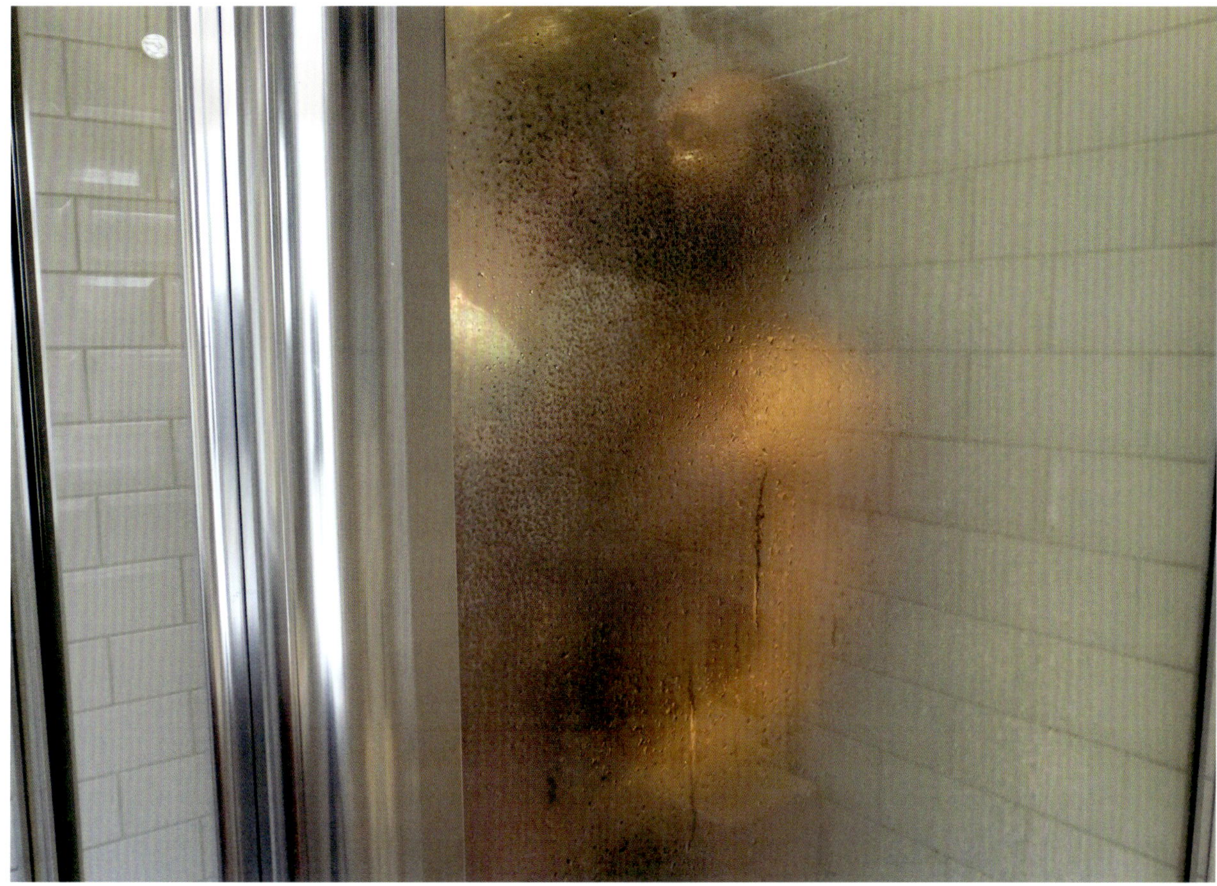

Sexual intimacy—unapologetic sexual intimacy—is an integral part of many human relationships. In the early days of my diagnosis, I was afraid of transmitting the virus to partners. Sex was overshadowed by risk, the body a vessel for fear rather than joy.

I am interested in depicting the body within a fledgling relationship, and what that means, in the context of HIV between the two of us, because David, my partner in these photos, is not positive. The photos I have taken are indicative of my desire to represent my HIV within a broader context of human intimacy, as healthy, erotic, and sensual, as playful and loving, as sacred and nurturing, because I am all of those things.

I have a lot of tattoos across my body. Many of these images gesture toward the love I have been gifted throughout my life. Some of the tattoos allude, metaphorically, to my journey with HIV. A man struck up a conversation with me in the changing room of my gym, asking me why so many of my tattoos reference the spiritual. And it dawned on me that, viewed as a whole, the most common theme written across my body is my divine connection to love. Once upon a time, I believed HIV would prevent me from loving and being loved. These photos capture a brief moment in time when the divine nature of love blossomed between me and David.

Gordon

I was brought up in chaos and, in my adult life, I didn't realize that I didn't need to repeat that. So creating order in chaos has been a long-term project of mine.

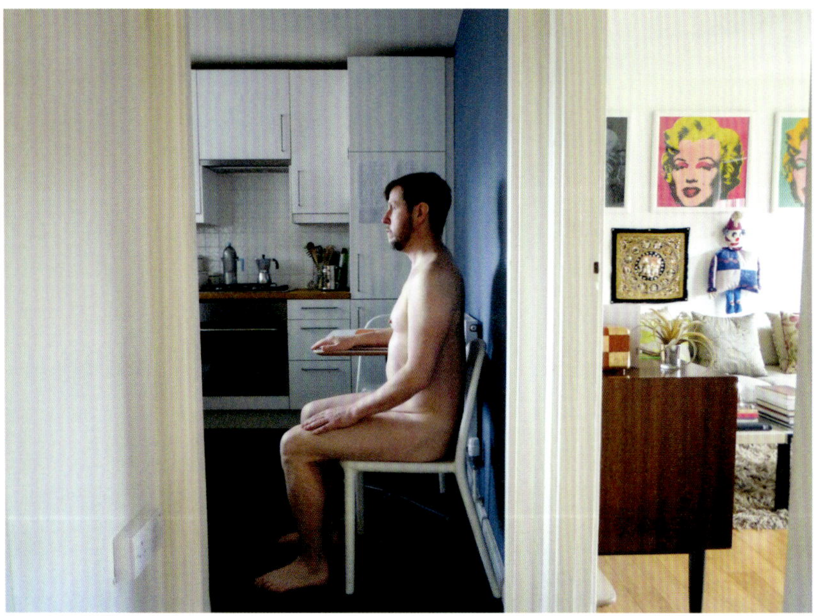

About ten years ago, my life imploded and I felt completely out of control. I was in a relationship that was killing me. My friends were telling me that I was going to die and I could not see it.

He pushed me into the bath. My head hit the taps. He was standing above me and there was blood running off his hands. Suddenly, I realized that he had scraped all the skin off his knuckles, on my head, and it was his own blood that was running down his hands.

He kept yelling if the HIV that he gave me didn't kill me that he was going to kill me.

I need to be clear that today I don't believe that anyone should be prosecuted for HIV transmission, as he was. I do love him and I do pray for him. Wherever he is, I hope that he's at peace.

I made a commitment to myself this year to reconnect with my own creativity. In making my "Bag of Shame," I realized that someone has to give me that label and I can choose whether I take it and stick it on myself. I come from chaos. I was brought up in chaos and, in my adult life, I didn't realize that I didn't need to repeat that. So creating order in chaos has been a long-term project of mine. It is really important for me to quiet my head because I felt that my head was killing me, and in trying to make sense of my life and my journey, I had distanced myself from humanity quite a lot. In the last few years I have come out of that.

I realized that I have way more choices than I thought I had and I can choose moving forward.

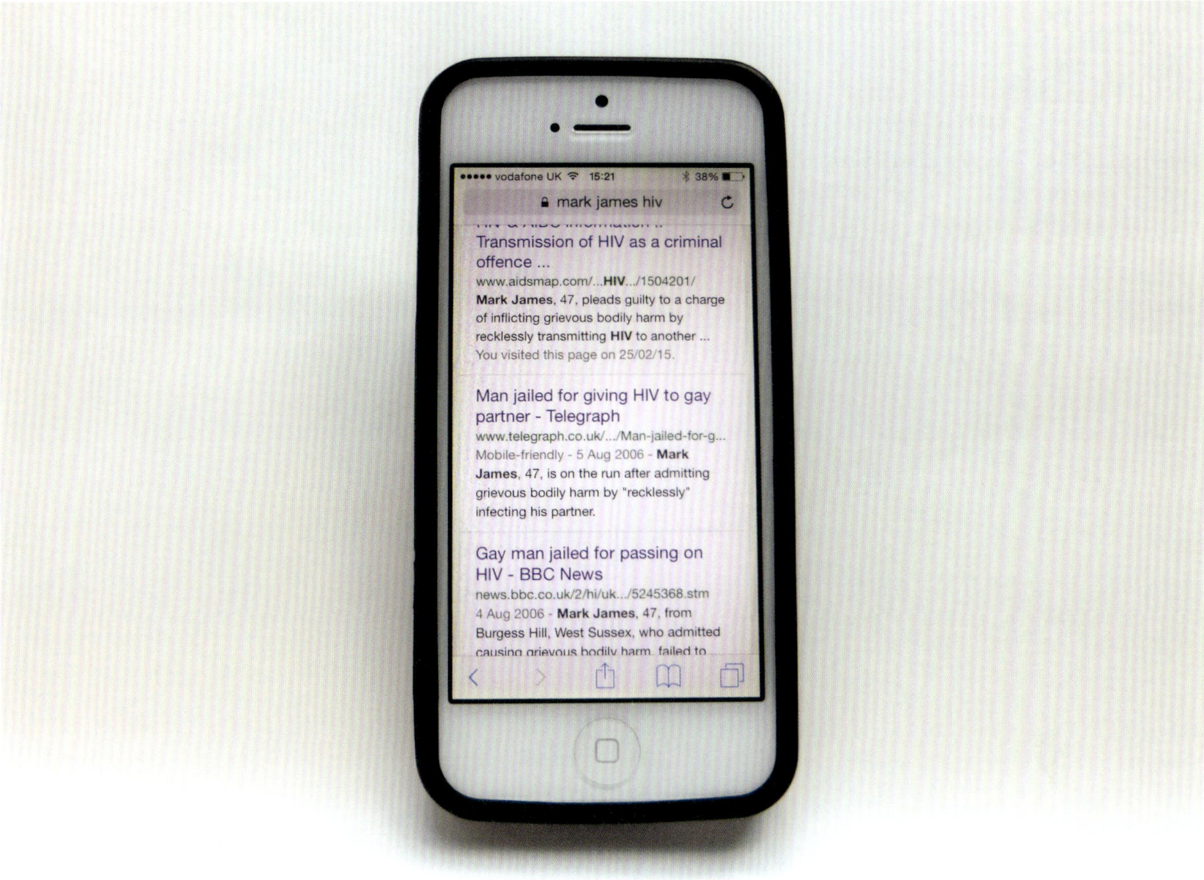

vodafone UK 15:21 38%
mark james hiv
Transmission of HIV as a criminal offence ...
www.aidsmap.com/...HIV.../1504201/
Mark James, 47, pleads guilty to a charge of inflicting grievous bodily harm by recklessly transmitting HIV to another ...
You visited this page on 25/02/15.
Man jailed for giving HIV to gay partner - Telegraph
www.telegraph.co.uk/.../Man-jailed-for-g...
Mobile-friendly - 5 Aug 2006 - Mark James, 47, is on the run after admitting grievous bodily harm by "recklessly" infecting his partner.
Gay man jailed for passing on HIV - BBC News
news.bbc.co.uk/2/hi/uk.../5245368.stm
4 Aug 2006 - Mark James, 47, from Burgess Hill, West Sussex, who admitted

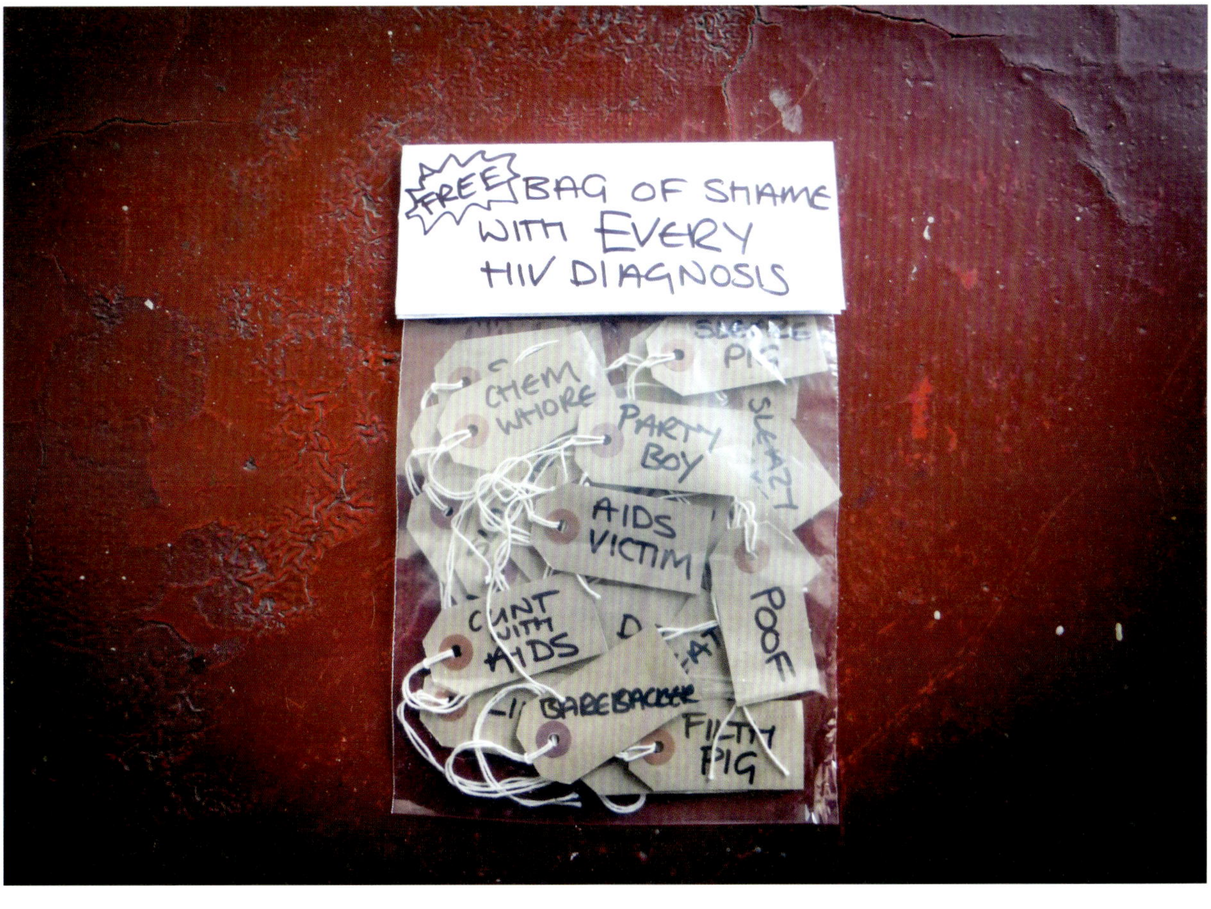

FREE BAG OF SHAME WITH EVERY HIV DIAGNOSIS
CHEM WHORE
PARTY BOY
AIDS VICTIM
CUNT WITH AIDS
POOF
BAREBACKER
FILTHY PIG

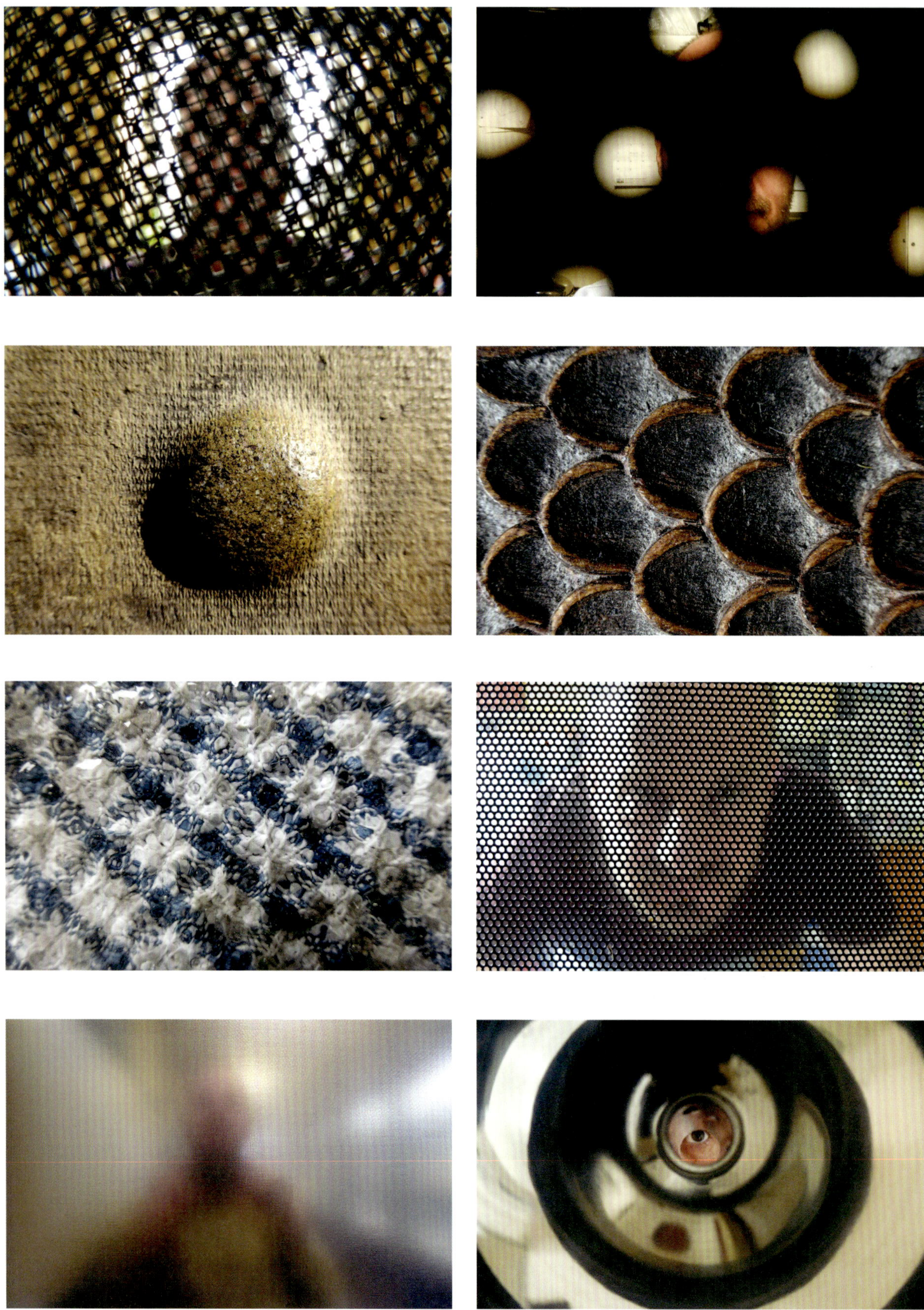

Keith

Living in London, in a big modern city in today's world, as a gay man, people don't want to see the cracked or broken me. But there are many days when this is exactly how I feel.

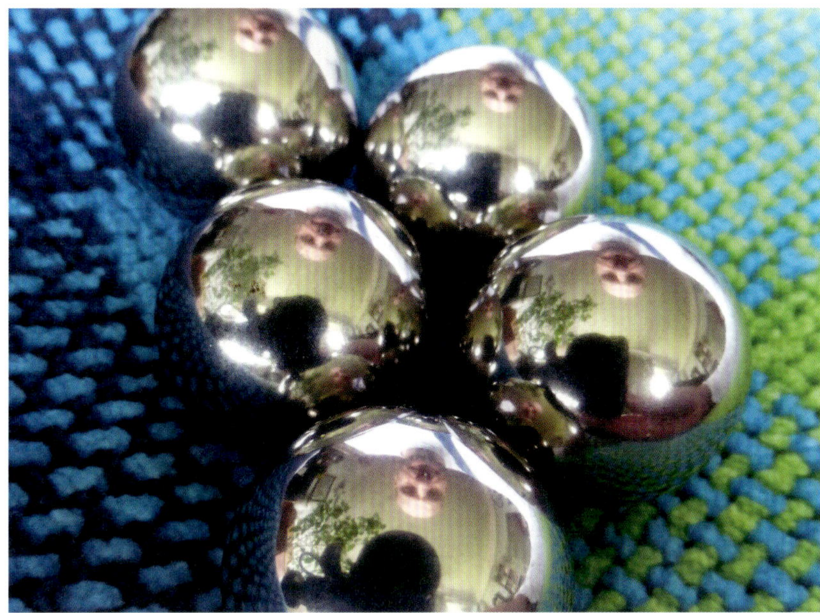

I am an openly gay man who happens to be HIV-positive, but I'm not so open about my HIV status. In my photos, I remain anonymous. I don't really reveal myself. I'm there but I'm hiding, I suppose. Actually, at times I feel very isolated and very alone.

Living in London, in a big modern city in today's world, as a gay man, people don't want to see the cracked or broken me. But there are many days when this is exactly how I feel. I am not perfect. I am damaged, and I am somewhat broken.

I'm projecting a veneer, because it can be painful and hurtful to show all of yourself, if it is something as personal as being HIV-positive.

I take up to ten or twelve pills a day, including my antiretrovirals and medication to deal with the side effects. I also have to take pills for depression and pills for aches and pains, which are linked to HIV.

This is an essential part of my daily life. It keeps me healthy. I mean, ultimately, it keeps me alive. Still, I don't enjoy it and it brings all sorts of unique pressures, particularly, you know, because I'm not open about my status. I don't want to hide my HIV status, I want to be comfortable about it, but it's not easy.

Virginia

I volunteer for a charity and I teach gardening classes. I try to encourage people to reconnect with their food through learning how easy it is to grow.

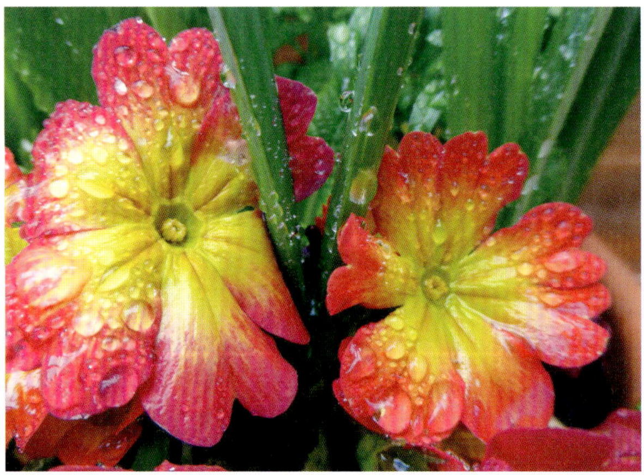

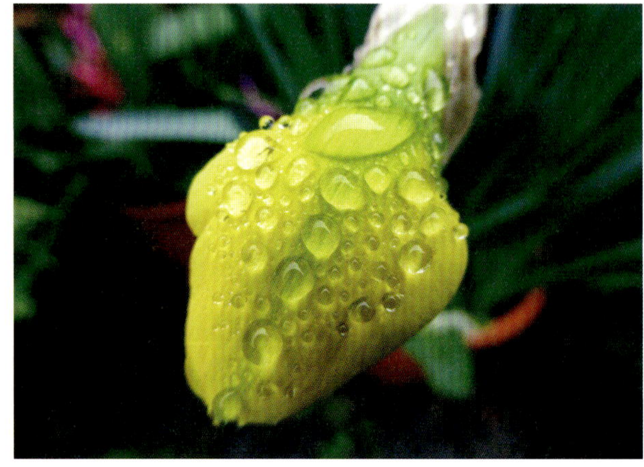

I was born in Argentina. I live in London now because my husband is a Londoner, London-Irish. We met in 1993 in India. We sent letters for three years and then, when we met again, they diagnosed me with HIV. He said that nothing had changed in our relationship, and that is why I'm here now.

I am very close to my family. When I said I was going to be part of this project, my sister said, "How can we be involved?" And I said, "Try to send me a picture."

I volunteer for a charity and I teach gardening classes. I try to encourage people to reconnect with their food through learning how easy it is to grow. Ever since I learned how to walk, my granddad used to bring me to the botanical gardens in Buenos Aires. In London, I work with nature every day of my life. There is beauty in nature.

This is what I say to people: You think you will not recover, but you must always hold on to hope. Being an immigrant, the network I have built up in London is very important to me, including people at the clinic, at the gym, or at the place where I volunteer. Beautiful things make me smile, but it is the other things too that you cannot photograph, all the kindness and support you experience through relationships with people.

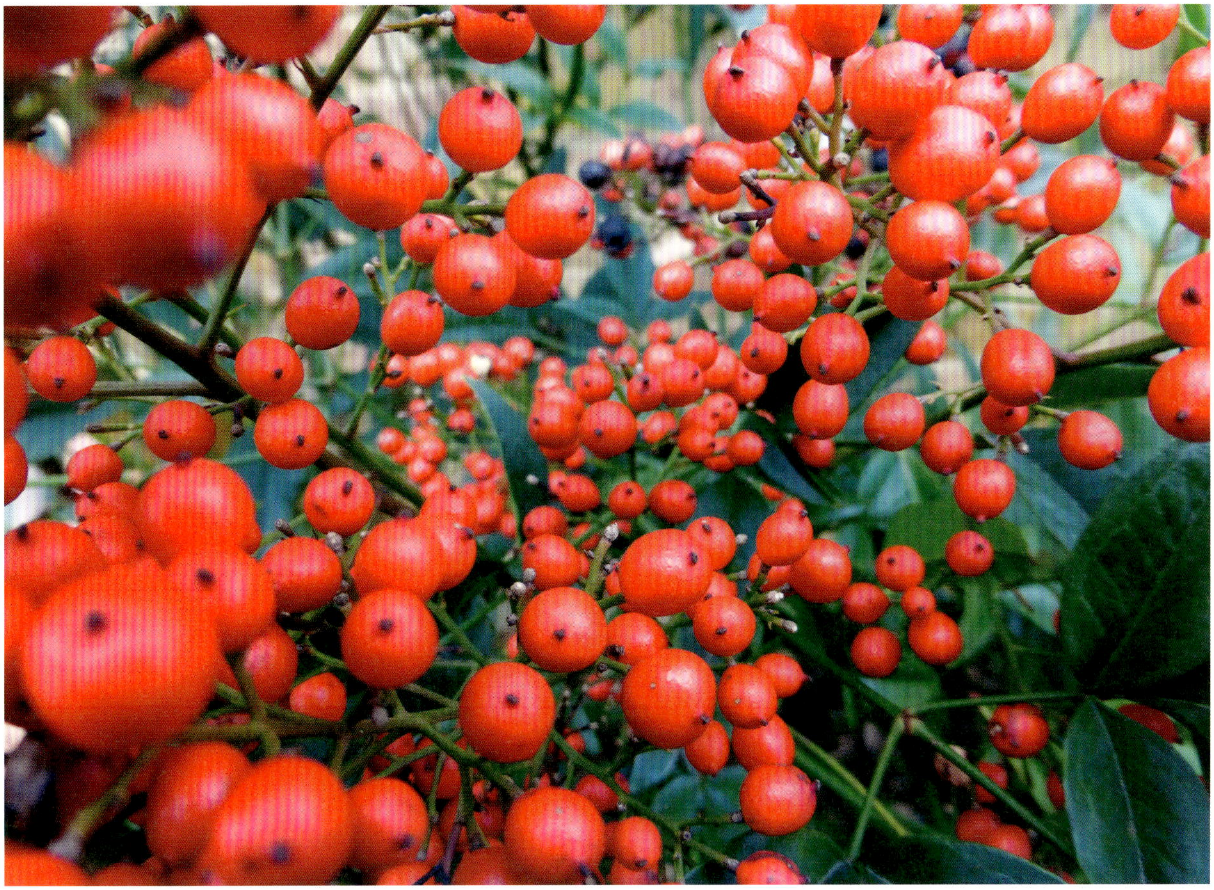

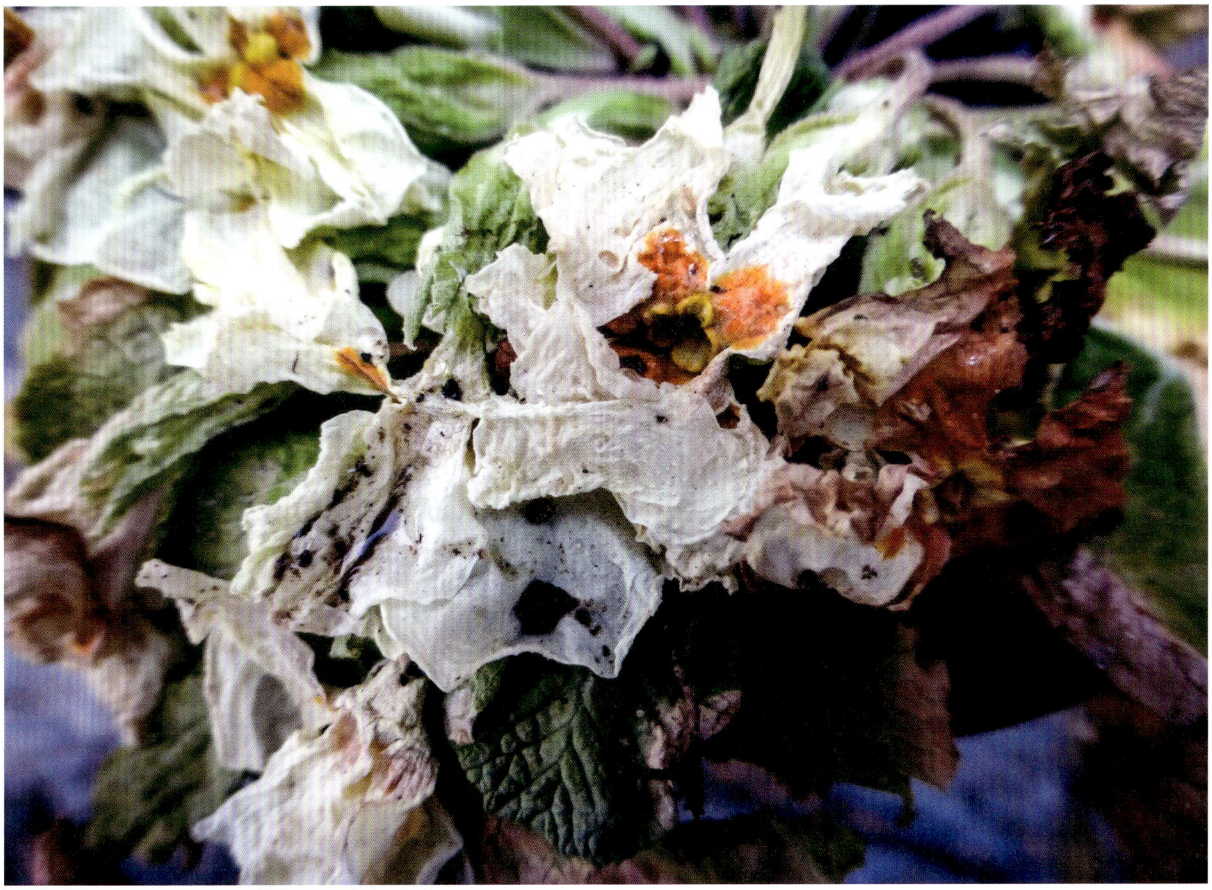

Michael

If I weren't HIV-positive, I probably would have been sitting in an office typing away at a computer, day in and day out. Living with HIV has helped me bring out the creative side of myself.

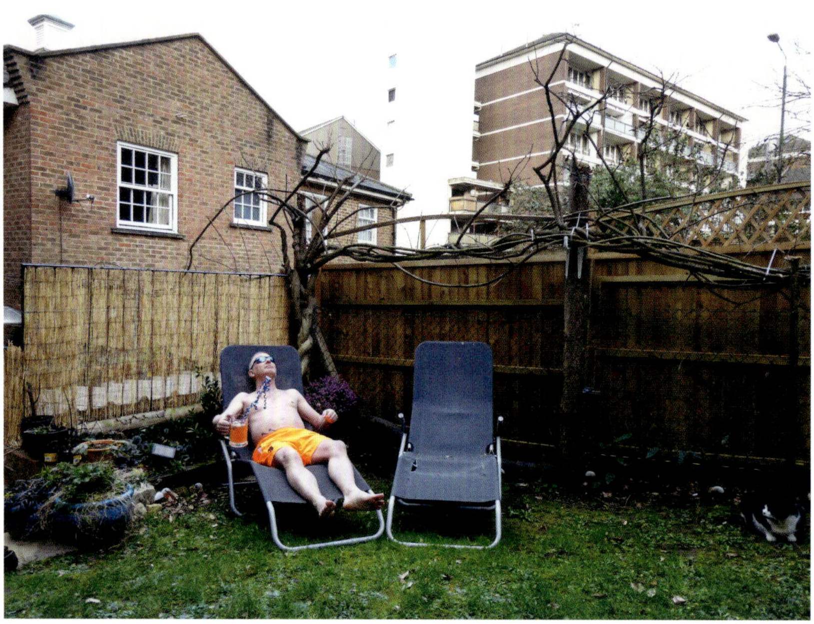

I moved from Liverpool to London in the late '80s, looking for a different life and excitement and somebody to love. When I arrived, I found what I was looking for in abundance. It was everywhere.

I was quite promiscuous. I'd gone to the clinic to be checked for gonorrhea, which I had passed on to my partner. While I was there, I decided to go for an HIV test. The doctor basically turned around and said, "I'm afraid to tell you this, but you're HIV-positive." My head was so mixed up, I wasn't sure what was happening to me and where I was going. I thought I was going to die. I ended up on the streets for a while. I had nowhere to live.

I came across an organization for people living with HIV and AIDS that put me back on my feet. It was the best thing I ever did. Coming out to my family was one of the hardest things I ever did, because you're telling them basically that you've got a death sentence, which HIV was in 1992. Luckily enough, I'm still here. I managed to see life through and I've had such a fantastic time getting here. My family has all been so supportive.

Being optimistic about my HIV has been something that helped me through my life. It has given me the ability to go out and live a fruitful life. If I weren't HIV-positive, I probably would have been sitting in an office typing away at a computer, day in and day out. Living with HIV has helped me bring out the creative side of myself.

HIV makes you become a different person. I'm HIV-positive and I love myself for being HIV-positive. It has made me who I am today.

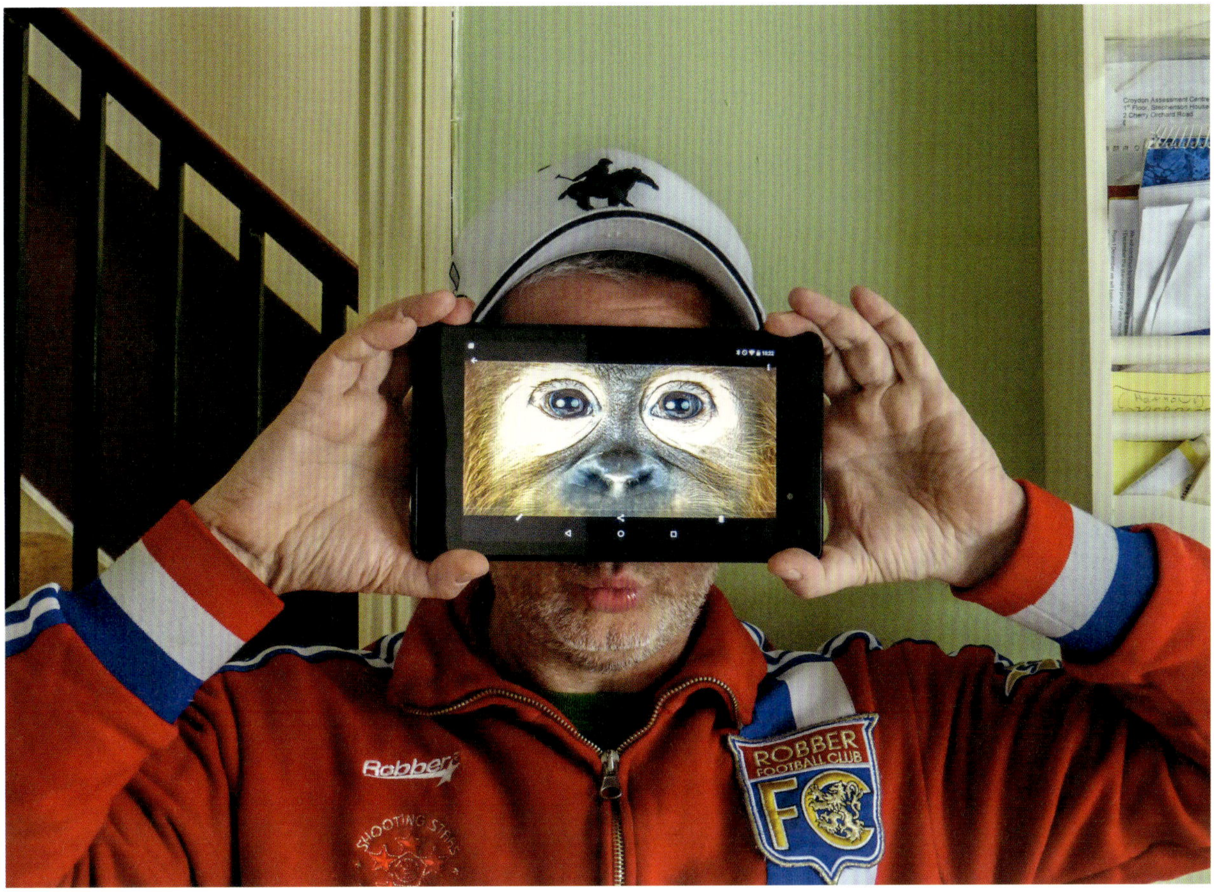

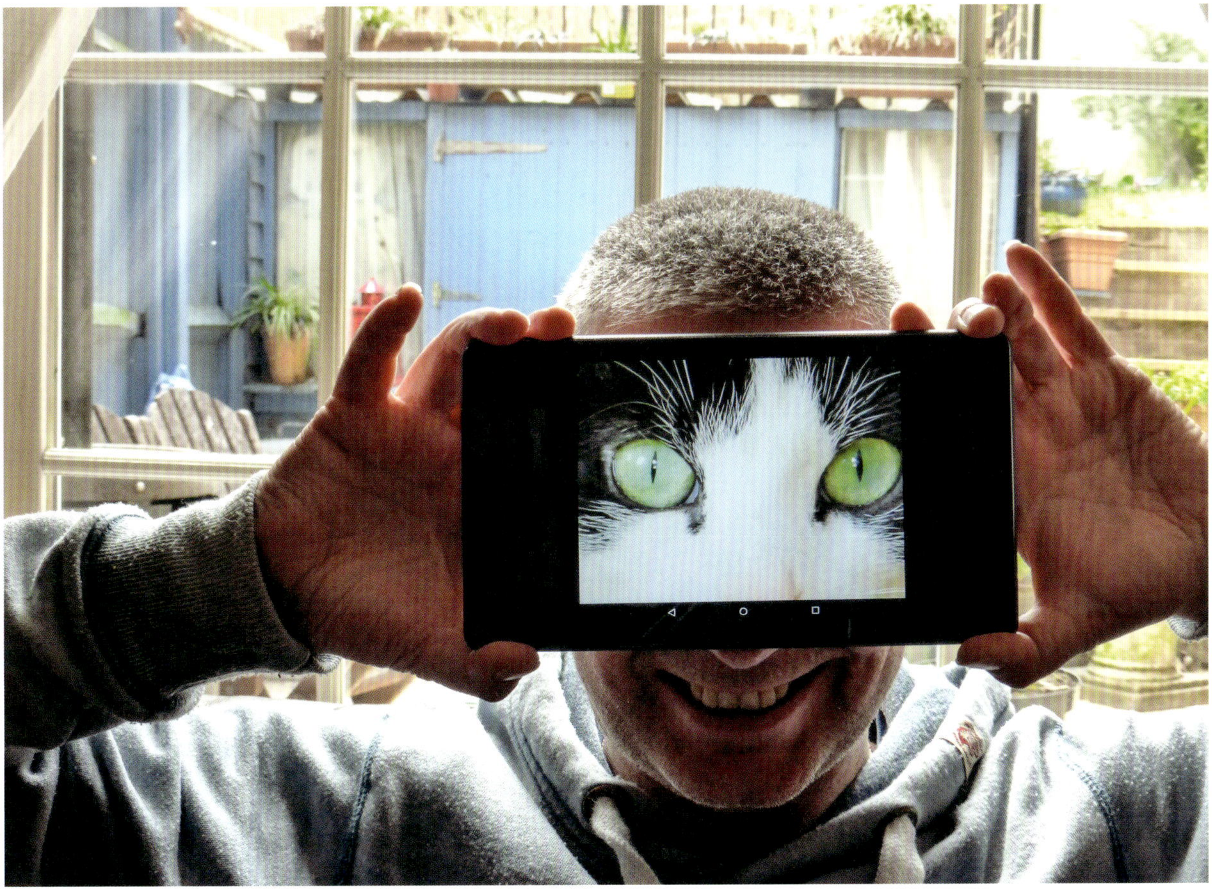

Darren

We're a fun, fun family. We are always either dancing or singing. There's a lot of love. We are not short of love in our home.

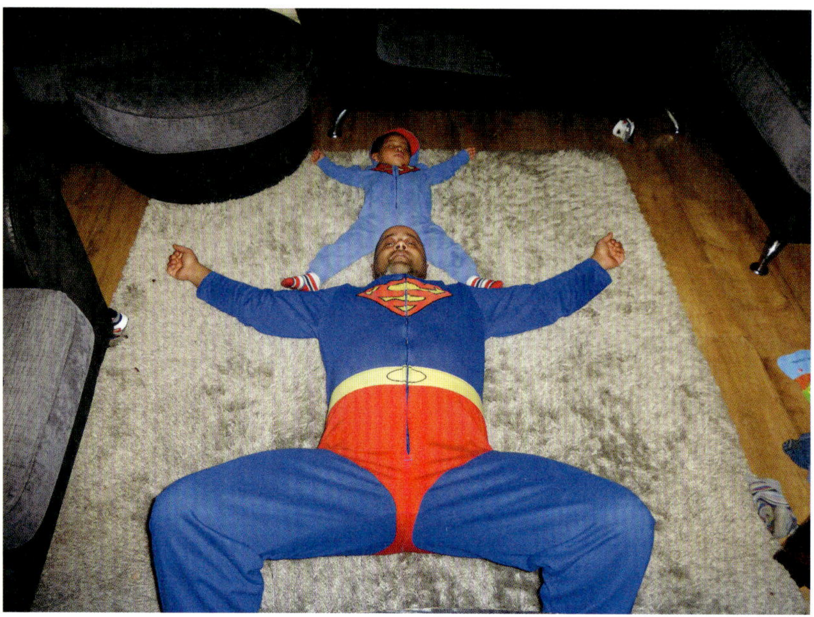

My life is very much focused on family and my responsibilities as a parent of eight children. HIV is a very small part of my life and it is not something that dictates how I move or how I view myself. I have a very supportive family. They all know about my HIV status and it has never been an issue for them. We were able to plan to have our babies safely, so thankfully all of them were born negative.

I am a full-time dad at the moment. I am not working. I haven't been working for some time. I was diagnosed with osteoporosis of the spine, which causes a lot of problems for my mobility. That is one area of my life that is very dark. It is very depressing. Especially being an African man, I've always been used to being the provider. There is a need for me to go out every day, just to free myself of any pain or burdens or issues, so that when I walk back into my home it's happy days.

Religion plays a very big part in our family. My closeness to Christianity has given me a lot of courage. It has given me the direction and comfort that I've needed during the difficult times in my life.

We're a fun, fun family. We are always either dancing or singing. There's a lot of love. We are not short of love in our home.

When I was behind the lens taking pictures of my little kids, somewhat morbid thoughts were going through my mind that if I did die before my time with my HIV diagnosis, at least there would be this album —beautiful pictures to remember me by.

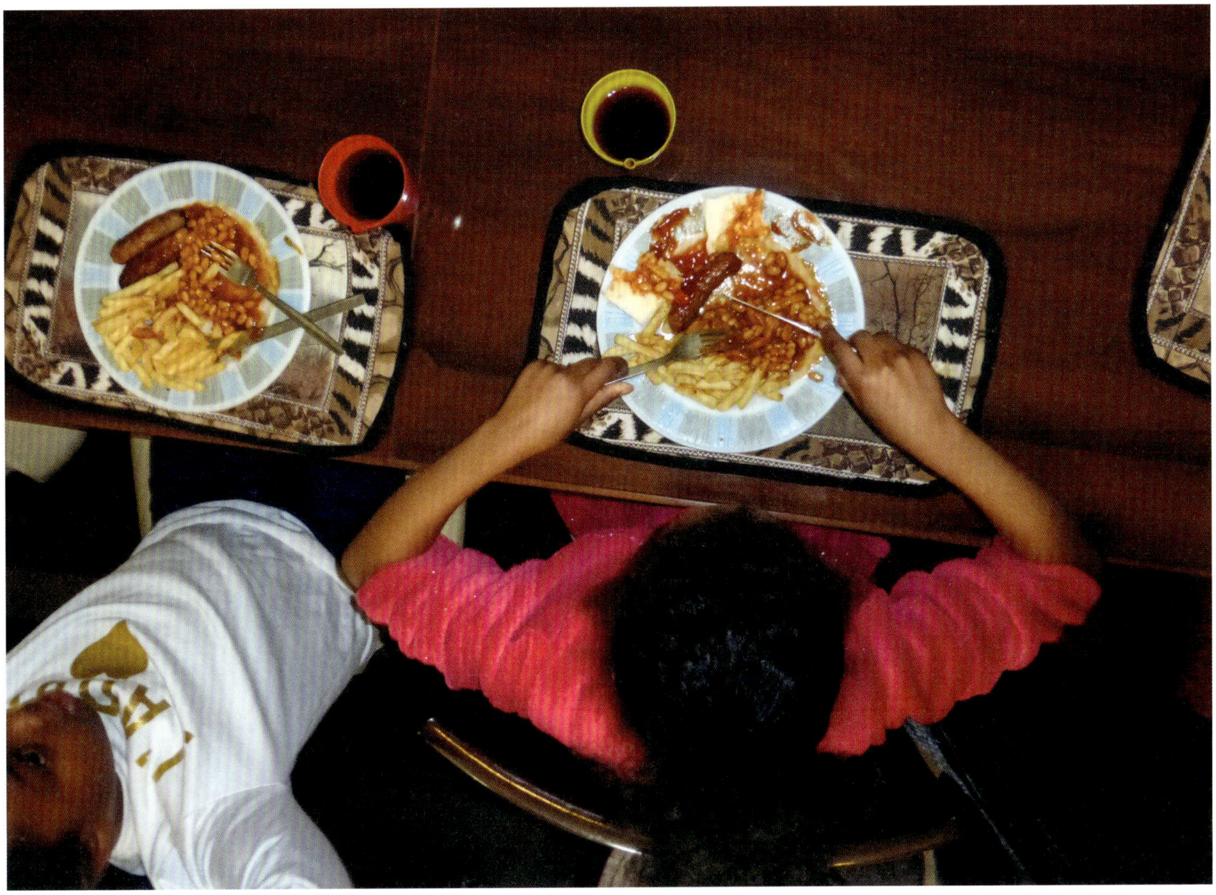

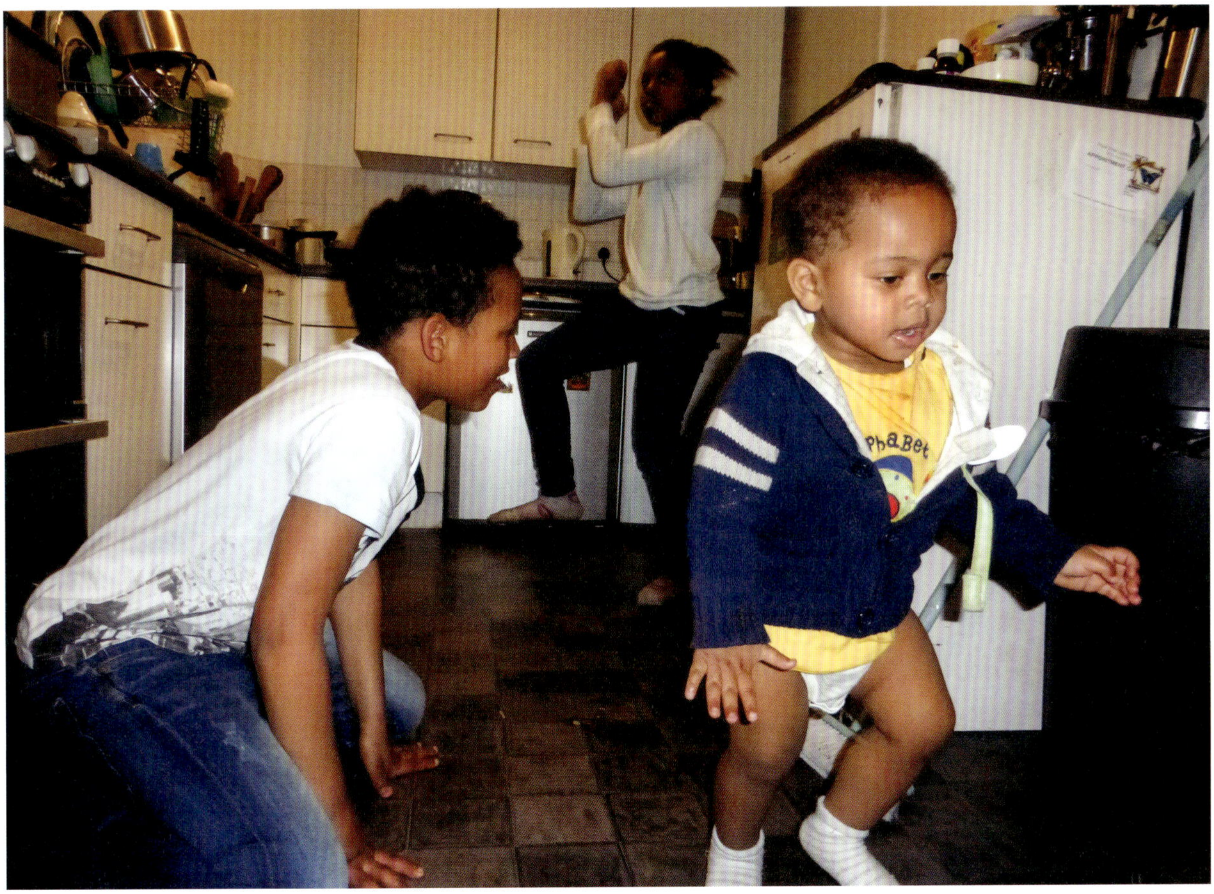

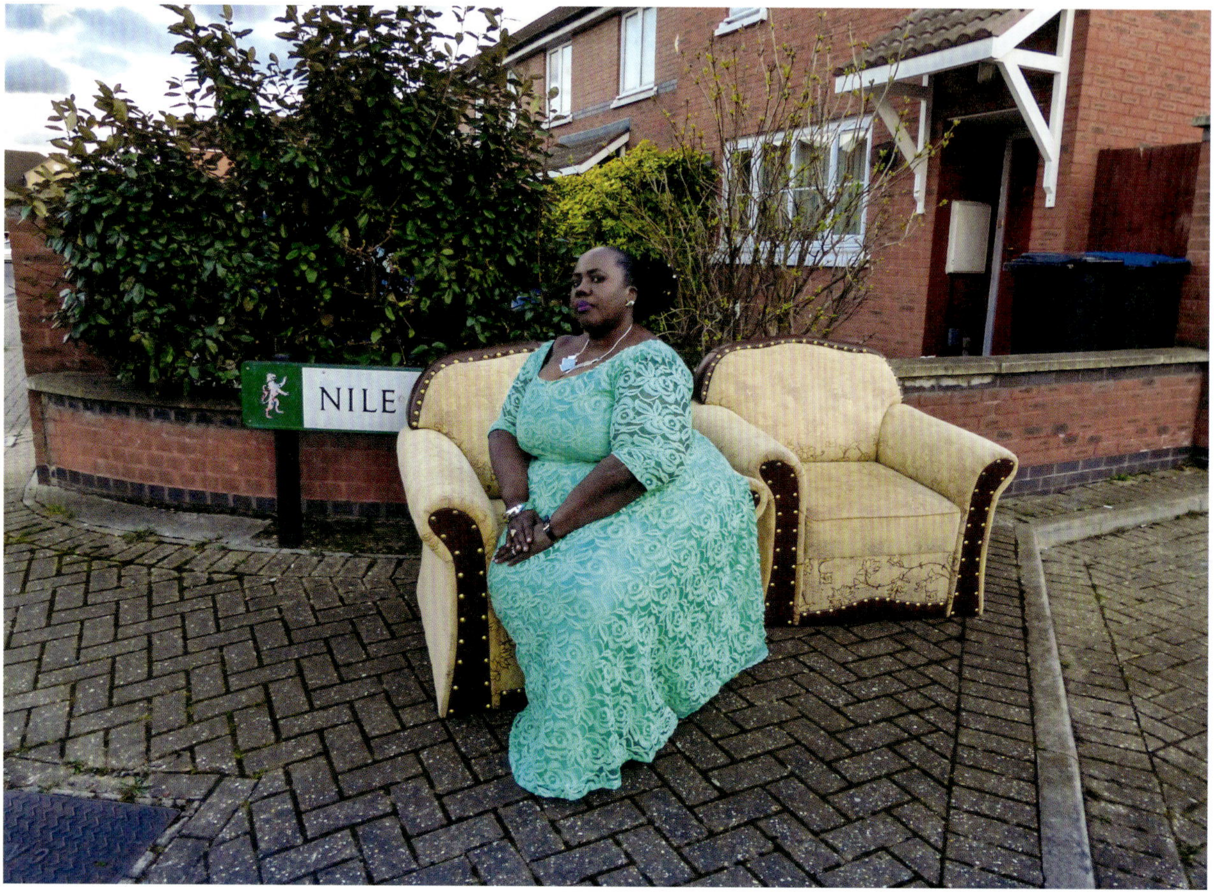

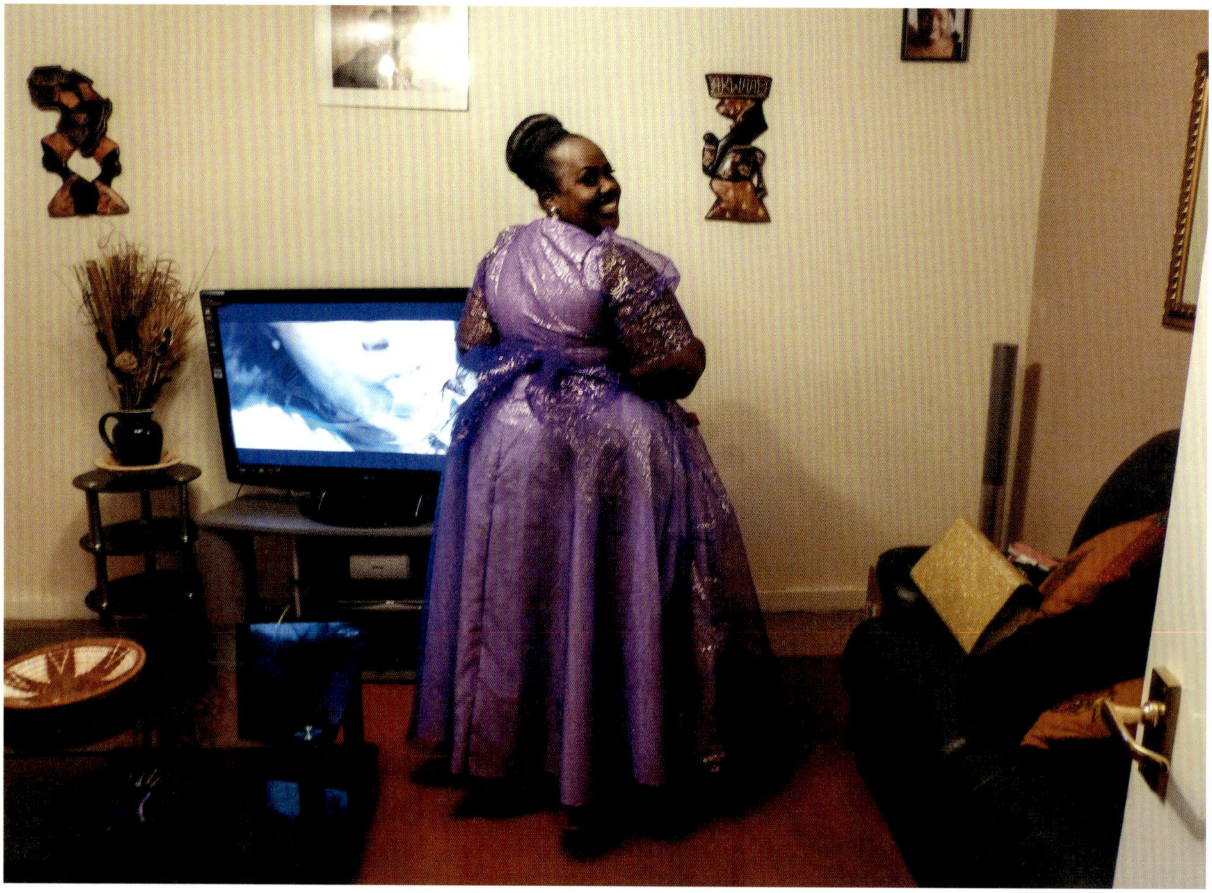

Maureen

People used to think someone who was HIV-positive should be skinny and miserable and all that. No, no, no, things have changed. Now we're looking good.

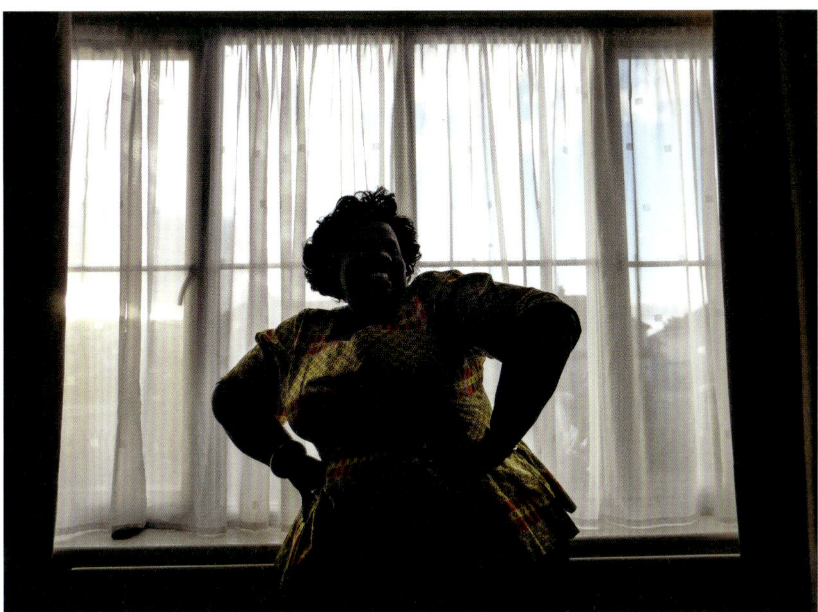

I come from Zimbabwe. But now I live in London and I'm British.

When I came to the UK, I started losing weight and having fevers. Something was suspicious. I collapsed in my house and was taken to the hospital, where they discovered I had pulmonary tuberculosis. To my shock, they also told me I'm HIV-positive.

My room was facing the Thames River. One day I thought I should jump through the window and just die. I couldn't take the shame, the stigma within my community, the stigma within my family.

Then I was introduced to an HIV support group in Enfield and the people there were all looking so good. With all the confidence that I was gaining, from meeting people living with HIV, I started to discover myself. I started speaking openly about HIV. I set myself free and discovered that within me there is the passion to work with other people living with HIV.

With the antiretroviral treatment that we take, the skin changes, especially for people of color. I said no, I have to change the way I look.

I love fashion. I mean, I'm big and there is no way I can walk into Harrod's and get a dress of my size, so I make my own clothes. Everything I do, I do it myself. Before I leave the house, no matter how late I am, I have to run and peer into the mirror and see how I look. Only then do I step out.

I never thought I would make it till now. I received my diagnosis when I was thirty-nine, but now I'm fifty-one. People used to think that someone who was HIV-positive should be skinny and miserable and all that. No, no, no, things have changed. Now we're looking good. We can do everything. I always tell people, the only thing I can't do is donate blood.

If you are bitter, everything just doesn't coordinate. I love smiling. To me that's my medicine.

Chris

The Lazarus effect is not instant. It takes time. But I want to show that, after being diagnosed with HIV, people can recover and live full, active lives.

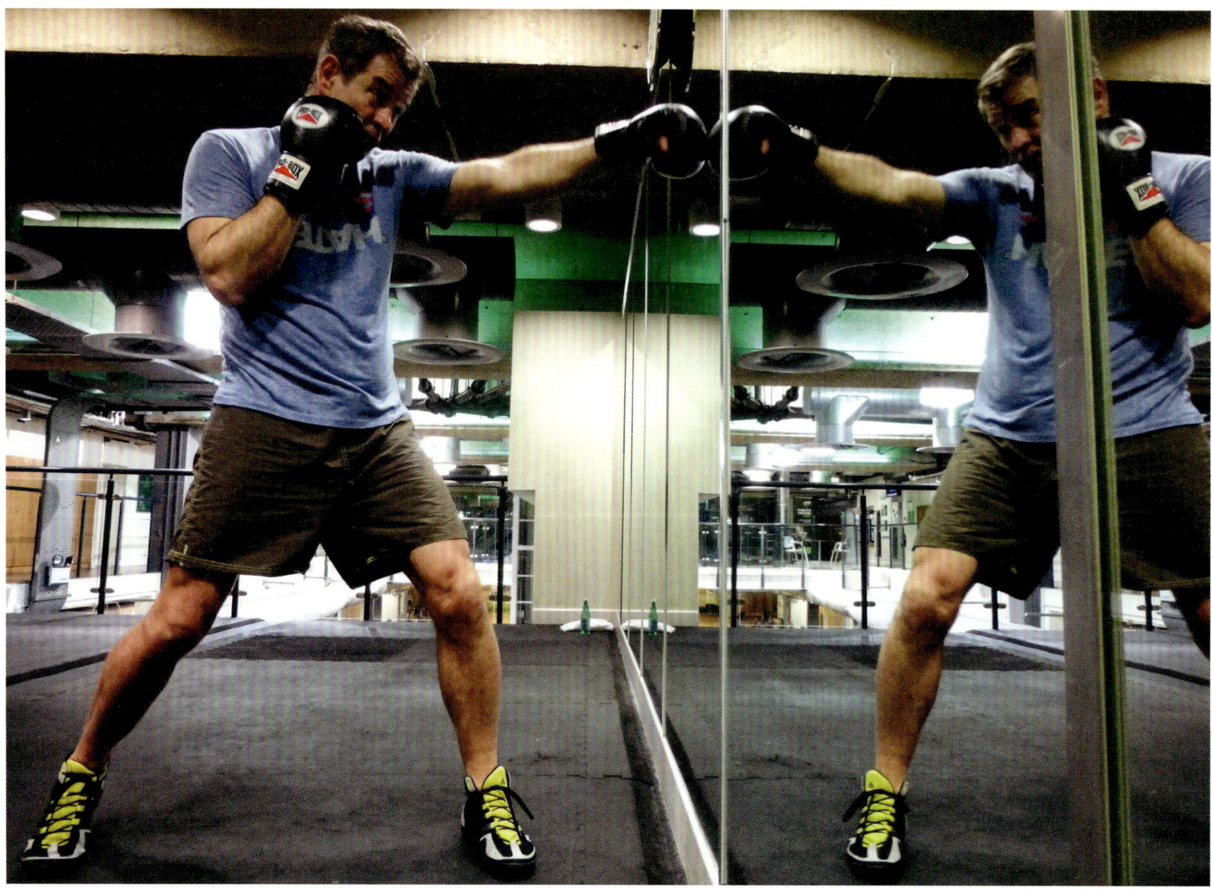

I was already ill when, in short order, I contracted a whole host of opportunistic infections: pneumonia, esophageal candida, herpes, thrush. It was like when you see those nature films where you have a log in a forest, and you speed up the film to watch it decay. That's what it felt like. It felt like I was drowning.

A year after my diagnosis, I was in the hospital weighing sixty-five kilos [143 pounds]. I had double pneumonia, diarrhea, and night sweats. I was told I had just a couple of months to live.

I was not long married. You talk about my life with HIV, it's our life with HIV, my wife's and mine together. She's been through all the processes of dealing with me when I was really ill, and dealing with me when I was recovering, and dealing with me when I didn't know what to do. She's the glue that has kept me together.

I've had doctors say, "Well, isn't this like diabetes?" But it isn't. I've never come across a diabetic who was reluctant to tell his mother and father that he's diabetic, who can lose a job because he's diabetic, who doesn't know how to tell a prospective girlfriend that he's diabetic.

Regardless of the stigma, I have been given the gift of grace. I'm not frightened anymore.

Loads of guys got ARVs—antiretroviral treatment—and still didn't make it. It was too late for them. It hasn't been straightforward, coming back from the brink. The Lazarus effect is not instant. It takes time. But I want to show that, after being diagnosed with HIV, people can recover and live full, active lives.

Aaron

I was diagnosed in 2004 when I was living in Spain. (I was born in Mexico and have been living in London now for eight years.) I was quite shocked and said, "How long do I have?" I was still full of outdated information from the 1980s and 1990s. I remember going back home on the bus, looking at all these old people, and thinking, "Oh my gosh, I am never going to grow old like them." I felt stupid for having made the wrong decisions. But the reality is that, I mean, at twenty-six you are very sexual. You like to have fun and you like to have sex.

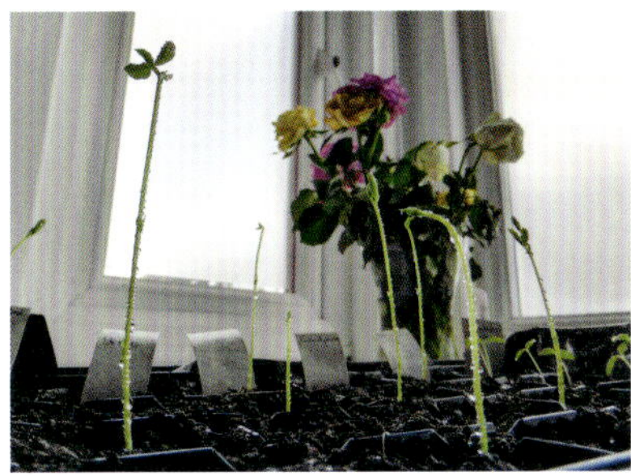

Nowadays, HIV has become a minuscule thing for me. You just talk about which pills you take, and that sort of stuff, but it's not a death sentence anymore for us. There is not really drama around HIV for me anymore. The only thing I worry about now is the mundane: looking after the bills, getting a job. I have to worry about the mortgage and things like that. Pensions.

Alongside these problems, there's hope. I'm living a quintessentially British life in London. I'm trying to pretend I'm creative. I am really into gardening. I love seeing how something grows from a seed. Sometimes you can see the whole meaning of life in miniature things like this.

HIV has affected me, but the great medication that we have now allows me to just live my life as normally as everybody else, which is fantastic.

Graeme

I was diagnosed in the very early days of the epidemic. I wasn't aware of anybody else in my circle having HIV. It did seem like a death sentence then. You literally didn't know whether you had weeks, months, or if you could even think about years to live. And I was thirty-two, relatively young, and the thought of dying was quite scary really. So between my diagnosis in 1985 and 1996, when effective medication became available, a lot of my friends died. But I was very lucky that I was a slow progressor, so by 1996, when my CD4 count had dropped to 200, the threshold for treatment, I was able to get on the medications.

Some people think that life post-medication is a piece of cake, but it isn't. In two years' time, when I'm sixty-four, I will have spent half my life with HIV.

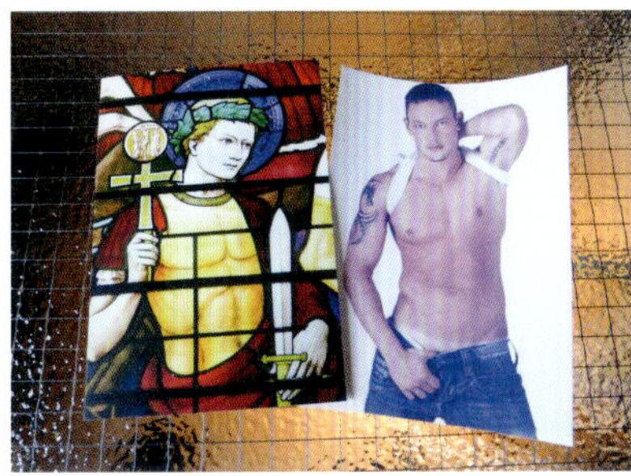

My own church is known as liberal Catholic, all embracing. We have a diversity policy where everyone is welcome. I always felt able to come out about my sexuality in church, but I didn't generally come out about my HIV status. So as part of a special church program, I gave them my life history in forty minutes with musical tracks in between. I was totally honest about my life, my being gay and my becoming HIV-positive. At the end, when I finished, there was silence for a few seconds and then there was applause. I went forward closer to them and people stood up and hugged me, which is a really tremendous affirmation of the love in the church.

Isaac

My life revolves around four little creatures. I love my dogs dearly, but they also really annoy me. Bella is my baby. She has been the stability within my unstable life, living with HIV.

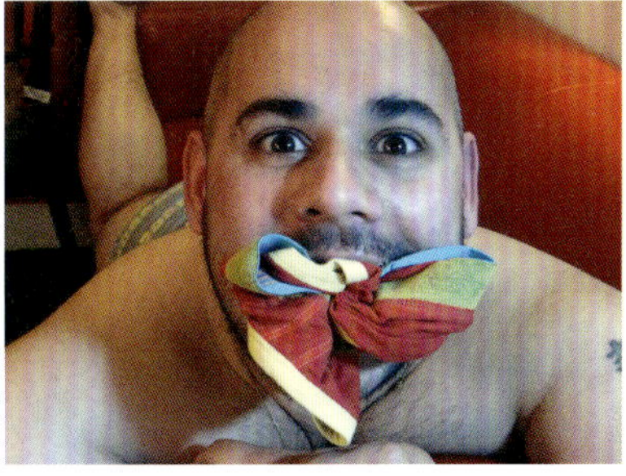

I've always had a very artistic flare and I like to experiment with things.

I love the fact that I'm an openly HIV-positive man who doesn't care what people think about my status. I became HIV-positive by having great condom-less sex, with somebody who was positive. Nothing more, nothing less. You can actually never wash away HIV. For me, the attempts that I've made to wash away HIV have just brought me closer to it.

I take twenty-nine tablets a day as a result of being HIV-positive. I have a very difficult relationship with medication, but I'm also very grateful. I struggle with the fact that, as a spoiled westerner, I have access to medication and some people in the world don't.

I wish that, along my journey as a young person, somebody would have spoken to me about being able to negotiate sex. I think that being positive has changed my life. I feel like I'm a better person. I just want to say to everybody out there, if you have preconceived ideas about positive people, just forget them. We are sexual beings with rights. I choose not to be stigmatized. I say pants-in-the-mouth to stigma.

Joshua

In London, a lot of gay men use Grindr, which is a dating app. A lot of people use it for casual sex. You look at the profiles of people on there, and they all say, "Clean, STI free," which means no sexually transmitted infections, including HIV. Everyone is so scared of getting it, that they look down on people who do have it. Yet, they still engage in sexual activity that will expose them to the virus quite easily. I was diagnosed on Halloween 2014. It was horrific. In my head I had all these ignorant preconceptions about the sort of person who would get it, or the type of behavior that you'd be engaged in to get it.

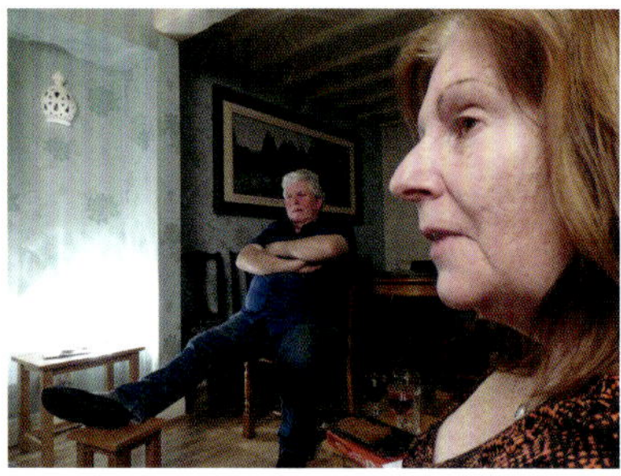

There was no way I could accept it at that stage. I was using language like, "I have been told that I have...," not, "I have HIV," because it just wasn't real. I never thought I would be saying those words to my mom. The only way I can describe it is that we were joined as one, just hugging each other. I've never felt someone's heart beat so strongly as I did when we were hugging, both hysterically crying.

It's gotten a lot easier. I don't cry anymore. I live with my brother and his wife, and they've been my pillars since I was diagnosed. He was sort of my psychologist and she was my social worker, and if I was living on my own without them, I don't know if I would have coped the same as I did. I think the cherry on top of the cake of my story so far with HIV is having all of my family be together and everyone accepting me as being HIV-positive.

When I first went to the clinic I was just gob-smacked about how much money they must have spent on it to make it appealing to people, to want to go there. No one in my family would want to see me experiencing something like an HIV diagnosis alone.

I would like to think that, although there may be a lot of shock for some people, from their families or friends, the reward for going through it and talking about it and normalizing it is just incredibly beneficial for you and for the people you love.

Marc

I tried to remember what it felt like to be negative as a young gay man and couldn't. I probably had a year of living gay and HIV-negative. You know, I was seventeen when I was diagnosed. I had had three boyfriends.

I was very fortunate in that I was able to tell my mom, who was the most unbelievable support. I remember sitting down at the table in floods and floods of tears, trying to get the words out, and she leaned over and calmly said, "You might be knocked over by a bus tomorrow, but with this I know what to do, I know that I can take care of you. So stop your tears, stop your crying, we'll get through it." I come from a very strong Jamaican background. You have to be a man. You have to stand up. And I kind of stood up to HIV. That's what I did. It's not going to take me out.

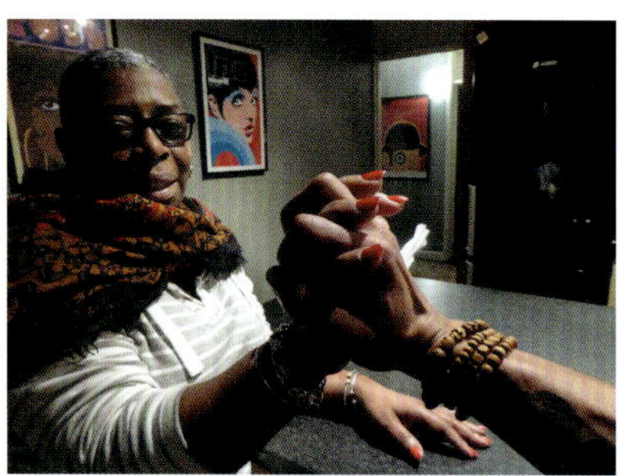

I run a peer-mentoring program. I recruit, train, and manage other people who live with HIV to provide one-to-one support to positive people. It is challenging and it's really, really rewarding. It's a passion of mine. I love it. I feel like I've got some sort of balance in my life now. Day-to-day life is pretty chill. I've got a really close-knit circle of friends, black gay men of a certain age, who have all been together for twenty-odd years.

Most days I spend time with my special tree. I noticed it a couple of years ago when it was in full bloom. It touched me because it wasn't perfect, yet it was so beautiful. I share that space with my dog, Travis, who really did save my life from going down a rabbit hole of drinking and drugs. He just filled my life with happiness. We're up every single morning. Rain or shine, 365 days a year. We're in the park and we're walking.

I like being solo right now because I'm finding myself and I'm quite happy in that space. It's not a bad space to be.

Durban

The June 2016 *Through Positive Eyes* workshop in Durban—epicenter of South Africa's AIDS epidemic in the province of KwaZulu-Natal—attests to the uneven progress toward curbing HIV and AIDS in the country with the highest number of cases in the world. In 2016, 19% of South African adults between the ages of fifteen and forty-nine were HIV-positive. In KwaZulu-Natal, the percentage was even higher: 30%. In response, massive efforts have been made to bring KwaZulu-Natal's epidemic under control. In Durban in 2016, for example, 89% of the 621,000 individuals infected with HIV were already receiving antiretroviral treatment. Leaving statistics aside, the participants in the Durban workshop demonstrated through their stories that too many young people, especially young women, are becoming infected with HIV at the very start of their sexual lives. This revelation underlines the need for gender-sensitive early sexual health education and intervention, not only in South Africa but around the world.

Durban's AIDS epidemic, as of 2016

Number of people living with HIV:	621,000

(this is 8.2% of all South Africans living with HIV)

HIV prevalence

Adults (15–49 years):	22.6%
Female sex workers:	53.5%
Men who have sex with men:	48.2%

Treatment

% of people living with HIV who know their HIV status:	74%
% of those needing treatment who are receiving it:	89%
% of those with undetectable viral load:	67%

Two conferences

Two international AIDS conferences have been held in Durban. In 2000, treatment activists demonstrated in the street against the HIV denialism of South African president Thabo Mbeki. By the time of the 2016 conference, South Africa had the largest treatment program in the world, with 3.4 million people receiving free antiretroviral therapy, largely in the public sector.

Through Positive Eyes in Durban was organized in partnership with the AIDS Foundation of South Africa. Major funding was provided by The Herb Ritts Foundation, with additional support from The Andy Warhol Foundation for the Visual Arts, Electronic Theatre Controls (ETC), The Ford Foundation, Gere Foundation, UNAIDS, and UCLA.

Xoli

My first boyfriend played a fatherly role. He was my "blesser." I wanted to hate the guy for infecting me with HIV, but, at the end of the day, he also gave me life because, with his financial support, I managed to finish school.

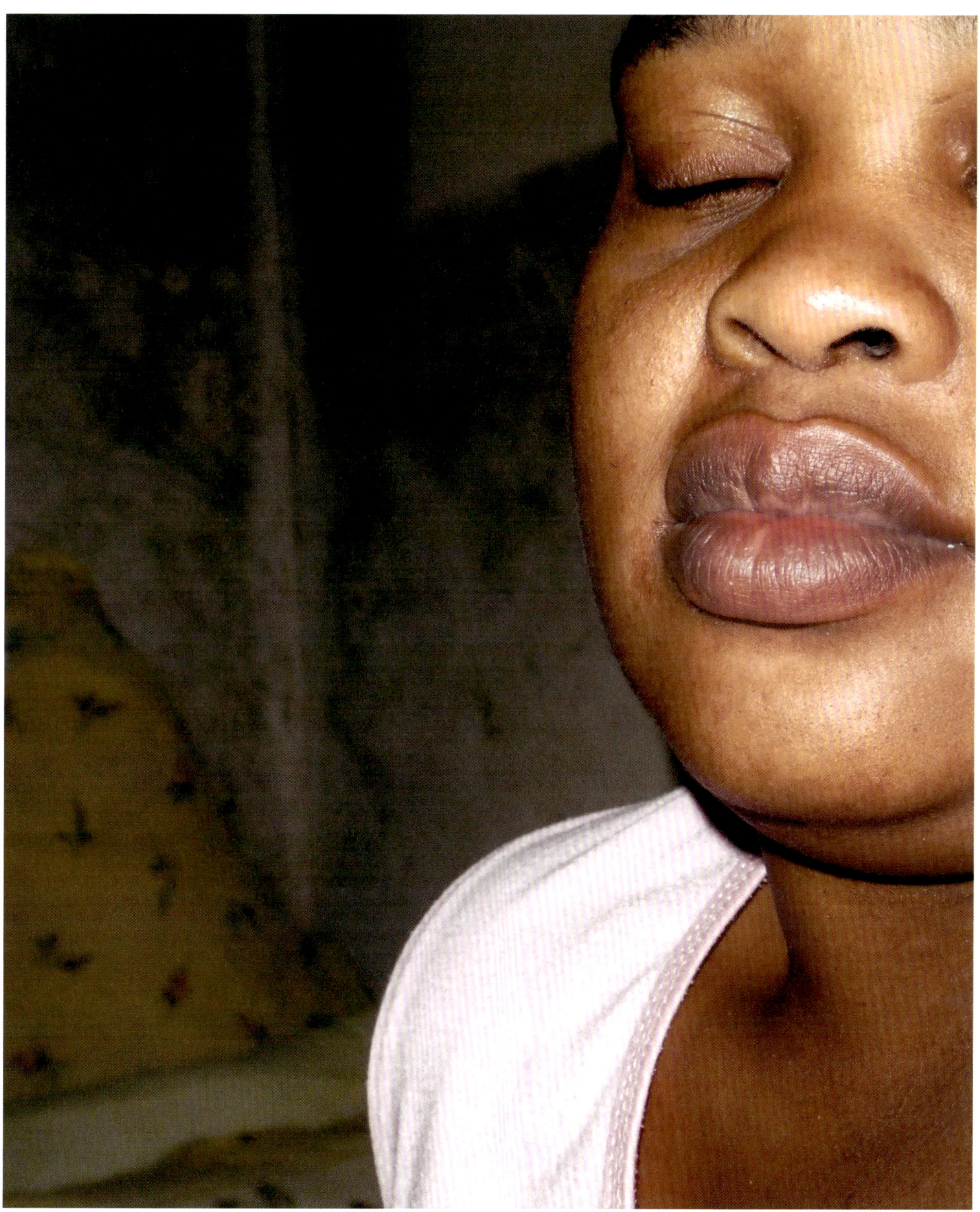

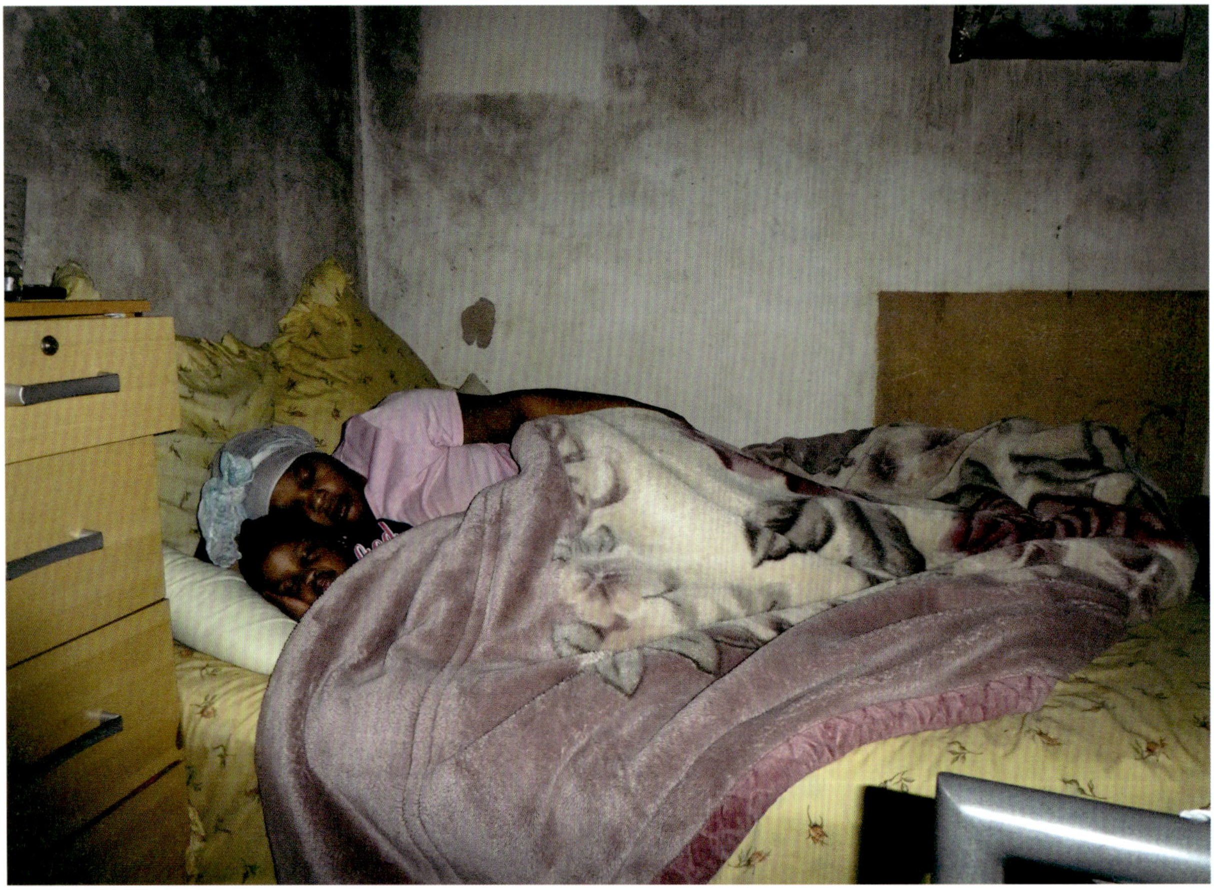

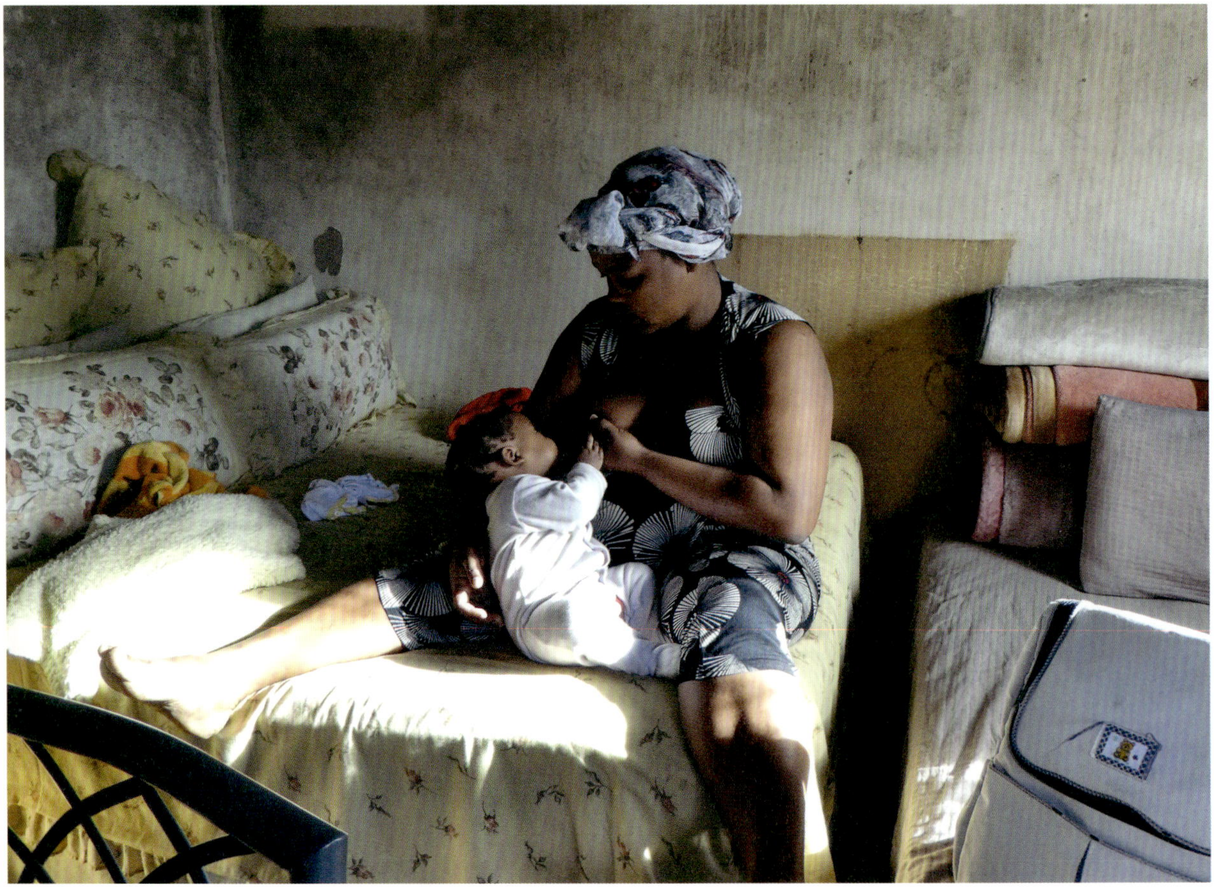

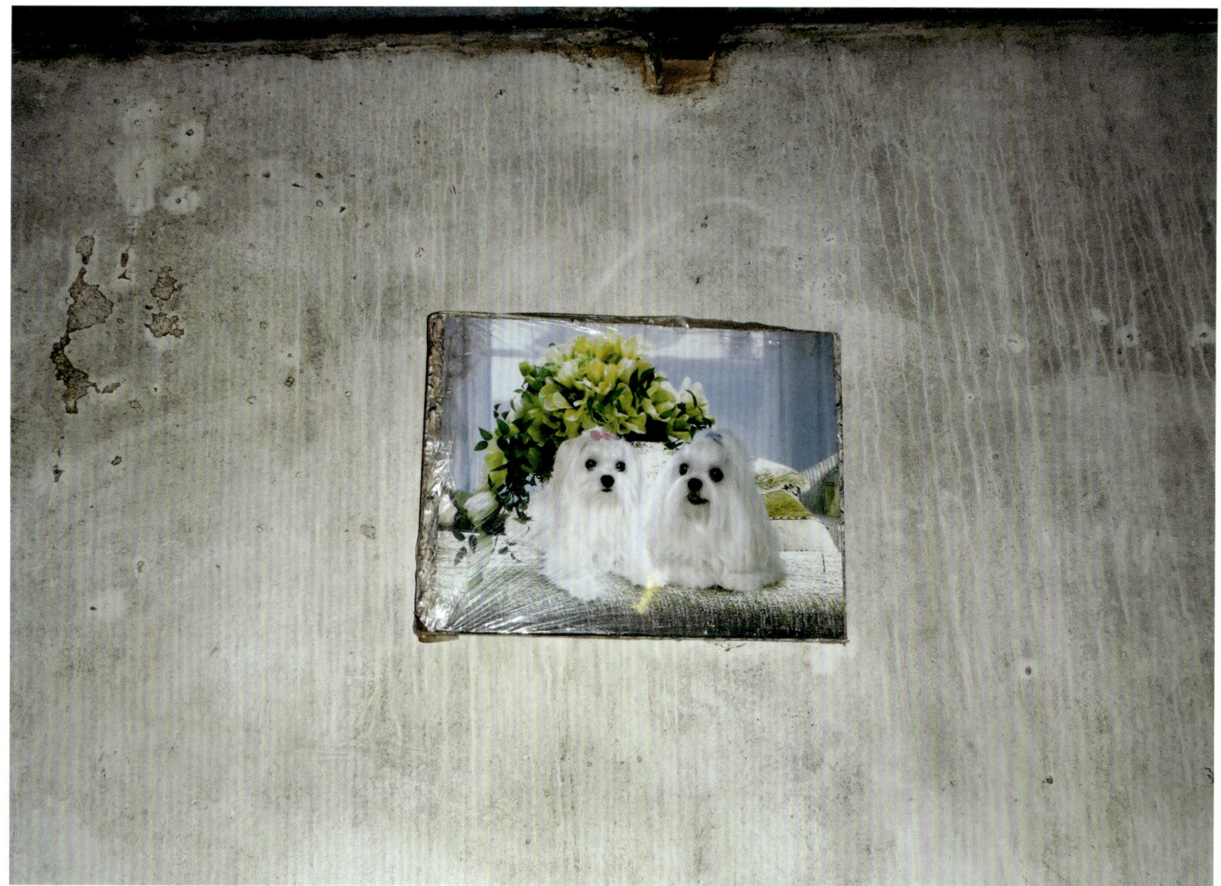

I was born and raised in Lindelani, a village in KwaZulu-Natal, by my grandma and my granddad. Due to the absence of my parents, I grew up in a dysfunctional family. I knew I wanted to finish school, but as a girl, I didn't have that support.

As a kid I was quite beautiful. I was big-boned, which resulted in me attracting older guys. As a result of attracting all the wrong guys, I fell pregnant at the age of sixteen. I lost that baby and, at the same time, discovered I was HIV-positive. So the pain was double.

My first boyfriend did everything for me. He played a fatherly role. He was my "blesser," my sugar daddy. I wanted to hate the guy for infecting me with HIV, but, at the end of the day, he also gave me life because, with his financial support, I managed to finish school.

He did all the good things for me, I had the good life.

As much as I wanted to hate him, I couldn't. Instead, I started resenting my parents because I thought if they were there for me I wouldn't have been in this situation. I wouldn't have had the need for a blesser.

After finishing school, I had so many emotions, I was uncontrollable. I just wanted to live my life so fast, to get it over and done with because I knew that, at the end of the road, HIV was going to kill me. I was scared. And I felt like trash.

I had to stop and think and really find out, Why am I alive? What do I want out of my life? And what I found was that I still had hope, and that I wanted to live. I wanted to have everything my parents couldn't give me. I wanted a family. I wanted to be bigger than HIV.

I started my ARVs, not because I was sick, but because I wanted to have a child. He's a healthy boy, seven years old now. And I had two more after that. So I have three beautiful children. I call them my Nevirapines, because I had to take the drug Nevirapine in order for them to be HIV-negative.

Imagine, now I have a husband and three kids. They're all negative. I'm the only one who's positive. They give me all the support that I need.

A final piece of advice to all the parents out there: Treasure your daughters. Give them all the love you can.

Simiso

When I disclosed to her after maybe a year of dating, she gave me a hug and she said, "Shame, you poor thing," and she gave me a kiss.

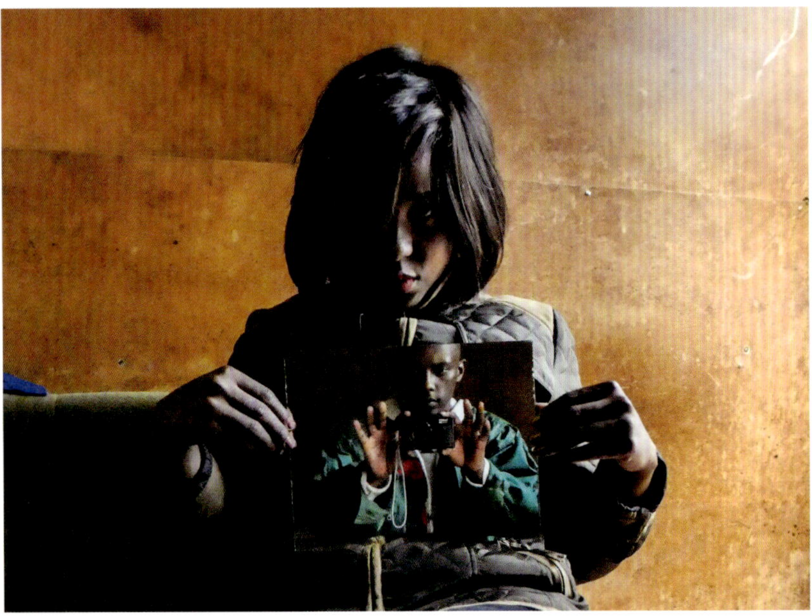

Prior to actually finding out about my status, I was riding on the assumption that HIV is for old people. I looked at it as something far away from me. It was never even close to crossing my mind.

I knew that we had something called condoms. And I knew that we had HIV in this country. I had seen people who had gotten ill and eventually lost their lives. But I was very ignorant about it. I never pictured myself having it.

So once the diagnosis came, I realized that actually there are a lot of young people who have the same mentality I had. This is one of the leading factors of why the youth of this country keep on getting infected.

I had a girlfriend who was regularly testing, so, she convinced me to go and test as well. We had 100% certainty that she was negative. When I came back and I told her the results, that I'm positive, both of us were shocked and confused. So obviously she went to her best friends, who all came up with this idea that she should break up with me because I'm HIV-Positive. She actually listened to her friends rather than following her heart.

I felt like a failure, a disappointment to myself, family, and friends. This was totally the opposite of how I used to look at life and feel.

I started looking at everything that happens, anything that goes wrong in my life, it was always related to HIV. So, I could be walking and I could bump my toe and then I'd be sitting down, feeling like crying, thinking, "Ah goddamnit, this HIV is making me trip and fall now." HIV was Simiso and Simiso was HIV.

Back to normal life, I found another girl. I don't disclose right away. I like to let the person know me for who I am. Turns out, her grandmother was one of the very few people, when the outbreak happened in South Africa, who was chosen to lead the task force in the fight with HIV. So her grandmother has been teaching her about HIV and making her understand HIV. So when I disclosed to her after maybe a year of dating, she gave me a hug and she said, "Shame, you poor thing," and she gave me a kiss.

Sometimes people talk about destiny and fate. Even though I'm not completely sold on it, I'm almost buying into it now.

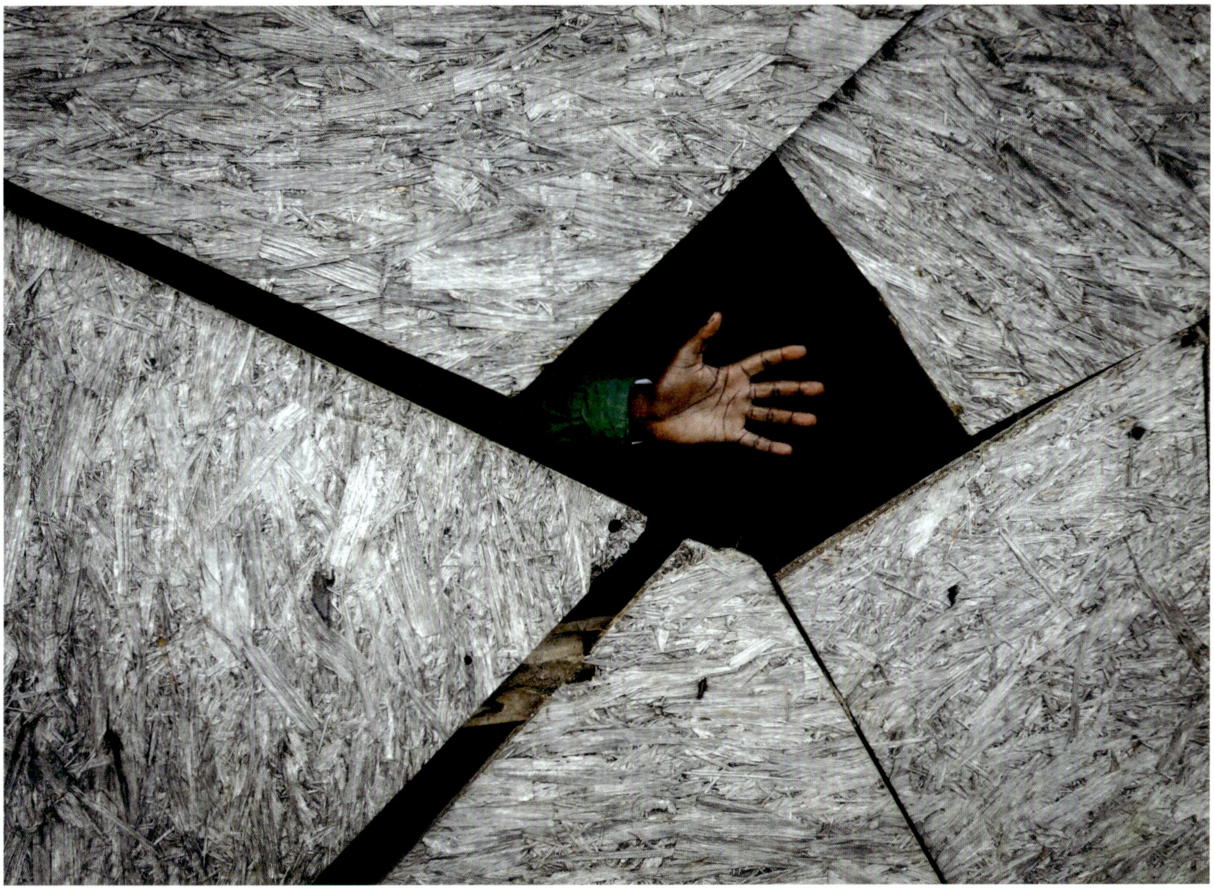

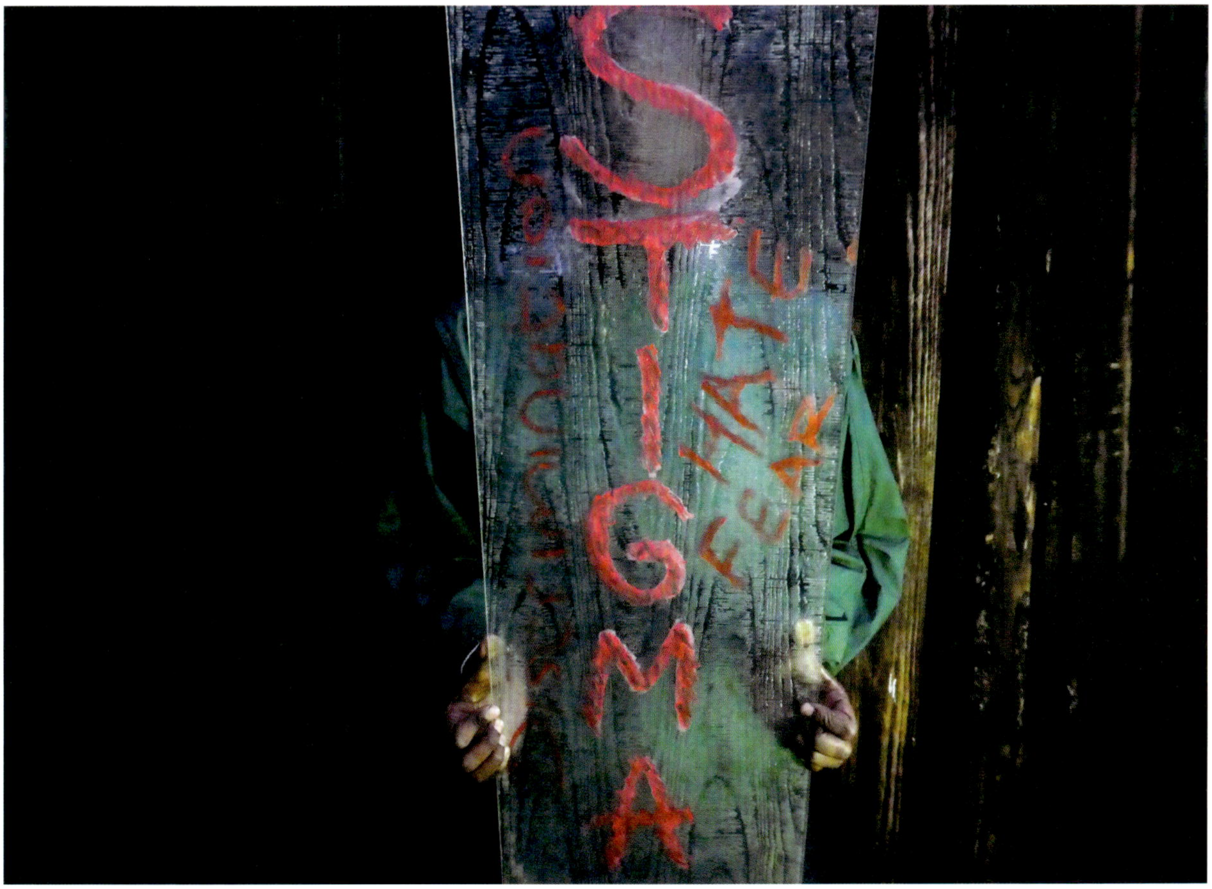

Jennifer

I decided to disclose my status to my partner. But he didn't take it well. He blamed me. And we fought, a lot.

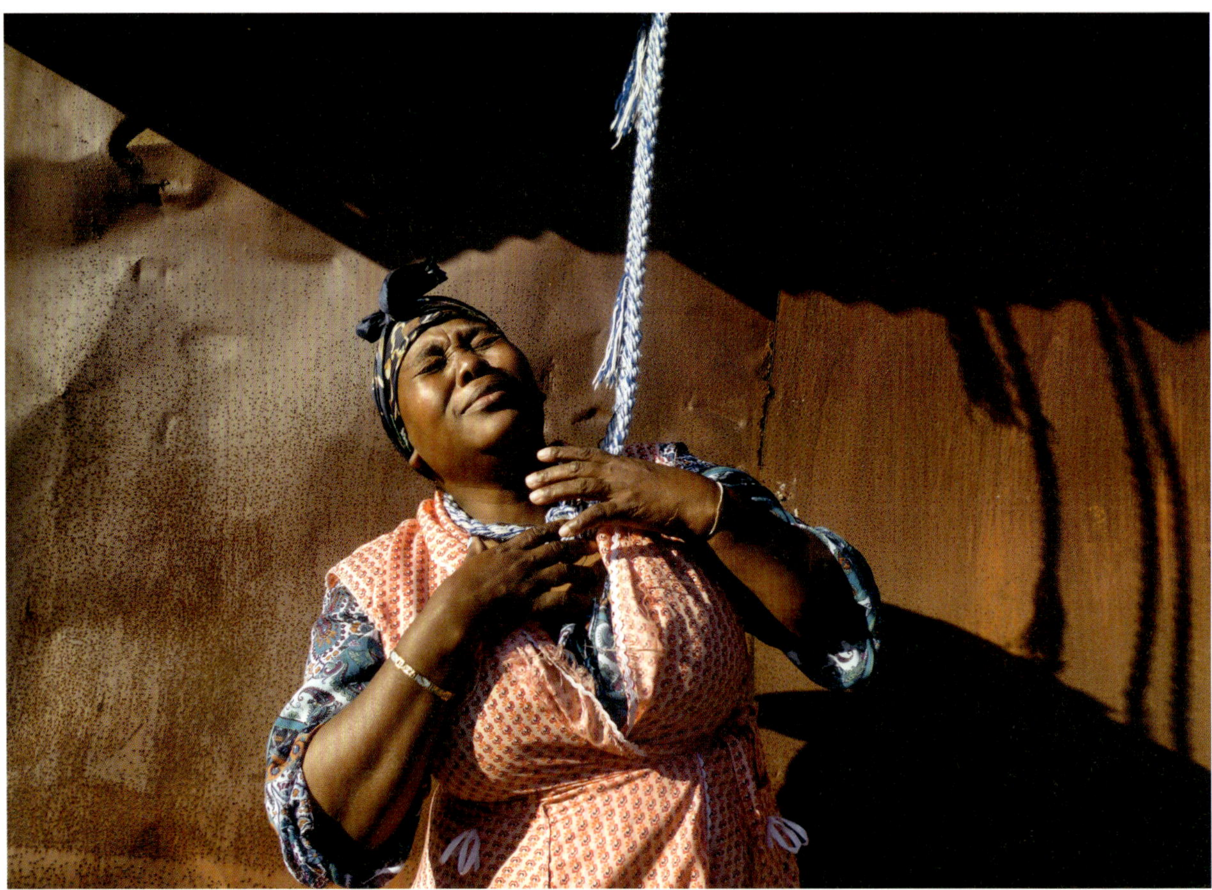

I was a beautiful young girl with a charming smile. All the men loved me. When I was nineteen, I had a strange feeling in my wrist. I went to the clinic to get treatment and the doctor told me that I have a sexually transmitted infection, caused by unprotected sex. I was shocked because I didn't know what an STI was. And then the assistant nurse told me I needed to take a blood test for HIV. That's when I found out that I'm HIV-positive.

I decided to disclose my status to my partner. But he didn't take it well. He blamed me. And we fought, a lot. I made a decision then to use a rope to take my life, but God was there for me. I didn't do it. I decided to go to my grandmother and disclose my status to her. After that, I started my life afresh.

I found a project near my home and worked there as a caregiver. I got the opportunity to take a course of study called "Home-based Care and Counseling." I disclosed my status to my chair lady. She was a good listener. She gave me good support. And thereafter, I went back to the clinic and started the medication called ARVs. I lived a healthy lifestyle and I joined an ongoing program with a support group.

After that, my partner realized that I'm still alive. He came back to his senses. And then he too went to take the test. I gave him my support to do that, and to start the ARVs when he received the news about his own HIV. Now, we are both on the medication. We are happy together with our family. So everything is going well.

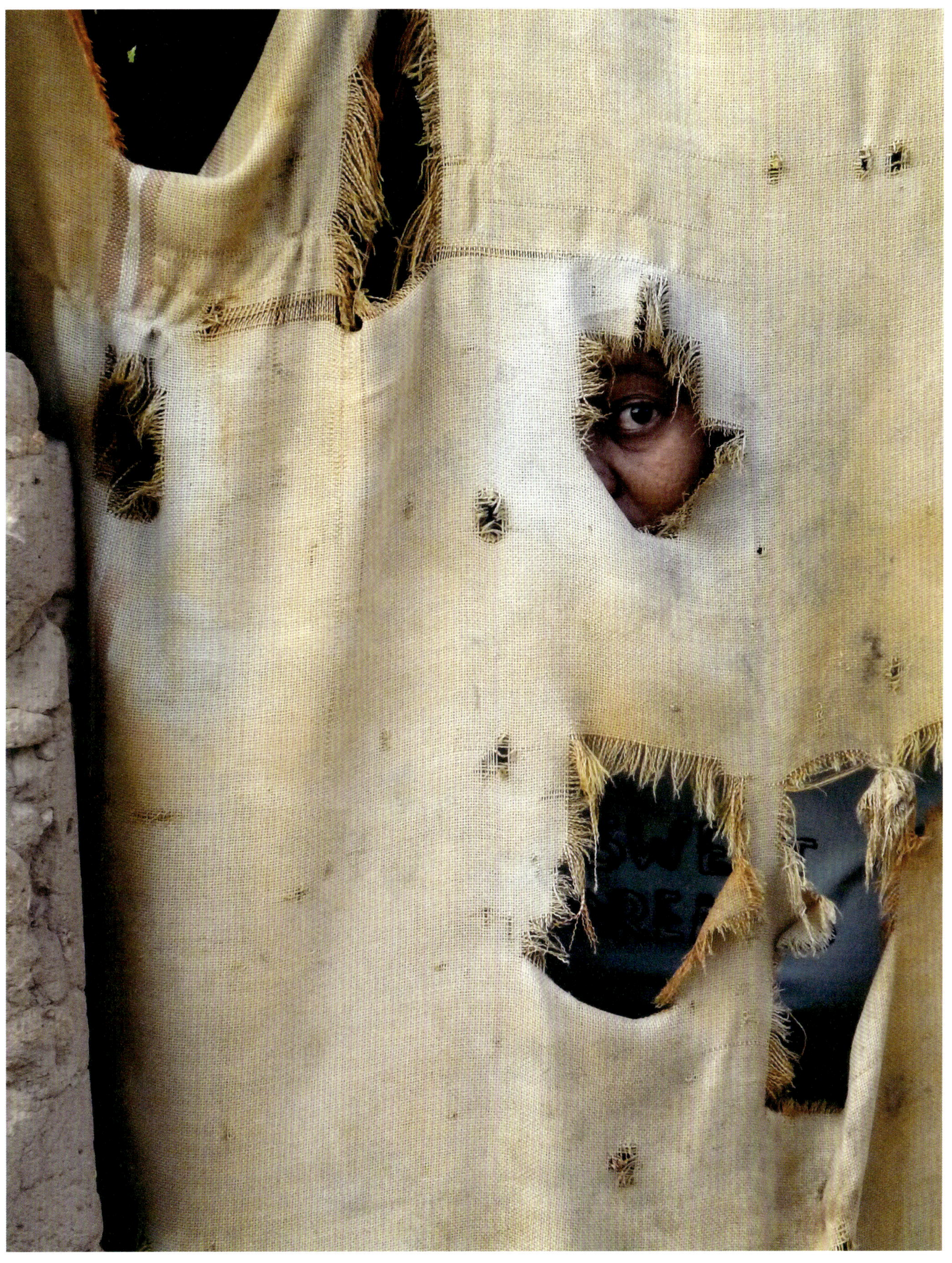

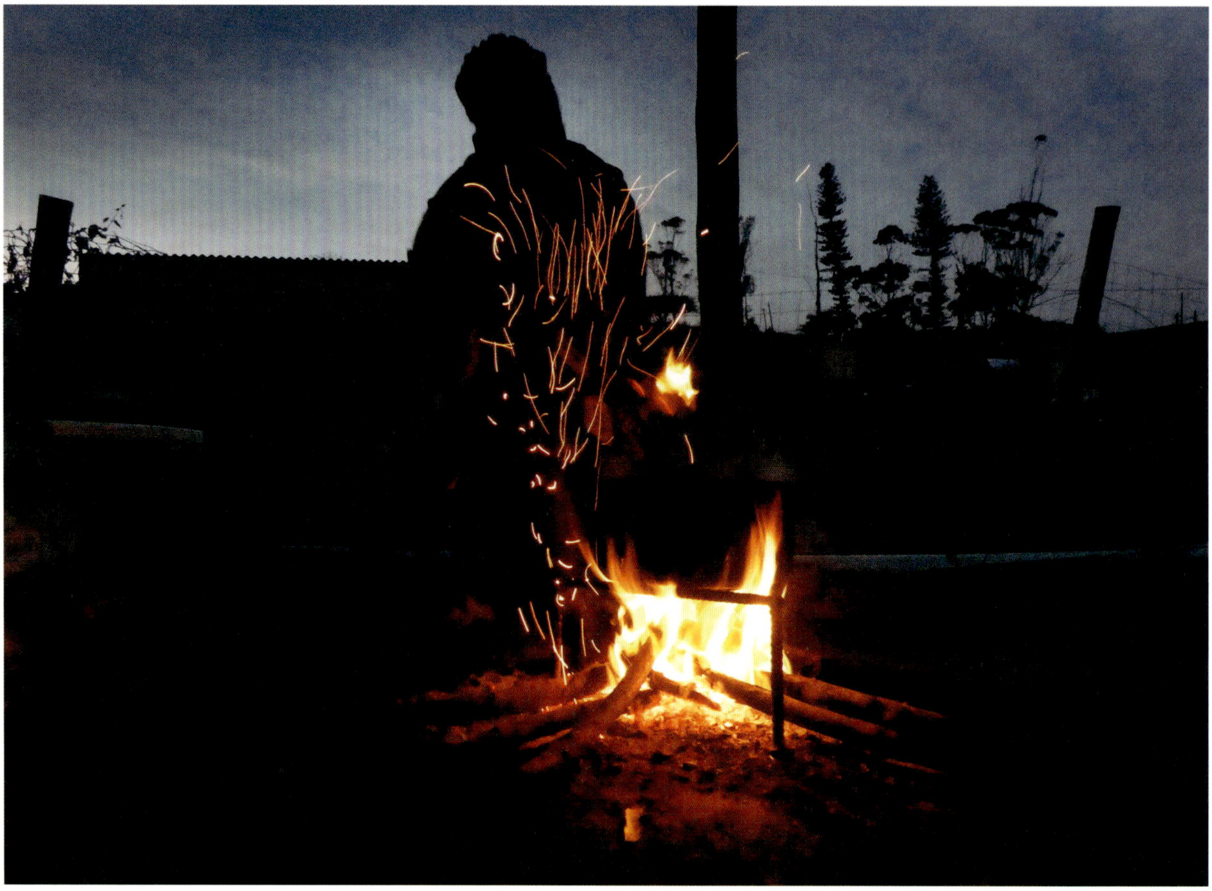

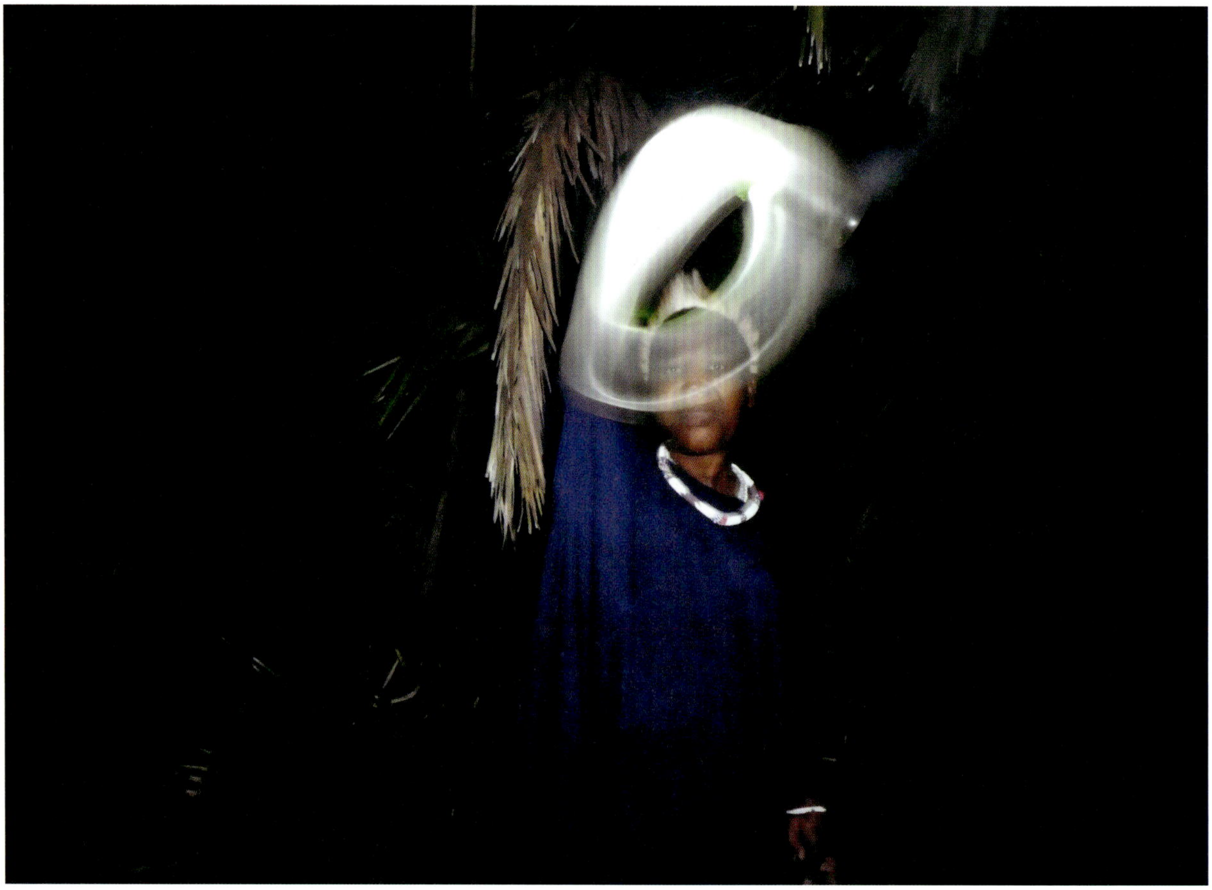

Gogo

One day, the woman neighbor who used to stigmatize me, she called and asked me to visit because she was sick. At that moment I said, "Wow, God, you have answered my prayers."

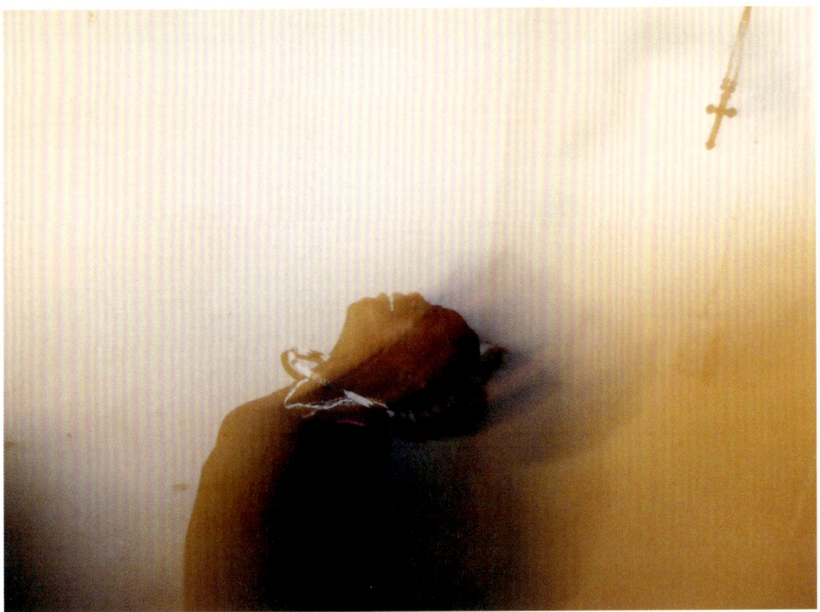

I am a traditional healer. I am a mother and grandmother. I am an HIV and AIDS human rights activist. I work with young people and that's where my passion is, especially for young girls.

When I tested HIV-positive, I thought that was the end of my life. I prayed, "God, please be with me. Help me to be able to face this monster in my life," as I was still young back then.

Two years later, I decided to disclose my HIV-positive status in public—guess what?—on the radio. Everybody learned about my HIV-positive status at once.

Those days, one of my neighbors, when I passed by her place, she would come out of her house and taunt me, which made me angry. I was angry with myself. I was angry with the community. I was angry with everything that was around me. But I used my anger to make sure that the community knows about HIV.

I then went straight to the Department of Health and told them that I was available. I said, "Let's partner and do something in my community." We began to train peer educators. We raised awareness on HIV and AIDS. I made sure that everybody was informed.

Since then I'm educating different communities through radio and media to raise awareness.

One day, the woman neighbor who used to stigmatize me, she called and asked me to visit because she was sick. At that moment I said, "Wow, God, you have answered my prayers." On my arrival at her place, she asked me to give her her handbag. She took out a piece of paper from the bag and guess what? It was the result of her HIV test, showing the HIV-positive result. And then I laughed, I don't want to lie.

I laughed, I laughed until I was done. Then I counseled her. We talked about everything. We talked about her feelings. And then from that day forward, we became friends. Now she is leading one of the powerful support groups in my area.

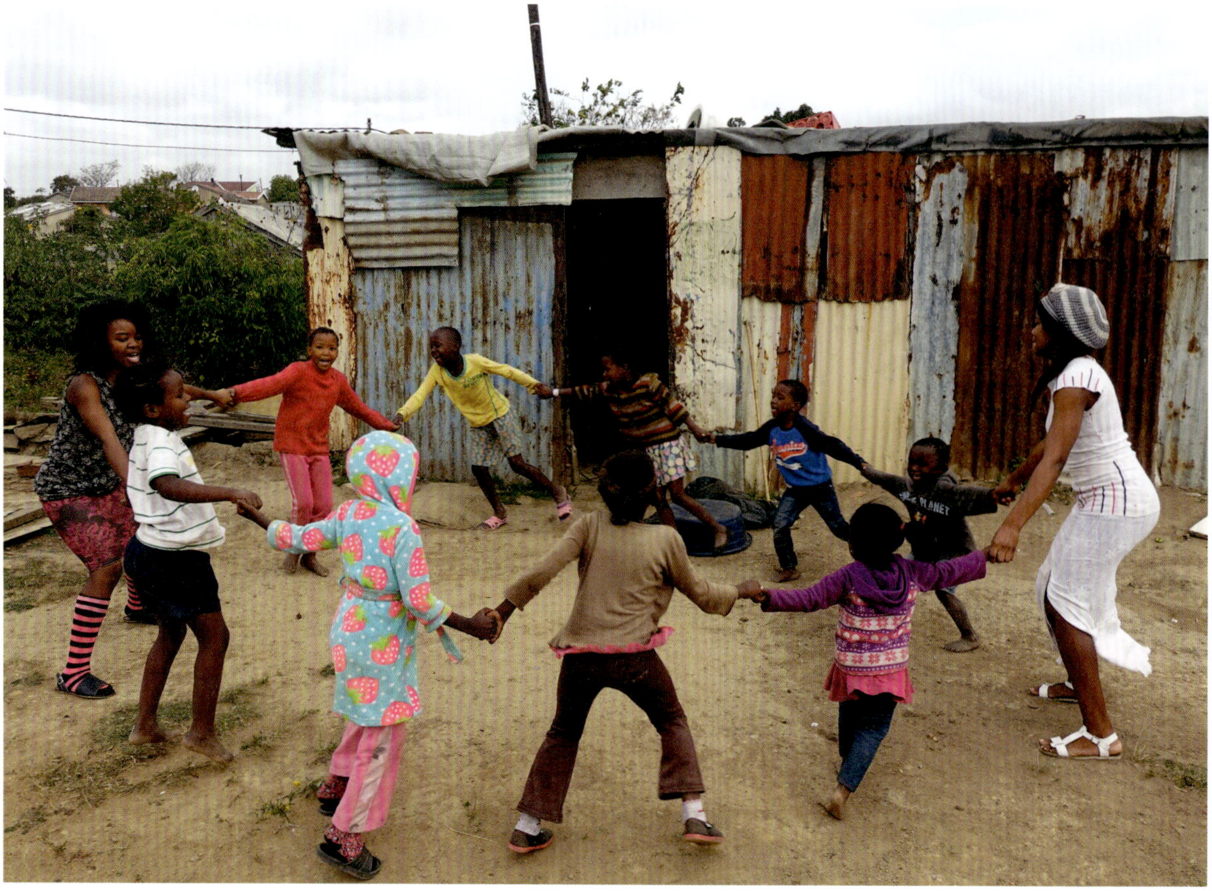

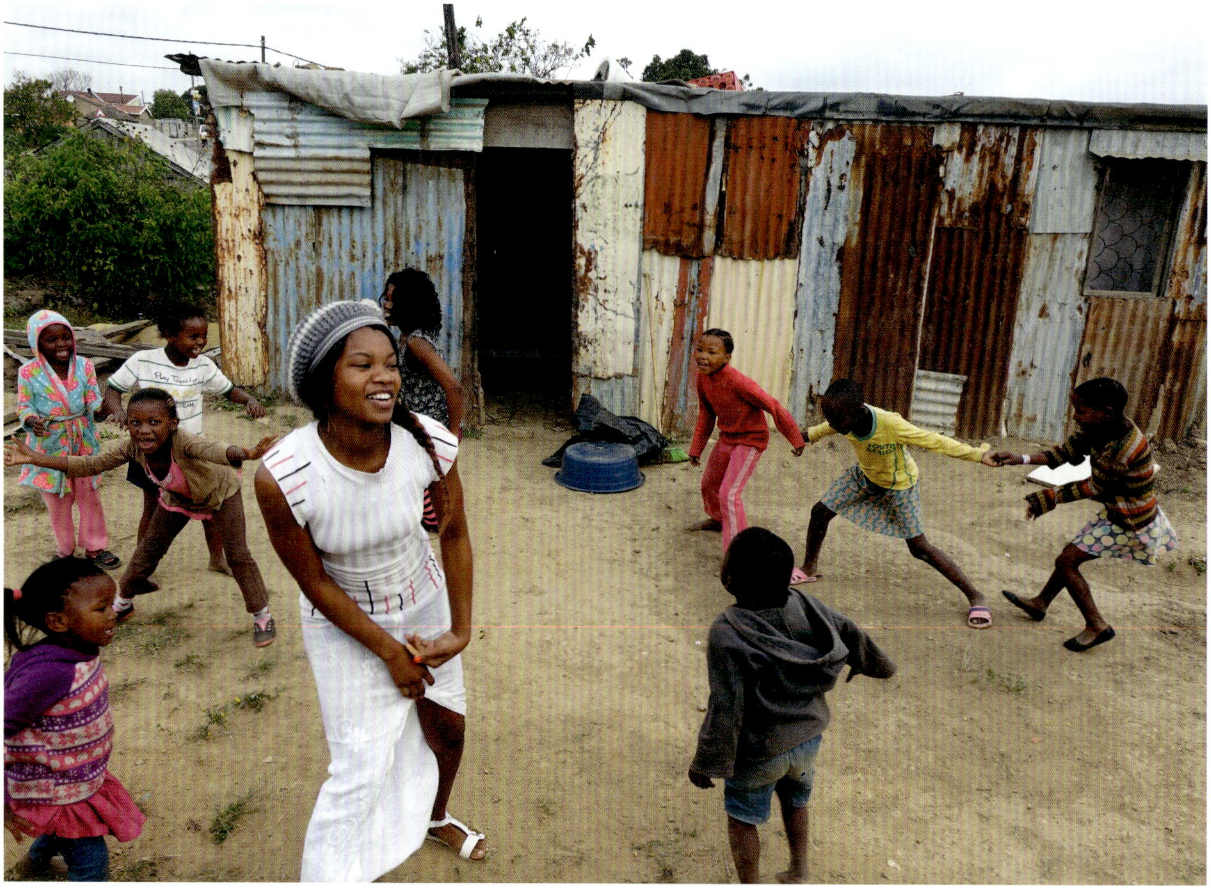

Yvonne

Because of Gugu Dlamini, I'm a strong woman. I know that I deserve treatment. I must look after myself, look after my family, and stay healthy. And I do.

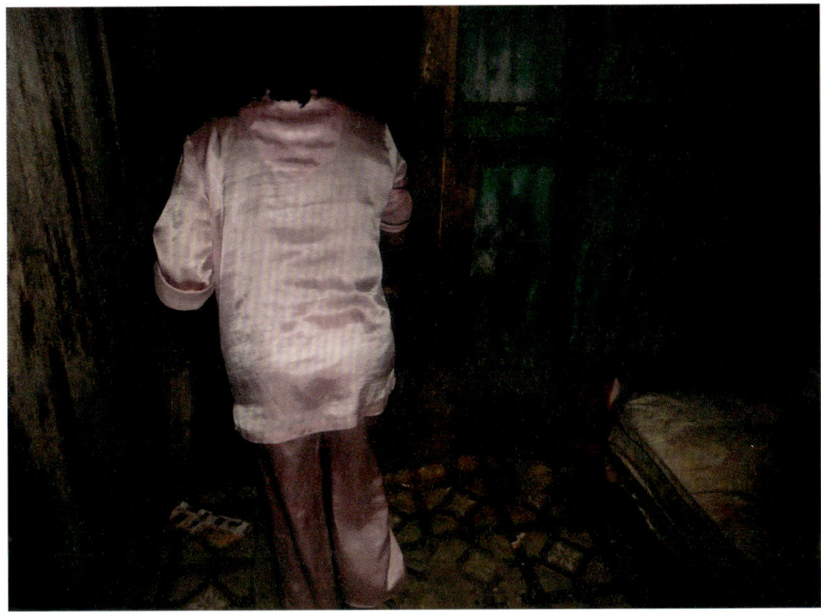

When I started working as a volunteer, and then as a cleaner, for the Gugu Dlamini Foundation, I was scared, because I knew the story about what had happened to her. In 1998, a young South African woman named Gugu Dlamini went on the radio, on World AIDS Day, to disclose that she was HIV-positive. The next day, her neighbors killed her. She was stoned and stabbed to death for speaking the truth about HIV and AIDS.

When I began working at the Foundation, I was scared because I was HIV-positive too, but I didn't feel comfortable speaking openly about it. My husband had passed away. I had three children and three grandchildren. I felt protective of them. And one more thing: I'm deaf, so when I speak, oftentimes people don't understand me. Especially men, they often undermine me. When a man sees a woman who's sick, he doesn't care about her.

I have got HIV and I'm not happy about it. But because of Gugu Dlamini, I'm a strong woman. I know that I deserve treatment. I must look after myself, look after my family, and stay healthy. And I do. I'm healthy and beautiful. And now I am also open about telling people that I am HIV-positive.

Today I say to Gugu Dlamini, thanks a lot. I'm happy to work at the foundation named after you because, when I go there, your daughter, Mandisa, who runs the organization, treats me like a sister. When I go to work I feel like I'm going home, I'm going to my family.

I'm happy today. I'm healthy. I feel wonderful. I wish those who have HIV will see me and be happy like me and enjoy family like me. I'm so thankful.

And I hope those who have HIV, as I do, will take treatment and look after themselves. And that they will use condoms to protect their bodies and other people's bodies.

Those who don't have HIV, they should go and test, to protect themselves and their future. Mainly what I want to say is, look after yourself.

Elizabeth

I grew up in group homes. At quiet moments, I used to stare out the window and think where I'd be in the next five or ten years' time.

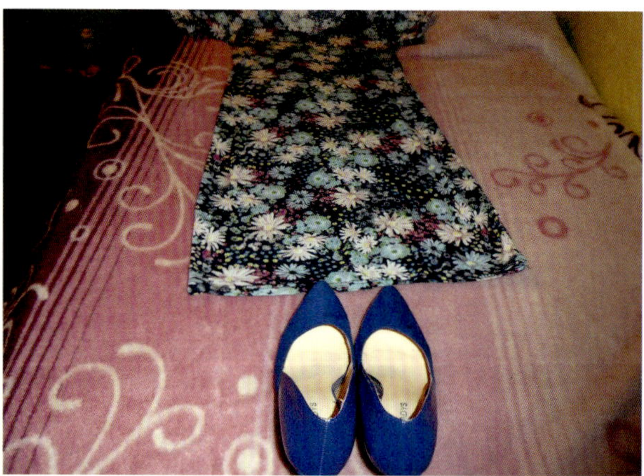

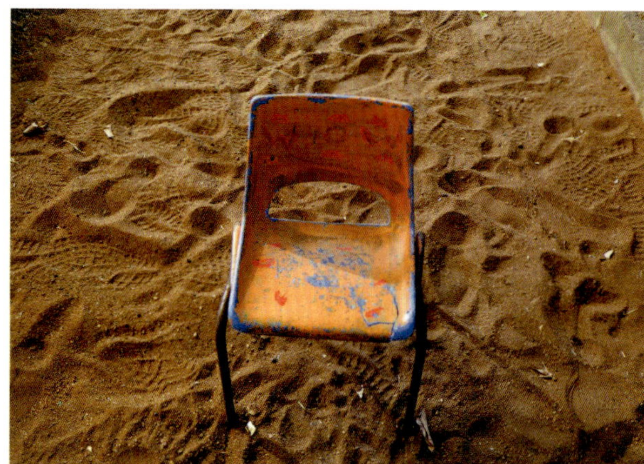

I'm an outgoing person. I love ice cream. I love to dress up. I love high heels. I love to dance. And I am HIV-positive.

At birth I was taken away from my mother, due to the fact she was mentally unstable. I grew up in group homes. It was fun living with my own age group, with only one or two housemothers around. We had lots of fun. At quiet moments, I used to stare out the window and think where I'd be in the next five or ten years' time.

As time went on, I was put in a foster home where I was badly abused. It was a difficult time for me, the hardest of my life. I felt like my childhood had been taken away from me. Eventually I was taken out of that home and placed into another. Luckily, my new foster mother treated me like a real daughter, like I was a precious egg.

Then, sadly, she passed away, and my life turned upside down. I was put in another foster home where, once again, I was met with abuse. In my fear, anxiety, and depression, I turned to drugs and alcohol. I just took it until I couldn't take it anymore. Eventually I spoke up and was removed from that home.

That is when, in 2008, I found out I was HIV-positive. I continued using alcohol and drugs, and I had two children. The first one I gave up for adoption because I felt my life was so upside down I couldn't look after her. The second one I decided to keep because I was a bit more mature. And I saw life from a different perspective. The day the doctor put her in my arms, I fell in love with her.

On the first of January 2016, I decided to change my life. I decided to give my heart to the Lord. Many things changed for me. Now I have so many opportunities to do things I've never done before. I feel like it's just been a turnaround in my life and I'm so excited to tell my story, I'm so excited to just get it out there.

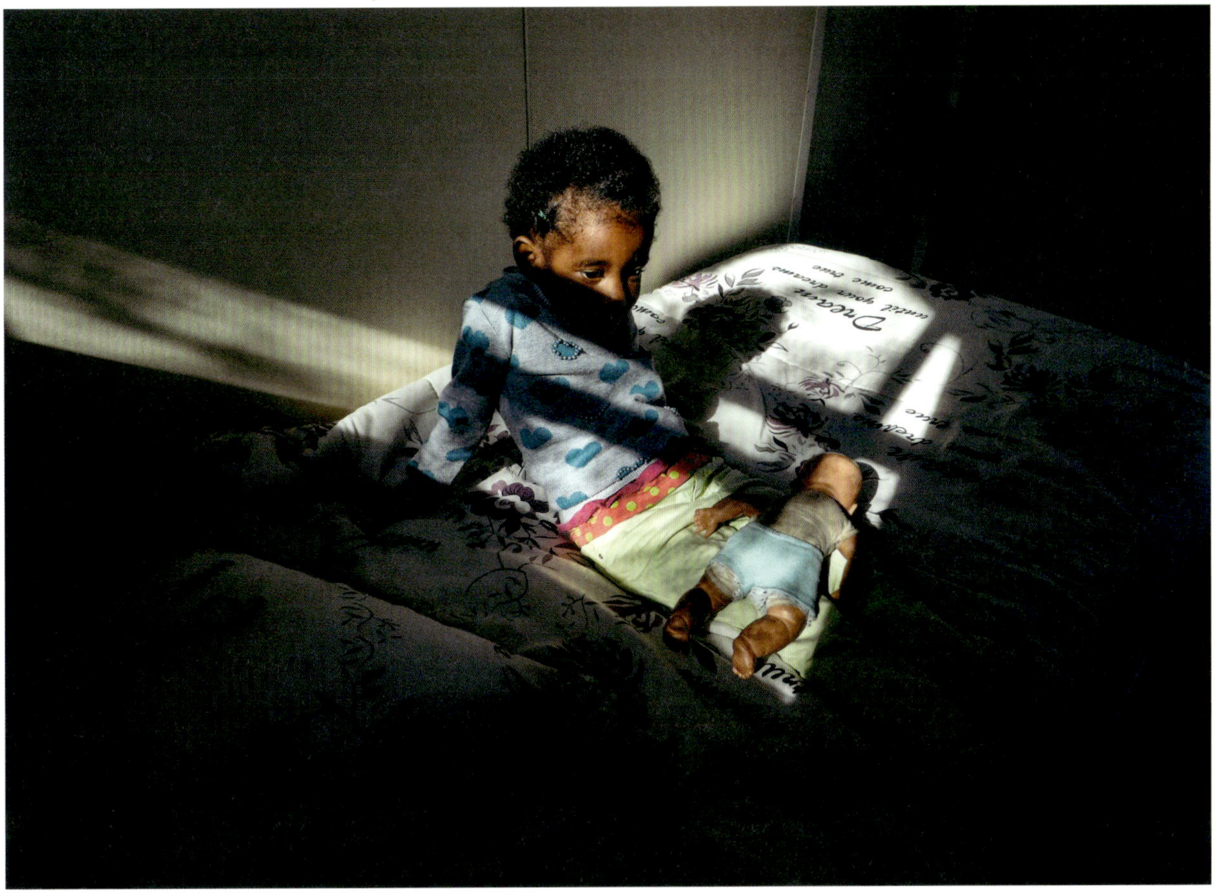

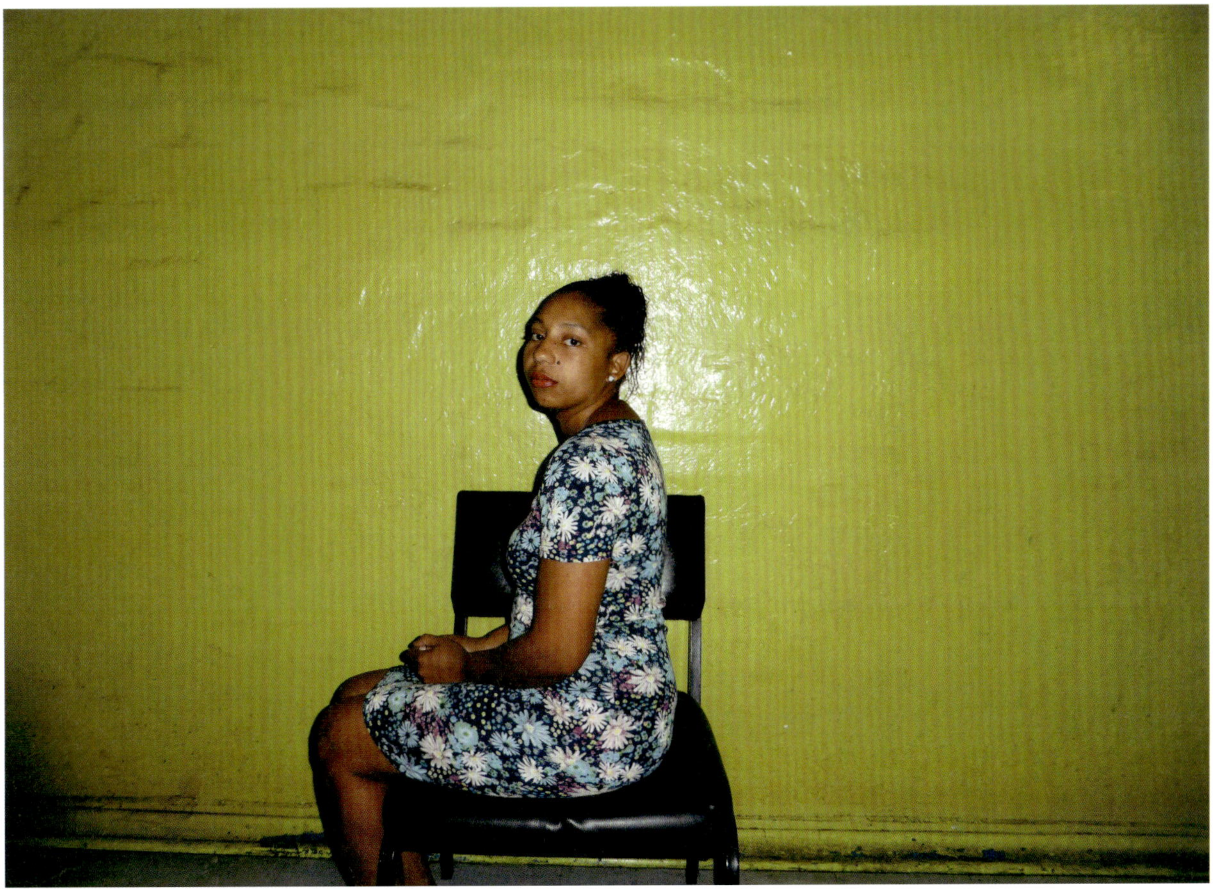

Sanele

When I was a teenager, I started to smoke and drink and have sex without wearing a condom. I had three children, with two different mothers. Some would say that I was a normal Zulu man.

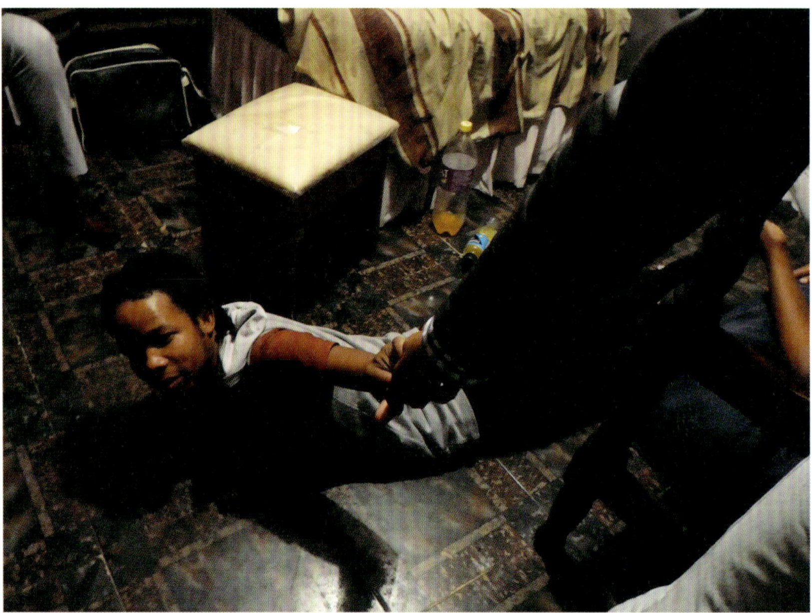

I'm a Zulu man from a rural area of KwaZulu-Natal. You can't be a real man in our culture without having more than one girlfriend. In general, being a man means having lots of children and not looking after them very well. For many, being a man also means not sharing your feelings with others.

I'm not that kind of a man, but in the past I've been like that. I want to be different. I want to be different, in our culture.

When I was not yet ten years old, my sister became very ill and I had to take care of her. One day, my sister offered me a banana and I broke off pieces to share with my cousin. Our mother told us, "No, never share food with your sister because she has AIDS." This made me very angry because no one had told me that my sister had AIDS.

It makes me angry even now. No one can be infected with HIV or AIDS by sharing food or sleeping in the same bed or providing care for a sick person. HIV only comes from having unprotected sex or from sharing needles as part of injecting drugs, or from mother-to-child in the womb. We are so uneducated, and that needs to change.

When I was a teenager, I started to smoke and drink and have sex without wearing a condom. I had three children, with two different mothers. Some would say that I was a normal Zulu man. But last year I decided to change, to restart my life, to become a new kind of a man.

I went to get tested for HIV. And I prepared myself for the fact that the test could be positive. Until this project, only my partner and two friends have known the results. May I share with you? I am HIV-positive, and I am now the man I want to be.

I have one partner who knows my status. I look after my children, making sure they grow up and know all about life. I'm loving and caring with them. I want them to look at me as a friend. I don't need to take medication yet but, when the time comes, I'll take medication and look after my health.

My name is Sanele. I'm a twenty-four-year-old man, from a rural area of KwaZulu-Natal. And I'm HIV-positive.

Thulile

Every time I fall ill, I always tell the virus that this is my body, you are a tenant, so behave well. Because if you don't I will die and you will die, because you will have no place to live.

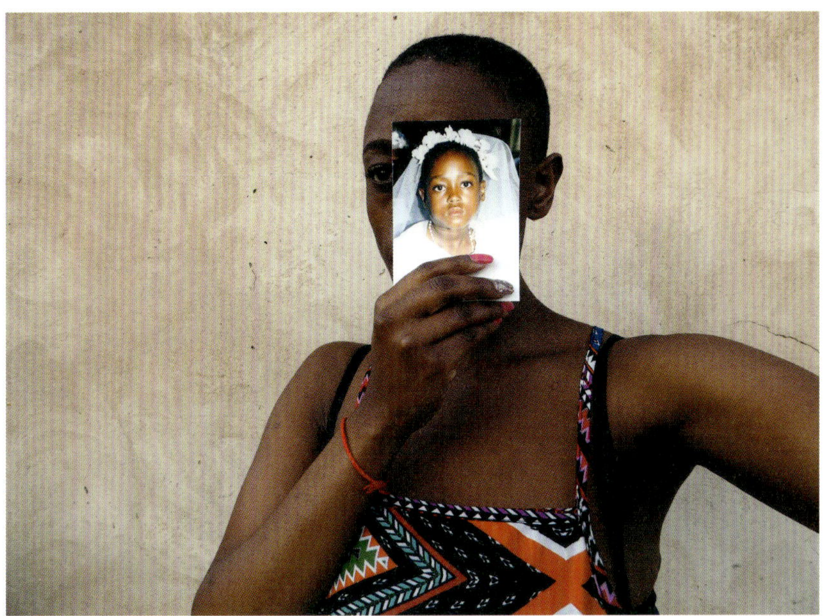

I was born with the virus. I have been living with it for about twenty-five years now. I am strong. I am beautiful. I am a positive woman, in all senses of that word. And I won't let anyone discriminate against me.

When I was a little girl, I heard the doctor talking to my granny and predicting that I wouldn't make it to my seventh birthday. During that time, there was no medication for the virus and I was so very ill. So when I reached seven, they said I wouldn't make it to ten. So when I made it to ten, they said I wouldn't make it to thirteen.

Even at thirteen, I was still a child, but my neighbors already knew that I was living with the virus, because my granny told them. As a result, some of my neighbors wouldn't let their kids play with me. I was so lonely, I was so ashamed, I just didn't know what was happening. I was so angry with my granny for sharing my information.

Since then, I've learned that my granny was just trying to protect me. Because she thought that if she died no one would take care of me. She wanted to let the neighbors know so that if she passed away, they would do it.

After that I thought, why not take care of myself, and go to my doctor, and schedule my checkups, and take my medication? Because this medication, it's mine.

That's why I have survived. Every time I fall ill, I always tell the virus that this is my body, you are a tenant, so behave well. Because if you don't I will die and you will die, because you will have no place to live.

Recently, I thought that I would start an organization. I call it The Angels' Light. I came up with the name because of the kids who are born with the virus. They are the angels, shining bright for the future.

Together, we are strong. We are beautiful. We are positive. And we will not allow anyone to discriminate against us.

Major funding for *Through Positive Eyes* has been provided by The Herb Ritts Foundation, led by board chair Erik Hyman and executive director Mark McKenna. We thank them for their sustained and passionate commitment to photography by people living with HIV and AIDS.

Additional support provided by:

The Ford Foundation; The Andy Warhol Foundation for the Visual Arts; Teiger Foundation; Gere Foundation; U.S. President's Emergency Fund for AIDS Relief; Brazilian Ministry of Health STD/AIDS Prevention Department; International AIDS Society; UNAIDS; University of California Institute for Mexico and the United States (UC MEXUS); City of Los Angeles AIDS Coordinator's Office; Heroes Project; National Endowment for the Arts; Electronic Theatre Controls (ETC); UCLA AIDS Institute; UCLA International Institute; UCLA School of the Arts and Architecture; UCLA Office of the Chancellor

Directors/Editors: Gideon Mendel and David Gere

We would like to acknowledge our partners and children, who support us in this work—even when it takes us far from home.

Photo Educator: Crispin Hughes
with support from Ricardo Funari and Luciana Saldanha (Rio de Janeiro), Mikhael Subotzky (Johannesburg), Parthiv Shah (Mumbai), Vinai Dithajohn and Apichart Sritakae (Bangkok), Marie Arago and Tatiana Mora Liautaud (Port-au-Prince), Simanga Konstant Zondo (Durban)

UCLA Text Editors: Gabrielle Bonder, Elisabeth Nails, Hanni Ress, Ariel Stevenson

Gideon Mendel Studio: Maria Quigley, Alice Mann

Community Organizer: Hanni Ress

Education Consultant: Timothy Kordic

Exhibition Curators: Carol Brown, David Gere, Stan Pressner

Infographics: Lesley Lawson

Website Design: Andy Brockie, Isaiah Baiseri

Website Video: Cut + Cue, Mo Stoebe, Katja Kulenkampff, Jesse Phinney

UCLA Art & Global Health Center Staff (2004–19): Noel Alumit, Marcia Argolo, Isaiah Baiseri, Brij Mohan Singh Bhandari, Gabrielle Bonder, Cathryn Dhanatya, David Gere, Kelly Gluckman, Bobby Gordon, Lauren Gould, Susana Hernandez, Lakhiyia Hicks, Carol Hobson, Claire Hoch-Frohman, Amanda Hoskinson, Ivy Hurwit, Kristin Killacky, Adrian Meza, Sebastian Milla, Veline Mojarro, Meena Murugesan, Elisabeth Nails, Phillip T. Nails, Lisa Park, Hanni Ress, Ariel Stevenson, Arianna Taboada, Luz Maria Torres, Rajeev Varma

Workshop Producers: Janna Shadduck-Hernandez (Mexico City co-director), Alejandro Brito-Lemus, Julia Arnaut (Mexico City); Cristina Pimenta (Rio de Janeiro); Pholokgolo Ramothwala (Johannesburg); Timothy Kordic, Nancy Ramos (Los Angeles); Ryan Hill, Anna Kassinger, Dan Solberg (Washington, D.C.); Vinitha Venkatraman (Mumbai); Nym Korakot Punlopruksa, Michael Sakamoto, Waewdao Sirisook, Scott Weeks (Bangkok); Marie Arago, Tatiana Mora Liautaud (Port-au-Prince); Jane Bruton, Lesley Lawson, Marc Thompson (London); Paul Browde, Carol Brown, Deborah Ewing, Mabusi Kgwete, Zinhle Khumalo, Stan Pressner (Durban)

Translators and Transcribers: Janna Shadduck-Hernandez (Mexico City); Ana Paula Höfling, Marina Magalhães, Luciana Saldanha (Rio de Janeiro); Katie Boot (Johannesburg, Los Angeles, Washington, D.C.); Kavita Nair Bhatia, Crystal Hues, Ahilya Kaul, Anuradha Kishore, Gopal Nair, Sreelesh Nambiar, Pooja Pottenkulam (Mumbai); Nym Korakot Punlopruksa (Bangkok); Rodolph La Pointe, Tatiana Mora Liautaud, Karl Pétion, Jeff St. Dic (Port-au-Prince); Patrick Phan (London); Maria Quigley (Durban)

Title page: Gugu/Johannesburg

throughpositiveeyes.org

Designer: SMITH

"And so they said" by Mary Bowman printed with permission. The infographics pages, authored by Lesley Lawson, draw on publicly available reports prepared by UNAIDS, Avert, and other reputable sources, all of which are published online.

First published by Aperture, 2019

Printed by Conti in Italy
10 9 8 7 6 5 4 3 2 1

Library of Congress Control Number: 2019909340
ISBN 978-1-59711-476-9

To order Aperture books, contact:
+1 212.946.7154; orders@aperture.org

For information about Aperture trade distribution worldwide, visit: aperture.org/distribution

aperture

Aperture Foundation
547 West 27th Street, 4th Floor
New York, N.Y. 10001
aperture.org

Aperture, a not-for-profit foundation, connects the photo community and its audiences with the most inspiring work, the sharpest ideas, and with each other—in print, in person, and online.